Handbook of Pulmonary Medicine

Handbook of Pulmonary Medicine

Edited by June Middleton

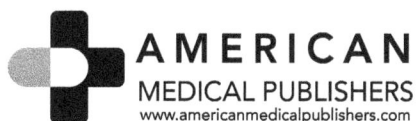

AMERICAN
MEDICAL PUBLISHERS
www.americanmedicalpublishers.com

American Medical Publishers,
41 Flatbush Avenue,
1st Floor, New York,
NY 11217, USA

Visit us on the World Wide Web at:
www.americanmedicalpublishers.com

ISBN: 978-1-63927-459-8

Cataloging-in-Publication Data

Handbook of pulmonary medicine / edited by June Middleton.
p. cm.
Includes bibliographical references and index.
ISBN 978-1-63927-459-8
1. Lungs--Diseases. 2. Respiratory organs--Diseases. 3. Pulmonary manifestations of general diseases. I. Middleton, June.
RC756 .H36 2022
616.24--dc23

Table of Contents

Preface

Pulmonary medicine refers to a medical specialty that is concerned with the diseases affecting the respiratory tract. It falls under the umbrella of internal medicine. Some common diseases treated under this domain are asthma, pneumonia, emphysema, tuberculosis, etc. Pulmonary medicine also provides patients with life support and mechanical ventilation. The diagnosis of pulmonary diseases focuses on hereditary diseases, exposure to toxicants, infectious agents, etc. Some other clinical procedures for detection of diseases are spirometry, bronchoscopy, CT scanning, scintigraphy, etc. Bronchodilators, steroids, antibiotics, leukotriene antagonists are some of the medications that are used in treating respiratory diseases. The topics covered in this extensive book deal with the core aspects of pulmonary medicine. It aims to shed light on some of the unexplored aspects and the recent researches in this field. This book will serve as a reference to a broad spectrum of readers.

This book unites the global concepts and researches in an organized manner for a comprehensive understanding of the subject. It is a ripe text for all researchers, students, scientists or anyone else who is interested in acquiring a better knowledge of this dynamic field.

I extend my sincere thanks to the contributors for such eloquent research chapters. Finally, I thank my family for being a source of support and help.

Editor

Treatment patterns, resource use and costs of idiopathic pulmonary fibrosis in Spain – results of a Delphi Panel

Ferran Morell[1], Dirk Esser[2], Jonathan Lim[2], Susanne Stowasser[2], Alba Villacampa[3*], Diana Nieves[3] and Max Brosa[3]

Abstract

Background: Idiopathic pulmonary fibrosis (IPF) is a form of chronic fibrosing interstitial pneumonia characterized by progressive worsening of dyspnea and lung function, with a poor prognosis. The objective of this study was to determine treatment patterns, resource use and costs of managing Spanish patients with IPF.

Methods: A three-round Delphi consensus panel of 15 clinical experts was held between December 2012 and June 2013 using questionnaires to describe the management of patients with IPF. A cost analysis based on Delphi panel estimates was made from the Spanish National Health System (NHS) perspective, including the direct costs of IPF diagnosis and management. Unit costs were applied to Delphi panel estimates of health resource use. Univariate sensitivity analyses were made to evaluate uncertainties in parameters.

Results: The Delphi panel estimated that 20, 60 and 20 % of IPF patients presented with stable disease, slow and rapid disease progression, respectively. The estimated annual cost per patient with stable disease, slow and rapid disease progression was €11,484, €20,978 and €57,759, respectively. This corresponds to a weighted average annual cost of €26,435 with itemized costs of €1,184 (4.5), €7,147 (27.0), €5,950 (22.5), €11,666 (44.1) and €488 (1.9 %) for the diagnosis of IPF, treatment, monitoring, management of acute exacerbations and end-of-life care, respectively. The parameter that varied the annual cost per patient the most was resource use associated with acute exacerbations.

Conclusions: The management of patients with IPF in Spain, especially patients with rapid disease progression, has a high economic impact on the NHS.

Keywords: Costs, Delphi technique, Idiopathic pulmonary fibrosis, Spain

Background

Idiopathic pulmonary fibrosis (IPF) is a specific form of chronic, progressive fibrosing interstitial pneumonia associated with the histopathological and/or radiological pattern of usual interstitial pneumonia (UIP) [1]. A diagnosis of IPF requires the exclusion of other forms of interstitial lung disease (ILD) such as those associated with environmental exposure, medication or systemic disease [1]. IPF usually affects adults aged >50 years; the prevalence is higher in males and most patients have a history of smoking [1–3].

IPF is characterised by progressive worsening of dyspnoea and lung function, with a poor prognosis, but the natural history of the disease is variable and unpredictable in the individual patient [1]. In most patients, IPF worsens slowly but steadily ("slow progression"), in some it remains stable ("stable") and in some it worsens rapidly ("rapid progression") [1]. In addition, some patients experience acute exacerbations, defined as episodes of acute respiratory worsening of unknown cause [4].

In the past, IPF was considered to have an inflammatory origin and, consequently, anti-inflammatory and immuno-suppressive drugs have been used [5, 6]. However, the central event currently considered to be involved in the development of IPF is repeated alveolar epithelial cell injury resulting in an impaired repair process with development of fibrosis with inflammation now considered less important [7]. This scenario has encouraged the development of new drugs with antifibrotic properties [8].

* Correspondence: alba.villacampa@oblikue.com
[3]Oblikue Consulting S.L., Avenida Diagonal 514, 3°-3a, 08006 Barcelona, Spain
Full list of author information is available at the end of the article

The overall economic burden associated with IPF in Spain remains unknown. Studies analysing the cost of illness could help to define the magnitude of economic burden associated with IPF and its impact on Spanish society. The objective of this study, which used a Delphi panel, was to determine treatment patterns, resource use and the associated costs of managing patients with IPF in the Spanish healthcare system.

Methods

Delphi panel

A three-round Delphi panel of clinical experts was held between December 2012 and June 2013 using postal questionnaires to describe the treatment patterns and resource use associated with IPF. The first questionnaire included questions on the clinical management of patients with IPF in Spain and open questions that investigated several aspects of the disease. The second questionnaire sought to study specific issues in greater detail and to resolve any doubts about questions asked in the first questionnaire. The third questionnaire was carried out to reach a consensus among the experts. An aggregate of the three questionnaires is available on the journal website (Additional file 1). In each round, the participants were asked the questions individually. All participants remained anonymous until the end of the process.

Fifteen pulmonologists who were experts on ILD were recruited from the Spanish respiratory community to ensure that the findings of the Delphi panel were credible and reflective of clinical practice in Spain. Pulmonologists were recruited from different Spanish Autonomous Communities to guarantee that regional differences were captured (Andalusia, Asturias, Castile-La Mancha, Castile-Leon, Catalonia, Community of Madrid, Valencian Community, Galicia) (see Acknowledgements). The study sponsor did not influence selection of the panelists and was unaware of their identity until study completion. Study panelists were unaware of the identity of the study sponsor. The study did not require approval from an ethics committee due to its design [9].

Cost analysis

A cost analysis was made from the Spanish National Health System (NHS) perspective, based on data obtained through a systematic literature review and the Delphi panel estimates of the number of patients with IPF in Spain and their resource use during diagnosis, treatment (pharmacological and non-pharmacological) and management (medical visits, tests, other resources). All costs were estimated per patient per year, and were specified with respect to the different types of disease course. To calculate an overall annual cost per patient, the estimated cost associated with each type of disease course was weighted by its proportion of all patients. Costs were expressed in 2013 euro.

Unit costs

Unit costs were obtained from Spanish databases (see Additional file 2: Table S1, Table 1). Pharmacological costs were obtained from the Spanish database of the Consejo General de Colegios Oficiales de Farmacéuticos, and all costs included were ex-factory price [10]. Unit costs related to medical visits, tests, hospital admissions, etc. were obtained from the eSalud Spanish health costs database [11]. Diagnostic-related group costs were obtained from the Spanish Ministry of Health database [12].

Types of disease course in IPF

The expert panel estimated the proportion of patients with IPF with stable disease, slow and rapid disease progression, according to the types of disease courses described in the ATS/ERS/JRS/ALAT Statement [1]. Treatment and monitoring costs were estimated according to the type of disease course. The costs associated with an acute exacerbation were assumed to be the same for all types of patients. The annual cost for each type of disease course was calculated by weighting the cost according to the number of exacerbations per each type of patient per year. A similar approach was used to estimate costs associated with end-of-life care. The cost per year associated with end-of-life care was weighted by the survival rates observed per type of disease course.

Epidemiological approach

The cost of illness analysis was performed using a prevalence-based approach, as this method allows disease-

Table 1 Cost of management of adverse events associated with the treatment of IPF

	Non-hospitalised grade 3 adverse events[a]	Grade 3 and 4 adverse events in hospitalised patients
Osteoporosis	€89.43	€3,495.47
Hyperglycaemia	€69.93	€3,898.39
Cushing syndrome	€74.66	€4,468.42
Compression fractures	€74.66	€3,495.47
Diabetes	€84.74	€3,898.39
Digestive intolerance	€68.14	€2,452.50
Opportunistic infections	€74.66	€7,085.52
Hepatotoxicity	€74.66	€2,739.44
Nausea	€68.14	€ 3,082.73
Digestive intolerance	€74.66	[b]
Nasal dryness	€27.95	€1,678.20
Asthenia	[b]	€3,082.73

Source: eSalud [11]
[a]Costs were estimated taking into account medical visits and tests undergone by patients for their management
[b]These adverse events were reported by <5 % of patients therefore these costs were not included

attributable costs that occur concurrently with prevalent cases over a specified time period (1 year in this case) to be measured [13]. To calculate the current number of patients with IPF in Spain, the median prevalence obtained through the Delphi panel was multiplied by the Spanish population obtained from the Spanish National Statistics Institute [14].

Diagnostic costs
To calculate the number of patients diagnosed with IPF, the diagnostic rate was assumed to be 85 %, based on a series of patients with clinical characteristics of ILD [15], This rate was applied to the number of Spanish patients estimated by the Delphi panel. To estimate the total cost associated with the diagnosis of IPF, the median number of medical visits or tests carried out to reach the diagnosis was multiplied by their mean unit costs. To determine the cost of diagnosis per year, the estimated total cost associated with the diagnosis of IPF was multiplied by the ratio of incidence over prevalence.

Treatment of patients with IPF by disease course
The cost associated with pharmacological therapies included drugs and the cost of drug-related adverse events. The mean cost per unit and the daily median dose administered were multiplied by the median treatment duration. Only drug-related adverse events affecting >5 % of patients were included and costs associated with Common Terminology Criteria for Adverse Events grade 1–2 (mild and moderate) adverse events were excluded [16]. The cost associated with grade 3 (severe) adverse events included the cost of patients hospitalised due to adverse events and resource use by non-hospitalised patients (Table 1). It was assumed that all patients suffering grade 4 (potentially life threatening) adverse events were hospitalised. To calculate the costs associated with non-pharmacological therapies, the percentages of patients undergoing lung transplantation or pulmonary rehabilitation were multiplied by their unit costs (see Additional file 2: Table S1).

Monitoring by clinical disease course per year
To estimate the cost associated with IPF monitoring, the mean unit costs of medical visits, tests and hospital admissions (see Additional file 2: Table S1) were multiplied by the median number of resources used per type of patient and year according to estimates from the Delphi panel.

Management of patients during acute exacerbations
The total number of acute exacerbations suffered per type of patient/year was calculated to estimate the costs associated with their management per year according to the estimates of the Delphi panel. Diagnosis, treatment, healthcare resource use and follow-up costs were

included. To calculate the cost associated with diagnosis, unit costs related to tests carried out to differentiate acute exacerbations from other causes of acute respiratory failure or clinical deterioration were multiplied by the percentage of patients undergoing each test as estimated by the Delphi panel. Treatment costs associated with acute exacerbations were included. To calculate the costs associated with each therapeutic regimen, the mean cost per unit and the daily median dose were multiplied by the duration of treatment. The associated costs of healthcare resource use and follow-up during an acute exacerbation were estimated, and the unit costs of medical visits and tests were multiplied by the percentage of patients receiving them. To estimate the overall cost per year associated with acute exacerbations for each type of disease course, the total cost of an acute exacerbation was multiplied by the number of acute exacerbations suffered per year by each type of patient.

End-of-life care
Treatment costs were calculated by multiplying mean unit costs, median doses administered and the duration of each treatment by the percentage of patients receiving each treatment according to Delphi panel estimates. To calculate the costs associated with outpatient visits, the median number of visits per patient was multiplied by their unit cost. To distribute end-of-life care costs annually, the annual mortality rate per type of disease course was multiplied by the total end-of-life cost, in order to weight this cost by the proportion of patients who receive end-of-life care per year. The annual mortality rate was calculated using a DEALE approximation (Declining Exponential Approximation to Life Expectancy) [17].

Sensitivity analysis
Successive univariate sensitivity analyses were performed on key values in the cost analysis to ascertain the circumstances under which uncertainty or lack of agreement about any estimate may significantly impact the results. Specific parameters were varied one at a time across a plausible range, while the remaining values were held at baseline values. The parameters varied were the prevalence and incidence estimates made by the Delphi panel (±25 %), resource use associated with the management of IPF derived from the Delphi panel (minimum and maximum values), and unit costs obtained from Spanish databases (minimum and maximum values).

Results
Delphi panel
The first round Delphi Panel was completed by 15 pulmonologists and the second and third rounds by 14. The degree of consensus in the third questionnaire was high, with 77–100 % agreement per question.

Epidemiological estimates by the Delphi panel suggested that the prevalence of IPF in Spain is 12 cases per 100,000 people/year and the incidence is 3 cases per 100,000 people/year. Based on a Spanish population of 46,039,979, it was calculated that there are 5,525 people with IPF in Spain.

Considering a diagnostic rate of 85 % [15], the number of diagnosed patients with IPF in Spain was estimated to be 4,696. The Delphi panel estimated that two primary care visits, three pulmonary medicine department visits, multiple laboratory tests and other tests such as chest x-ray, high resolution computed tomography (HRCT), bronchoscopy, bronchoalveolar lavage, transbronchial biopsy, surgical lung biopsy, blood gases and respiratory function tests were carried out to reach a diagnosis of IPF.

It was estimated that 20, 60 and 20 % of IPF patients presented with stable disease, slow and rapid disease progression, respectively, and that mean survival after diagnosis was 66, 42 and 15 months, respectively.

The Delphi panel estimated that most patients with IPF are administered N-acetylcysteine (Table 2). All patients with rapid disease progression also receive long-term oxygen therapy and half are treated with prednisone (Table 2). N-acetylcysteine does not induce grade 3–4 adverse events (Table 3). The main grade 3–4 adverse events associated with prednisone are osteoporosis, myopathy, hyperglycemia, Cushing syndrome and diabetes (Table 3). The main grade 1–4 adverse event associated with long-term oxygen therapy is nasal dryness (Table 3). Some patients are also treated with non-pharmacological therapies such as pulmonary rehabilitation (10 % of patients) and single-lung transplant (5 and 8 % of patients with slow and rapid disease progression, respectively) (Table 2).

Table 4 shows that patients with rapid disease progression used the most healthcare resources.

Table 2 Treatment of patients with IPF by clinical disease course

	Stable disease	Slow disease progression	Rapid disease progression
Pharmacological			
N-acetylcysteine	80 %	100 %	100 %
Anticoagulants	0 %	0 %	4.3 %
Prednisone	0 %	0 %	50 %
Long-term oxygen therapy	25 %	30 %	100 %
Omeprazole or pantoprazole	7 %	7 %	7 %
Pirfenidone (compassionate use /importation)	0 %	5 %	0 %
Non-pharmacological			
Single-lung transplant	0 %	5 %	8 %
Pulmonary rehabilitation	10 %	10 %	10 %

Table 3 Adverse events associated with IPF treatments

	% of patients		
	Grade 1–2	Grade 3	Grade 4
N-Acetylcysteine			
Epigastric pain	5 %	0 %	0 %
Digestive intolerance	8 %	0 %	0 %
Dyspepsia	5 %	0 %	0 %
Reflux	1 %	0 %	0 %
Nausea	1 %	0 %	0 %
Anticoagulants			
Haematoma	10 %	0 %	0 %
Systemic corticosteroids			
Osteoporosis	30 %	18 %	5 %
Opportunistic infections	10 %	5 %	1 %
Oedema	10 %	3 %	0 %
Myopathy	15 %	5 %	5 %
Hyperglycaemia	30 %	18 %	5 %
Cushing syndrome	20 %	10 %	5 %
Compression fractures	10 %	10 %	3 %
Diabetes	15 %	10 %	5 %
Hypertension	10 %	5 %	0 %
Cataracts	8 %	5 %	1 %
Digestive intolerance	10 %	7 %	3 %
Pirfenidone			
Photosensitivity	20 %	0 %	0 %
Epigastric pain	15 %	3 %	0 %
Skin reactions	15 %	0 %	0 %
Nausea	8 %	10 %	0 %
Asthenia	10 %	3 %	0 %
Digestive intolerance	10 %	8 %	0 %
Long-term oxygen therapy			
Nasal dryness	40 %	10 %	3 %
Epistaxis	10 %	0 %	0 %
Dry mouth	8 %	3 %	0 %

The Delphi panel estimated that the number of exacerbations per patient/year was 0.76 in patients with stable disease, 0.82 in patients with slow disease progression and 1.8 in patients with rapid progression. The panel estimated that 51 % of patients with IPF with an acute exacerbation die from this event. Of these, 69 die in the hospital and 31 % during the 6 months after hospital discharge. Tests performed in more than 50 % of patients with IPF to differentiate an acute exacerbation from other causes of acute respiratory failure or clinical deterioration included computed tomography, echocardiography and laboratory tests. Table 4 shows that, during an acute exacerbation and follow-up, patients use

Table 4 Median healthcare resource use for managing acute exacerbations and follow-up of patients with IPF

	Acute exacerbation and follow-up	Management and follow-up of patients with IPF (over a 3-month period)		
		Stable disease	Slow disease progression	Rapid disease progression
Outpatient visits				
General practitioner home visits	0.2	0.0	0.0	0.0
Pulmonary specialist	2.0	1.0	1.0	2.0
Nurse (or other healthcare professional)	0.6	0.0	0.0	0.0
Elective ambulance	0.3	0.0	0.0	0.0
Emergency				
Emergency room visits	1.0	0.0	0.0	1.0
Emergency ambulance	0.8	0.0	0.0	0.0
Hospital admissions				
Pulmonary department (days)	11.3	0.0	0.0	7.5
Intensive care unit (days)	2.5	0.0	0.0	0.8
Laboratory tests				
Complete blood count	3.0	1.0	1.0	1.0
Sedimentation rate	2.0	0.0	1.0	1.0
Liver profile	2.0	0.0	1.0	1.0
Creatine phosphokinase	1.5	0.0	0.0	1.0
Urinalysis	0.2	0.0	0.0	0.0
Microbiology	0.1	0.0	0.0	0.0
Respiratory function tests				
Spirometry	1.0	1.0	1.0	1.0
Body plethysmography	0.1	0.0	1.0	1.0
Diffusing capacity of carbon monoxide	1.0	0.0	1.0	1.0
6-min walk test	0.3	0.0	1.0	1.0
Other tests				
Chest X-ray	3.0	0.0	0.5	1.0
High-resolution computed tomography	1.0	0.0	0.0	1.0
Blood gases	3.0	0.0	0.3	1.5
Computed tomography pulmonary angiogram	0.3	0.0	0.0	0.0
Bronchoscopy	0.3	0.0	0.0	0.0
Sputum assessment	0.8	0.0	0.0	0.0
Bronchoalveolar lavage	0.2	0.0	0.0	0.0

considerable healthcare resources, including medical visits, hospitalisations and multiple tests. Treatments administered to treat acute exacerbations were corticosteroids (100 of patients), antibiotics (93), and anticoagulant drugs (79) and non-invasive (79) and invasive (71 %) mechanical ventilation.

The Delphi panel estimated that, during end-of-life care, most physicians initiate palliative care when patients with IPF develop uncontrollable dyspnoea. Annual mortality rates were 18.2, 28.6 and 80 % in patients with stable disease, slow and rapid disease progression, respectively. The median duration of palliative treatment was 4.5 months. The main active ingredients administered as palliative treatment were paracetamol (50 of patients), codeine (40), morphine (40) and corticosteroids (20 %).

Costs

The total cost of the diagnosis of IPF was €4,736 per patient. When this cost was distributed by the proportion of new patients diagnosed every year (by multiplying with the ratio of incidence over prevalence), there was an annual cost of €1,184 per patient (Table 5). The main cost drivers were surgical lung biopsy, bronchoscopy with bronchoalveolar lavage and transbronchial biopsy and pulmonary medicine department visits.

Table 5 Total cost per patient per year according to disease course

	Stable disease	Slow disease progression	Rapid disease progression	Total cost weighted by type of disease distribution
Diagnosis	€1,184.07	€1,184.07	€1,184.07	€1,184.07
Treatment	€722.26	€8,069.33	€10,802.52	€7,146.55
Monitoring	€453.94	€1,698.91	€24,199.00	€5,949.93
Acute exacerbations	€8,882.22	€9,646.21	€20,511.50	€11,666.47
End-of-life care	€241.28	€379.15	€1,061.62	€488.07
TOTAL	€11,483.76	€20,977.67	€57,758.70	€26,435.10

The mean associated cost of treatment per patient/year was €722 for patients with stable disease, €8,069 for patients with slow disease progression and €10,803 for patients with rapid disease progression (Table 5). The high cost in patients with slow disease progression and rapid disease progression was mainly attributable to the cost of lung transplantation. When total costs per patient were weighted by the proportion of patients with each type of disease course, an overall cost of €7,147 was obtained per patient/year (Table 5).

The annual mean costs associated with IPF monitoring were €454, €1,699 and €24,199 per patient with stable disease, slow and rapid disease progression, respectively (Table 5). The most costly resources were those associated with pulmonary specialist visits and spirometry tests for patients with stable disease, diffusing capacity of carbon monoxide and 6-min walk tests for patients with slow disease progression, and hospital admissions for patients with rapid disease progression. The cost weighted by types of disease course showed an overall cost of €5,950 per IPF patient/year (Table 5).

The cost of a diagnosis of an acute exacerbation was €339, the overall treatment cost was €305 (corticosteroids, antibiotics, and anticoagulants and non-invasive ventilation) and the cost of healthcare resource use and follow-up during an acute exacerbation was €11,074 per patient. Therefore, the total cost of an acute exacerbation was €11,718, with healthcare resource use and follow-up representing 95 % of the total cost. The overall cost associated with acute exacerbations per year was €8,882 per patient with stable disease, €9,646 per patient with slow disease progression and €20,511 per patient with rapid disease progression (Table 5). Weighting these costs per type of disease course showed a global cost of €11,666 per patient per year (Table 5).

The mean total cost of end-of-life care treatment was €463 per patient, regardless of the type of disease course. The cost of outpatient visits during end-of-life care was €864 per patient. Therefore, considering both treatment and medical visits, the total cost of end-of-life care was €1,327 per patient. Considering the annual mortality rate for each type of disease course, the mean associated cost of end-of-life care per year was €241 for patients with stable disease, €379 for patients with slow disease progression and

€1,062 for patients with rapid disease progression (Table 5). The cost weighted by types of disease course showed an overall cost of €488 per patient per year (Table 5).

Taking into consideration all the factors studied, a total cost of €11,484, €20,978 and €57,759 were obtained per year per patient with stable disease, slow disease progression and rapid disease progression, respectively (Table 5). Therefore, the cost in patients with rapid disease progression was about 5 times higher than that for patients with stable disease and 3 times higher than that for patients with slow disease progression. Weighting these costs by the proportion of patients representing each type of clinical disease course resulted in a mean cost of €26,435 per patient per year (Table 5; Fig. 1).

Sensitivity analysis

Univariate sensitivity analyses of the prevalence, incidence, resource use and cost data were made to calculate changes in total costs when these parameters were varied. The main parameters that the total cost was most sensitive to were resource use during the clinical management of exacerbations, treatment and monitoring. The costs associated with treatment (pharmacological and the cost of treating adverse events) also changed the results considerably (Table 6).

Discussion

This study aimed to assess treatment patterns, resource use and associated costs in Spanish patients with IPF. The results are of interest due to the lack of studies analysing the burden associated with IPF and may help to indicate medical needs in the management of patients with IPF and guide research and investment in health resources. Our study is the first detailed analysis of healthcare costs associated with the overall management of patients with IPF in Spain, from diagnosis until end-of-life care.

Our results show that the total annual costs per patient with stable disease, slow and rapid disease progression were €11,484, €20,978 and €57,759, respectively. Weighting these costs by type of disease course showed a mean cost of €26,435 per IPF patient per year. These results are comparable to those of a retrospective study of US claims databases that included 9,286 patients and

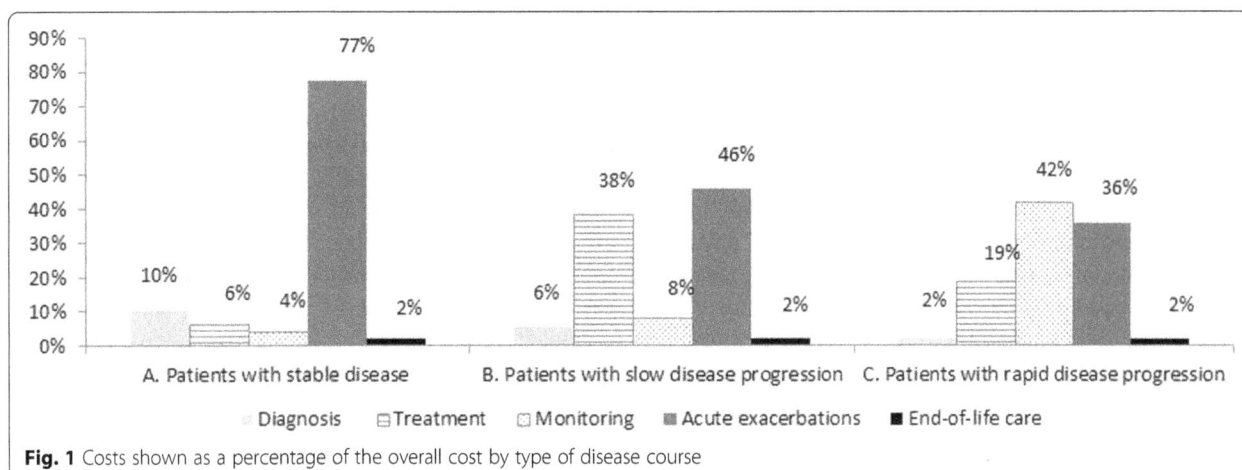

Fig. 1 Costs shown as a percentage of the overall cost by type of disease course

found that the total direct cost of IPF was $26,378 per patient per year [18]. However, there were methodological differences between this and our study. In the US study, two cohorts (patients with IPF and matched controls) were retrospectively identified from US claims databases in order to analyse the prevalence and incidence of pre-selected comorbidities and to collect data on healthcare resource use (hospital, outpatient, drugs) in each cohort; costs were not estimated according to type of disease course. As reflected by our results, the clinical course has a considerable impact on disease management and costs of treatment. We did not analyse the incidence and prevalence of comorbidities because we considered that they are not a direct or inevitable consequence of IPF.

In Spain, some studies have evaluated the cost associated with the management of chronic lung diseases such as chronic obstructive pulmonary disease (COPD). The

mean annual cost per patient with COPD (including hospital care, ambulatory care, oxygen therapy, usual drug therapy and drug therapy for exacerbations) has been estimated at around €2,000 [19–21], suggesting that the cost associated with the management of patients with IPF (€26,435 in our study) is considerably higher than other chronic lung diseases.

The sensitivity analysis showed that the parameters with the greatest impact on the results were those related to healthcare resource use during the clinical management of exacerbations, treatment and monitoring. The impact of these factors was due to variations in the estimates of resource use by the clinical experts (rather than estimated unit costs). This suggests differences in clinical practice between experts and variations in access to, or use of, healthcare resources between health centers. In addition, variations between published recommendations and clinical practice were found (for

Table 6 Univariate sensitivity analysis

	Mean cost per patient per year				
Base case	€26,435				
Parameter	Minimum	Maximum	Minimum. Difference from base case (%)		Maximum. Difference from base case (%)
Prevalence	€26,830	€26,198	1 %		−1 %
Incidence	€26,139	€26,731	−1 %		1 %
Resource use during disease diagnosis	€25,349	€27,745	−4 %		5 %
Resource use during treatment by disease course	€19,408	€83,145	−27 %		215 %
Resource use during monitoring by disease course	€21,882	€51,531	−17 %		95 %
Resource use during clinical management of exacerbations	€16,882	€93,113	−36 %		252 %
Resource use during end-of-life care	€25,975	€31,351	−2 %		19 %
Cost of medical visits	€24,772	€28,574	−6 %		8 %
Cost of hospitalizations	€24,926	€28,491	−6 %		8 %
Cost of treatment	€24,492	€35,522	−7 %		34 %
Cost of tests	€24,127	€28,938	−9 %		9 %

example, in the use of diagnostic tools such as broncho-alveolar lavage).

Our results may reflect true variability of the management of patients with IPF in Spanish clinical practice, likely due in part to the lack of effective pharmacological treatments. It remains to be seen how recently reported findings in IPF [22–24] and the availability of new therapeutic options will change treatment patterns in IPF. Nintedanib was not available at the time that this Delphi panel was carried out while pirfenidone had not been reimbursed and was only available through compassionate use; consideration of these treatments would probably increase the estimated economic burden associated with IPF.

Lung transplantation is the main determinant of treatment costs in patients with IPF. It might seem that the number of patients receiving lung transplantation in our study is low (5 and 8 % of patients with slow and rapid disease progression, respectively), but considering that 262 lung transplants were performed in Spain in 2014 [25] and that approximately one third of them are in patients with IPF [26], it can be extrapolated that approximately 1.3 % of patients with IPF receive a transplantation. It is also important to note that not all patients with IPF are candidates for lung transplantation [27].

The incidence and prevalence rates in our study (3 cases per 100,000 people/year and 12 cases per 100,000 people/year, respectively) are within the values in a recent review that estimated an annual incidence of IPF between 0.22 and 7.4 per 100,000 population and a prevalence between 1.25 and 23.4 cases per 100,000 population in Europe [28]. The true incidence and prevalence of IPF are difficult to estimate due to differences in coding, under- and misdiagnosis, e.g. a recent Spanish prospective observational study suggested that almost half of patients diagnosed with IPF may subsequently be diagnosed with chronic hypersensitivity pneumonitis [29].

One limitation of our study is that it was based on estimates from a Delphi panel and not on prospective or retrospective data. The Delphi panel consisted of 15 physicians who, although selected because of their ILD expertise, may not be fully representative of Spanish clinical practice. Nevertheless, it should be taken into account that experts were chosen from different regions in Spain, and since IPF is an orphan disease, the number of Spanish experts is limited. Indirect costs (e.g. work productivity) could not be determined because experts stated they lacked the information required to answer questions related to the impact of IPF on patients, relatives and caregivers. Studies assessing indirect costs would help to show the impact of IPF from the societal perspective. The study results were calculated on the basis of classifying patients as having stable disease, slow disease progression or rapid disease progression.

Although these groups correspond to different possible natural histories of IPF, there is no precise definition of these terms, which may be a limitation of our study. The Delphi panel estimates did not distinguish between the outpatient and inpatient costs associated with exacerbations, treatment, monitoring and end-of-life care. This might have led to double counting and an overestimate of the costs (the cost of hospital admissions, for example, already include the cost of tests, treatments and visits). In contrast, the calculation of the cost of drug-related adverse events excluded grade 1–2 adverse effects and grade 3–4 adverse effects affecting ≤5 % of patients. Therefore, there might have been an underestimation of the cost of adverse events. Finally, the number of exacerbations per year could have been overestimated because the questionnaires of the Delphi panel did not include a specific definition for an acute exacerbation of IPF and physicians may have included worsenings of IPF with an identifiable cause. This could explain why our results are higher than other data on acute exacerbations of IPF [30]. Despite these limitations, the similarities between our results and those of other studies on the impact of IPF [18] suggest that our study may provide a reasonable estimate of the cost of IPF in Spain.

Conclusions

The results of this study suggest that the management of patients with IPF in Spain, and especially patients with rapid disease progression, has a high economic impact on the NHS. The cost associated with acute exacerbations represents nearly half of the total cost of managing patients with IPF and therefore, the availability of new treatments that reduce the risk of acute exacerbations may reduce the economic impact of IPF. This study further supports the need for treatments modifying the course of IPF.

Abbreviations
COPD: Chronic obstructive pulmonary disorder; DEALE: Declining Exponential Approximation to Life Expectancy; HRCT: High resolution computed tomography; ILD: Interstitial lung disease; IPF: Idiopathic pulmonary fibrosis; NHS: National Health System; UIP: Usual interstitial pneumonia.

Competing interests
This study was sponsored by Boehringer Ingelheim. FM participated in the preparation of the study as a clinical expert and has been an Advisory Board member for InterMune. DE, JL and SS are employees of Boehringer Ingelheim. AV, DN and MB received funding from Boehringer Ingelheim to conduct the research.

Authors' contributions
FM was the main clinical advisor in the development of the questionnaires and participated in the writing and review of the manuscript. DE and JL were involved in the design of the study and interpretation of the results, and contributed to the writing and review of the manuscript. SS provided medical input during the development of the questionnaires and was

involved in the interpretation of the results and review of the manuscript. AV, DN and MB were involved in the design of the study, carried out data collection and analysis, and contributed to the drafting of the manuscript. All authors approved the final manuscript.

Acknowledgements
The following Spanish experts participated in the Delphi panel: Dr. Carlos Almonacid (Hospital Universitario de Guadalajara, Guadalajara), Dr. Julio Ancochea (Hospital La Princesa, Madrid), Dr. Miguel Arias (Hospital Universitario Central de Asturias, Oviedo), Dr. Adolfo Baloira (Complejo Hospitalario de Pontevedra, Pontevedra), Dr. Elena Bollo (Hospital Universitario de León, León), Dr. Esteban Cano (Hospital Xeral de Lugo, Lugo), Dr. Diego Castillo (Hospital de Sant Pau, Barcelona), Dr. Eusebi Chiner (Hospital Universitario San Juan de Alicante, Alicante), Dr. Pilar de Lucas (Hospital Universitario Gregorio Marañón, Madrid), Dr. Estrella Fernandez (Hospital Peset, Valencia), Dr. Pedro J Marcos Rodríguez (Hospital Juan Canalejo, La Coruña), Dr. Maria Molina (Hospital de Bellvitge, Barcelona), Dr. José Antonio Rodríguez Portal (Hospital Virgen del Rocío, Sevilla), Dr. Ana Villar (Hospital Vall d'Hebron, Barcelona), Dr. Antoni Xaubet (Hospital Clínic, Barcelona).

Editorial assistance, supported financially by Boehringer Ingelheim, was provided by Wendy Morris of Fleishman-Hillard Group, Ltd, London, UK, during the preparation of this article. The authors were fully responsible for all content and editorial decisions, were involved at all stages of development, and have approved the final version.

Author details
[1]Vall d'Hebron Institut de Recerca (VHIR), Respiratory Department, Hospital Universitari Vall d'Hebron and CIBER in Respiratory Diseases, Passeig de la Vall d'Hebron, 119-129, 08035 Barcelona, Spain. [2]Boehringer Ingelheim, Binger Str. 173, 55216 Ingelheim am Rhein, Germany. [3]Oblikue Consulting S.L., Avenida Diagonal 514, 3°-3a, 08006 Barcelona, Spain.

References
1. Raghu G, Collard HR, Egan JJ, Martinez FJ, Behr J, Brown KK, et al. An official ATS/ERS/JRS/ALAT statement: idiopathic pulmonary fibrosis: evidence-based guidelines for diagnosis and management. Am J Respir Crit Care Med. 2011; 183:788–824.
2. Ancochea J, Antón E, Casanova A. [Consensus for the diagnosis of idiopathic interstitial pneumonias]. Arch Bronconeumol. 2010;46 Suppl 5:2–21.
3. Fernández Pérez ER, Daniels CE, Schroeder DR, St Sauver J, Hartman TE, Bartholmai BJ, et al. Incidence, prevalence, and clinical course of idiopathic pulmonary fibrosis: a population-based study. Chest. 2010;137:129–37.
4. Collard HR, Moore BB, Flaherty KR, Brown KK, Kaner RJ, King Jr TE, et al. Acute exacerbations of idiopathic pulmonary fibrosis. Am J Respir Crit Care Med. 2007;176:636–43.
5. Ancochea J, Antón E, Casanova A. [New therapeutic strategies in idiopathic pulmonary fibrosis]. Arch Bronconeumol. 2004;40 Suppl 6:16–22.
6. Spagnolo P, Del Giovane C, Luppi F, Cerri S, Balduzzi S, Walters EH, et al. Non-steroid agents for idiopathic pulmonary fibrosis. Cochrane Database Syst Rev. 2010;9:CD003134.
7. King Jr TE, Pardo A, Selman M. Idiopathic pulmonary fibrosis. Lancet. 2011; 378:1949–61.
8. Lota HK, Wells AU. The evolving pharmacotherapy of pulmonary fibrosis. Expert Opin Pharmacother. 2013;14:79–89.
9. BOE [Spanish Official State Gazette] 2009. Available at: http://www.boe.es/diario_boe/txt.php?id=BOE-A-2009-20817 (accessed December 17, 2015).
10. CGCOF [General Spanish Council of Pharmacist] 2013. Available at: http://www.portalfarma.com (accessed May 1, 2013).
11. eSalud. Spanish Health Costs Database 2013. Oblikue Consulting. Available at: http://www.oblikue.com/bddcostes (accessed May 1, 2013).
12. MSSSI [Ministry of Health, Social Services and Equality] 2013. Available at: https://www.msssi.gob.es (accessed May 1, 2013).
13. Larg A, Moss JR. Cost-of-illness studies: a guide to critical evaluation. Pharmacoeconomics. 2011;29:653–71.
14. INE [Spanish Statistical Office]. Population projections in the short term. Resident in Spain on 1 January 2014. Available at: http://www.ine.es/inebmenu/mnu_cifraspob.htm (accessed July 1, 2013).
15. Morell F, Reyes L, Doménech G, De Gracia J, Majó J, Ferrer J. Diagnoses and diagnostic procedures in 500 consecutive patients with clinical suspicion of interstitial lung disease. Arch Bronconeumol. 2008;44:185–91.
16. National Cancer Institute. Common Terminology Criteria for Adverse Events v4.0. NCI, NIH, DHHS. May 29, 2009. Available at: http://evs.nci.nih.gov/ftp1/CTCAE/CTCAE_4.03_2010-06-14_QuickReference_5x7.pdf (accessed December 1, 2012).
17. Beck JR, Kassirer JP, Pauker SG. A convenient approximation of life expectancy (the "DEALE"). I. Validation of the method. Am J Med. 1982;73:883–8.
18. Collard HR, Ward AJ, Lanes S, Cortney Hayflinger D, Rosenberg DM, Hunsche E. Burden of illness in idiopathic pulmonary fibrosis. J Med Econ. 2012;15:829–35.
19. Miravitlles M, Sicras A, Crespo C, Cuesta M, Brosa M, Galera J, et al. Costs of chronic obstructive pulmonary disease in relation to compliance with guidelines: a study in the primary care setting. Ther Adv Respir Dis. 2013;7: 139–50.
20. Izquierdo-Alonso JL, de Miguel-Díez J. Economic impact of pulmonary drugs on direct costs of stable chronic obstructive pulmonary disease. COPD. 2004;1:215–23.
21. Miravitlles M, Murio C, Guerrero T, Gisbert R. Costs of chronic bronchitis and COPD: a 1-year follow-up study. Chest. 2003;123:784–91.
22. Richeldi L, du Bois RM, Raghu G, Azuma A, Brown KK, Costabel U, et al. Efficacy and safety of nintedanib in idiopathic pulmonary fibrosis. N Engl J Med. 2014;370:2071–82.
23. Idiopathic Pulmonary Fibrosis Clinical Research Network, Martinez FJ, de Andrade JA, Anstrom KJ, King Jr TE, Raghu G. Randomized trial of acetylcysteine in idiopathic pulmonary fibrosis. N Engl J Med. 2014;370: 2093–101.
24. King Jr TE, Bradford WZ, Castro-Bernardini S, Fagan EA, Glaspole I, Glassberg MK, et al. A phase 3 trial of pirfenidone in patients with idiopathic pulmonary fibrosis. N Engl J Med. 2014;370:2083–92.
25. ONT [Spanish Transplant National Organization]. Activity in 2014. Available at: http://www.ont.es/prensa/NotasDePrensa/13%20Ene%2015%20NP%20Balance%20Donacion%20y%20Tx%202014.pdf (accessed January 20, 2015).
26. Coll E, Santos F, Ussetti P, Canela M, Borro JM, De La Torre M, et al. The Spanish Lung Transplant Registry: first report of results (2006–2010). Arch Bronconeumol. 2013;49:70–8.
27. Román A, Ussetti P, Solé A, Zurbano F, Borro JM, Vaquero JM, et al. Sociedad Española de Neumología y Cirugía Torácica. Guidelines for the selection of lung transplantation candidates. Arch Bronconeumol. 2011;47: 303–9.
28. Nalysnyk L, Cid-Ruzafa J, Rotella P, Esser D. Incidence and prevalence of idiopathic pulmonary fibrosis: review of the literature. Eur Respir Rev. 2012; 21:355–61.
29. Morell F, Villar A, Montero MA, Muñoz X, Colby TV, Pipvath S, et al. Chronic hypersensitivity pneumonitis in patients diagnosed with idiopathic pulmonary fibrosis: a prospective case-cohort study. Lancet Respir Med. 2013;1:685–94.
30. Collard HR, Yow E, Richeldi L, Anstrom KJ, Glazer C. IPFnet investigators. Suspected acute exacerbation of idiopathic pulmonary fibrosis as an outcome measure in clinical trials. Respir Res. 2013;14:73.

2

IL-8 predicts early mortality in patients with acute hypercapnic respiratory failure treated with noninvasive positive pressure ventilation

Brynja Jónsdóttir[1,2,3*], Åsa Jaworowski[2], Carmen San Miguel[3] and Olle Melander[1,3]

Abstract

Background: Patients with Acute Hypercapnic Respiratory Failure (AHRF) who are unresponsive to appropriate medical treatment, are often treated with Noninvasive Positive Pressure Ventilation (NPPV). Clinical predictors of the outcome of this treatment are scarce. Therefore, we evaluated the role of the biomarkers IL-8 and GDF-15 in predicting 28-day mortality in patients with AHRF who receive treatment with NPPV.

Methods: The study population were 46 patients treated with NPPV for AHRF. Clinical and background data was registered and blood samples taken for analysis of inflammatory biomarkers. IL-8 and GDF-15 were selected for analysis, and related to risk of 28-day mortality (primary endpoint) using Cox proportional hazard models adjusted for gender, age and various clinical parameters.

Results: Of the 46 patients, there were 3 subgroup in regards to primary diagnosis: Acute Exacerbation of COPD (AECOPD, $n = 34$), Acute Heart Failure (AHF, $n = 8$) and Acute Exacerbation in Obesity Hypoventilation Syndrome (AEOHS, $n = 4$). There was significant difference in the basic characteristic of the subgroups, but not in the clinical parameters that were used in treatment decisions. 13 patients died within 28 days of admission (28%). The Hazard Ratio for 28-days mortality per 1-SD increment of IL-8 was 3.88 (95% CI 1.86–8.06, $p < 0.001$). When IL-8 values were divided into tertiles, the highest tertile had a significant association with 28 days mortality, HR 10.02 (95% CI 1.24–80.77, p for trend 0.03), compared with the lowest tertile. This correlation was maintained when the largest subgroup with AECOPD was analyzed. GDF-15 was correlated in the same way, but when put into the same model as IL-8, the significance disappeared.

Conclusion: IL-8 is a target to explore further as a predictor of 28 days mortality, in patients with AHRF treated with NPPV.

Keywords: Acute Respiratory Failure, Noninvasive Positive Pressure Ventilation, Short-time Mortality, Interleukin-8, Growth Differentiation Factor 15

Background

As Chronic Obstructive Lung Disease continues to be a leading cause of mortality and morbidity worldwide, the importance of choosing the most appropriate treatment for each patient is vital [1, 2]. In Acute Hypercapnic Respiratory Failure (AHRF) due to Acute Exacerbation of COPD (AECOPD), Noninvasive Positive Pressure Ventilation (NPPV) has been shown to reduce the need for endotracheal intubation, the length of hospital stay, and the in-hospital mortality rate, in patients who are unresponsive to acute appropriate medical therapy [3–8]. Sixty-day survival benefit has even been shown in patients with acute-on-chronic respiratory failure [9]. Patient selection is important, and the treatment is most effective in the early stages of acidosis [10–13]. Factors that have been show to predict NPPV failure in patients with AECOPD (resulting in endotracheal intubation or death) are severe acidosis (pH <7.25), low Glasgow Coma Scale scores, high respiratory rate and high

* Correspondence: brynjajo@gmail.com
[1]The Department of Clinical Sciences Malmo, Faculty of Medicine, Lund University, Lund, Sweden
[2]Department of Lung- and Allergy Medicine, Skåne University Hospital, Malmö, Sweden

APACHE-II score [14]. Even lack of improvement within the first hour after initiation of NPPV is a negative prognostic factor in patients with various underlying causes of AHRF [15].

NPPV is even effective in some other causes of respiratory failure, such as acute heart failure, pneumonia in COPD patients and infections in immunocompromised patients [16–20]. Berg et al. stated in a review article, that in patients with acute heart failure treated with nonvasive ventilation, many studies show some degree of benefit in regards to relief of respiratory distress, lower intubation rates or decreased mortality. There is no difference between NPPV and CPAP (continuous positive airway pressure), the latter being the first treatment option in acute cardiogenic pulmonary edema, but NPPV is recommended if there is any evidence of hypercapnia or if the patient remains in distress despite treatment with CPAP [21] Both NPPV and CPAP are also commonly used in exacerbations of obesity hypoventilation syndrome [22]. A comparison of NPPV treatment in patients with AHRF in AECOPD or Obesity Hypoventilation Syndrome (OHS) showed similar effectiveness regarding survival, in-hospital mortality, and length of hospital stay [23]. There is a lack of randomized clinical trials for OHS patients with AHRF, but the treatment is considered safe and effective, even if acidosis prevails generally longer than in patients with AECOPD [24].

COPD is associated with low-grade systemic inflammation. The search for biomarkers to predict outcome in COPD patients, both during exacerbations and in stable condition, has been extensive in the last few years [25, 26]. To our knowledge, no study has been published that has evaluated the roll of inflammatory biomarkers to predict short term mortality in patients with AHRF (with various underlying causes) treated with NPPV.

In order to improve risk stratification of patients with acute dyspnea, we recently assessed inflammatory biomarkers and their predicting value for mortality in patients that came to the ER with acute dyspnea, and found that in this group, Interleukin-8 (IL-8) and Growth Differentiation Factor 15 (GDF-15) strongly and independently predict 90-days mortality, individually and as an aggregated score [27]. IL-8 is produced by various cells in the inflammatory pathway. Among other things, it induces the migration of neutrophils to the airway [28]. GDF-15 is a regulatory protein in the inflammatory pathway and is also produced by various cells in response to oxidative and inflammatory factors [29]. Based on the strong association between IL-8 and GDF-15 and mortality in patients with acute dyspnea in our previously published study [27], we hypothesize that these two inflammatory markers may add clinically meaningful information regarding 28-day mortality in AHRF patients receiving NPPV treatment.

Methods

Study population

During the period January 2014 to June 2014 we enrolled adult patients with acute respiratory failure that had clinical indication for treatment with NPPV according to local clinical guidelines, in the Intermediate Emergency Care Department at Skane University Hospital in Malmö, Sweden. The hospital serves a catchment area of approximately 400,000 inhabitants. We did not perform a power calculation as no prior suggested effect size for the association between IL-8 and GDF-15 on 28-day mortality in AHRF patients on NPPV treatment exist, on which the power calculation could be based. Written informed consent was obtained from all patients or their next of kin.

We included all patients that received treatment with NPPV for AHRF, decided by the attending physicians and regardless of the underlying disease. Patients with neurological disease or sepsis as the main cause of respiratory failure were excluded. Participation did not intervene with the treatment itself and the research personal was not responsible for the medical treatment in any way. Thus, the study was observational and prospective. As the clinical value of NPPV treatment in AHRF is nonmistakable according to various studies, it was not possible to have a control group deprived of the treatment [5, 8, 9, 16, 19, 23].

The study was approved by the Regional Ethics Board of Lund, Sweden and followed the precepts established by the Declaration of Helsinki.

Clinical parameters and follow-up

Vital parameters were obtained before and during the treatment at several previously decided time points (0, 1, 4, and 12 h after the start of treatment and venous blood samples and arterial blood gases (ABG) were taken. Vital parameters recorded were body temperature, peripheral oxygen saturation (SpO_2), heart rate, blood pressure, respiratory rate and degree of consciousness according to the "Reaction Level Scale" (RLS) [30]. The ABGs were analyzed immediately on a ABL800 Flex (Radiometer, Copenhagen, Denmark), while the venous blood samples were frozen and stored at −80 °C for later analysis of biomarkers, after having separated serum and plasma.

All the patients received Bilevel NPPV treatment with Trilogy100 and a suitable NPPV mask (Respironics, Murrysville, Pennsylvania/USA), using S/T mode. Expiratory positive airway pressure (EPAP) was set to 5 cm H_2O. Inspiratory positive airway pressure (IPAP) was automatically regulated with average volume assured pressure support (AVAPS), so that a pressure between 10 and 25 cm H_2O was applied to obtain a goal tidal volume of 8 ml/kg. Backup respiratory rate was set to 10 breaths/min. Oxygen was applied as needed with a goal SpO_2 of 88–90%. The patients were monitored closely during the treatment. The treatment was only stopped for shorter periods, for example during meals. The physicians on call decided when the treatment was discontinued. Details about treatment length and installations was obtained from the Directview Program (Respironics, Murrysville, Pennsylvania/USA).

The patients consented to have their medical history and current medication obtained through the journal database of the hospital. Smoking habits, employment history and marital status was obtained through interview.

Biomarker measurement

Based on our previous findings in risk stratification of patients with acute dyspnea [27], we selected to study IL-8 and GDF-15 which were measured in frozen plasma samples using the Proseek Multiplex CVD 1 biomarker panel (Olink Bioscience, Uppsala, Sweden). The method is a multiplex immunoassay based on a Proximity Extension Assay [31]. All assay characteristics including detection limits and measurements of assay performance and validations are available from the manufacturer's webpage [32].

Endpoint

The primary endpoint in the current study was defined as death within 28 days after admission to the ER. We confirmed deaths and date of death using the Swedish National civil registry.

Statistical analysis

All statistical analysis was performed with IBM SPSS statistics version 21 (SPSS Inc., Chigago, IL, USA). In univariate analyses we used Kruskal-Wallis test to analyze continuous variables, and expressed data as medians and interquartile ranges. For categorical variables, Fishers exact test was used and data was expressed as numbers and percentages. We used Cox proportional hazards model to relate baseline variables to risk of death during 28 days of follow-up. Biomarkers levels were transformed with the natural logarithm and expressed as hazard ratios (95% confidence interval) on a standardized scale (per 1 standard deviation increment) as well as in tertiles, with the lowest tertile as the reference group. We adjusted for age and gender (model 1) and age, gender and C-reactive protein (CRP) (model 2) and also entered multiple potential confounders using backward stepwise Wald selection with a retention P-value >0.10 (model 3). Finally, crude Kaplan-Meier plots for tertiles of IL-8 levels were plotted. All tests were two-sided and a p-value of <0.05 was considered statistically significant.

Results

Patient characteristics

Fifty-one patients were enrolled during the study time, but five patients were excluded because of withdrawal of consent ($n = 3$), presence of neurological disease ($n = 1$) and sepsis ($n = 1$) as main underlying causes of AHRF, leaving forty-six patients in the analysis. No patient was intubated during the hospital stay. Chest radiographies were performed bedside on 39 patients (85%). 2 patients had radiological evidence of possible consolidation, both of which survived the follow up time of 28 days. There was no significant correlation between radiologial evidence of heart failure or consolidation, and 28 days mortality (data not shown). All patients were evaluated by attending physicians regarding vital status, and in 33 patients (72%), the "Do Not Resuscitate" order was made and recorded in the medical journal, according to local guidelines. Twenty-four patients (52%) were evaluated not to be eligible for ICU ward. Thirteen patients died within 28 days after admission (28%), of whom 10 patients died during the hospital stay. The median length of stay was 7 days (IQR 4–11 days).

Before analysis of data, the medical records were examined by an internist and a primary discharge diagnosis was made. There were 3 subgroups of patients in regards to primary diagnosis: Acute Exacerbation of COPD (AECOPD), Acute Heart Failure (AHF) and Acute Respiratory failure in OHS (AEOHS). To evaluate if there was difference between the groups, clinical characteristics were compared between the groups (Table 1). There were significant group differences in age, BMI and smoking status. While the difference between the subgroups lay within the basic characteristics of the group population, but not in regards of variables which determined NPPV treatment, the assumption was made that all results could be analyzed as one group of patients with AHRF. Analyses were nonetheless also made on the largest subgroup of patients with AECOPD, as described below.

IL-8 and GDF-15

The biomarkers IL-8 and GDF-15 at admission before treatment was started, showed significant association with 28 days mortality through adjusted Cox proportional hazard models 1 (age and gender adjusted) and 2 (age, gender and CRP adjusted) (Tables 2 and 3). Each 1 SD increment of IL-8 was associated with almost fourfold increased risk of 28 days mortality, and for GDF-15 the increase in risk was almost threefold (Tables 2 and 3). Even CRP alone (adjusted for age and gender) was analyzed in model 2, and was an independent risk factor for 28 days mortality (HR 1.61 (1.08–2.41), p 0.02). In model 3, where additional parameters (BMI and blood analysis (pH, pO_2, pCO_2, lactate) as well as respiratory rate at start of treatment and primary discharge diagnosis) were entered in a backward stepwise elimination model (data missing on $n = 13$), both IL-8 ($p = 0.015$) and GDF-15 ($p = 0.008$) remained significantly related to

Table 1 Characteristics of the patients, as a whole group and divided into subgroups

	Whole group	AECOPD	AHF	AEOHS	P value[b]
General characteristics					
Number of patients	46	34	8	4	
Age years: median (IQR)	77.1 (68.7–84.0)	76.9 (68.8–83.9)	82.3 (77.7–86.8)	65.4 (60.5–73.0)	*0.035*
BMI kg/m^2: median (IQR)	23.4 (20.5–36.1)	24.0 (18.8–28.2)	27.7 (21.7–39.2)	46.6 (39.3–55.2)	*0.004*
Gender female %	65% (30/46)	65% (22/34)	63% (5/8)	75% (3/4)	0.054
Active or ex-smokers %	87% (40/46)	97% (33/34)	63% (5/8)	50% (2/4)	*<0.001*
FEV1%: median (IQR)	31 (24–43)	29 (22–36)	47[a]	43[a]	0.058
Variables related to AHRF					
pH: median (IQR)	7.28 (7.24–7.36)	7.31 (7.24–7.37)	7.24 (7.10–7.31)	7.30 (7.25–7.35)	0.17
pO$_2$ kPa: median (IQR)	7.45 (6.33–8.73)	6.85 (6.10–8.48)	7.50 (5.60–9.58)	8.40 (8.23–10.68)	0.24
pCO$_2$ kPa: median (IQR)	8.75 (7.78–10.5)	8.90 (7.78–10.35)	8.05 (6.38–10.73)	10.05 (8.45–11.73)	0.30
Respiratory rate bpm: median (IQR)	26 (20–29)	26 (20–29)	24 (22–29)	25 (21–27)	0.89
CRP mg/L: median (IQR)	15.5 (8.3–76.5)	36.5 (9.7–93.0)	8.7 (6.4–11.0)	12.5 (7.5–37.0)	0.076
Lactate mmol/L: median (IQR)	1.40 (0.80–2.75)	1.10 (0.80–2.10)	3.80 (2.78–5.63)	1.20 (0.80–2.35)	0.09
NPPV use first 4 h: median (IQR)	3.57 (3.50–4.00)	3.67 (3.50–4.00)	3.50 (2.50–4.00)	3.75 (3.50–4.00)	0.67

IQR interquartile range, *AECOPD* acute exacerbation of COPD, *AHF* acute heart failure, *AEOHS* acute exacerbation of obesity hypoventilation syndrome, *BMI* body mass index, *FEV1* forced expiratory volume in 1 s, *CRP* C-reactive protein, *NPPV* noninvasive positive pressure ventilation
[a]variable number too small to analyse IQR
[b]We used Kruskal-Wallis test for all but gender and smoking status, there we used Fisher´s exact test

risk of 28-day mortality. The independent significant association between IL-8 or GDF-15 and 28-day mortality remained after exclusion of the two patients with consolidation on chest radiograph (data not shown).

IL-8 tertiles were entered into model 1 and 2 adjusted Cox proportional hazard model, patients in the highest tertile showed a significant 10-fold and 13-fold, respectively, increased risk of 28 days mortality, as compared to the lowest tertile (Table 2). The event rate in IL-8 tertiles according to a Kaplan-Meier plot is shown in Fig. 1. When GDF-15 tertiles were analyzed in the same manner, there was no significant association in model 1, but in model 2 there was a significant association with a 2,5 fold increased risk for mortality for the highest tertile as compared to the lowest (Table 3).

To evaluate if both IL-8 and GDF-15 were independent risk factors, we simultaneously entered them as continuous variables into model 1 and found that only IL-8

remained significantly associated, with HR 3.38 (95% CI 1.35–8.43, p = 0.009) per 1 SD increment.

Being the largest group, we then analyzed the group of patients with AECOPD as their primary diagnosis (n = 34) separately. Both IL-8 and GDF-15 at admission showed significant association with 28 days mortality in models 1–2 with approximately fourfold and threefold increased risk per 1 SD increment (Table 4). When simultaneously entered into model 1, only IL-8 remained significantly associated with HR 4.31 (95% CI 1.57–11.84, p = 0.005).

Discussion

Our findings suggest that IL-8 is a target to explore further as a biomarker in predicting 28 days mortality, in patients with AHRF (Acute Hypercapnic Respiratory Failure) and AECOPD (Acute Exacerbation of COPD) who receive treatment with NPPV (Noninvasive Positive Pressure Ventilation). The results were driven by COPD

Table 2 Relationship between Interleukin-8 (IL-8) and risk of 28-day mortality

IL-8 on admission vs 28 days follow-up death (Model 1 and 2)						
	Continuous IL-8 analysis (per SD increment)	P-value	Tertile 1	Tertile 2	Tertile 3	P for trend
N/N events[b]	46/13		15/1	16/3	15/9	
HR (95% CI) (age and gender adjusted)	3.88 (1.86–8.06)	*<0.001*	1.0 (ref)	2.79 (0.29–26.89)	10.02 (1.24–80.77)	*0.009*
HR (95% CI) (age, gender and CRP adjusted)[a]	3.76 (2.02–7.03)	*<0.001*	1.0 (ref)	3.11 (0.32–29.93)	13.47 (1.70–106.91)	*0.003*

SD standard deviation, *HR* hazard ratio, *CI* confidence interval, *CRP* C-reactive protein
[a]Backward elimination model
[b]death within 28 days from admission

Table 3 Relationship between Growth Differentiation Factor 15(GDF-15) and risk of 28-day mortality

GDF-15 on admission vs 28 days follow-up death (Model 1 and 2)

	Continuous GDF-15 analysis (per SD increment)	P-value	Tertile 1	Tertile 2	Tertile 3	P for trend
N/N events[b]	46/13		15/1	16/3	15/9	
HR (95% CI) (age and gender adjusted)	2.76 (1.37–5.56)	0.004	1.0 (ref)	1.21 (0.19–7.77)	3.48 (0.54–22.34)	0.124
HR (95% CI) (age, gender and CRP adjusted)[a]	3.48 (1.78–6.80)	<0.001	1.0 (ref)	1.14 (0.16–8.21)	2.65 (0.36–19.41)	0.036

SD standard deviation, HR hazard ratio, CI confidence interval, CRP C-reactive protein
[a]Backward elimination model
[b]death within 28 days from admission

patients, so further studies are needed not only to replicate our findings but also to test if the our findings are valid in the comparably small subgroup of non-COPD patients.

NPPV is a well-known treatment option for patients with AHRF. Earlier studies have shown that in patients with AECOPD, NPPV can reduce the risk of intubation, reduce in-hospital mortality and shorten the hospital stay [3–7]. Its use has been growing and more data has appeared supporting the positive effects of the treatment, even in other types of respiratory failure [21]. The treatment is costly in terms of technical equipment and surveillance, and not all patients can tolerate the treatment or benefit from it [17]. Even if there are clinical tools that have been shown to help in predicting the outcome of NPPV treatment, the search for parameters that can provide additional help in treatment decisions is important, both in regard to costs and patient comfort [12–14, 33].

Because of its predictive value in relation to short term mortality, our findings imply that the inflammatory biomarker IL-8 could potentially be used in the initial evaluation of the patient with AHRF, to help choose the most appropriate treatment. This potential clinical use can be used on patients with AECOPD and even maybe in other types of AHRF (Acute Heart Failure or Acute Exacerbation of OHS). This is clinically important, as the main cause for the AHRF is not always clear when the patient arrives to the ER. GDF-15 showed similar results as IL-8, but our analysis implies that it is not an independent factor but dependent of IL-8 in this clinical setting. CRP did not influence the correlation between IL-8 and 28 days mortality, and it was even not effected by the confounding factors age, gender, BMI, blood analysis (pH, pO_2, pCO_2, lactate) as well as respiratory rate at start of treatment or primary discharge diagnosis (Table 2). A high value of IL-8 might thus prompt the physician to choose more invasive treatment such as intubation. As many forms of acute and chronic illnesses are characterized by enhanced inflammation, it is likely that high baseline values of IL-8 and GDF-15 reflects not only a more severe acute condition but most likely also more severe chronic illness.

IL-8 is a chemokine that induces the migration of neutrophils to the airway and affects degranulation [28]. Both sputum and serum IL-8 have been targets for

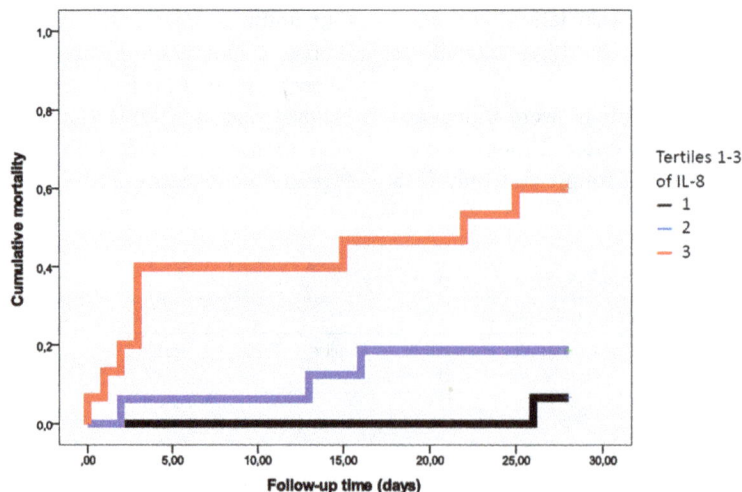

Fig. 1 Kaplan-Meier plot showing cumulative mortality during 28 days of follow-up. Tertile 1 denotes the lowest values of IL-8; and Tertile 3 the highest values

Table 4 Relationship between IL-8/GDF-15 and risk of 28-day mortality in a subgroup of patients with AECOPD

IL-8 and GDF-15 on admission vs 28 days follow-up death – AECOPD subgroup

	IL-8		GDF-15	
	Continuous analysis (per SD increment)	P-value	Continuous analysis (per SD increment)	P-value
N/N events[b]	34/11		34/11	
HR (95% CI) (age and gender adjusted)	4.16 (1.84–9.39)	0.001	3.10 (1.30–7.40)	0.011
HR (95% CI) (age, gender and CRP adjusted)[a]	4.34 (2.05–9.19)	<0.001	3.28 (1.56–6.88)	0.002

AECOPD acute exacerbation of COPD, SD standard deviation, HR hazard ratio, CI confidence interval, CRP C-reactive protein
[a]Backward elimination model
[b]death within 28 days from admission

research in regards to COPD mortality and exacerbations. A review by Koutsokera et al. summarized that IL-8 levels in spontaneous sputum in patients with AECOPD can be predictive of clinical severity, symptomatic recovery and even presence of bacterial infection and its eradication [34]. Agusti et al. identified 6 inflammatory biomarkers (including IL-8) that were related to systemic inflammation, and patients with COPD in which those biomarkers were elevated in serum showed increased all-cause mortality and exacerbation frequency, during three-year follow up time [35]. Lastly, Shafiak et al. showed that in patients with AECOPD, serum IL-8 had higher levels in non-responders of NPPV vs. responders, where failure was defined as termination of NPPV trial and initiation of invasive mechanical ventilation. IL-8 was however not correlated to presence of bacterial infection [36]. To our knowledge, that is the only prior study that has studied IL-8 levels and its correlation to AECOPD and NPPV treatment. The combination of these results support that IL-8 can possibly be used as a clinical predictor of response to NPPV treatment in patients with AECOPD, although to our knowledge, no prior study has focused on correlation between IL-8 in serum and short-term mortality in this patient group.

The GDF-15 protein is also a member of the inflammatory pathway, and is produced by multiple cells in response to oxidative and inflammatory factors. In recent years, studies have shown that GDF-15 levels can help in predicting mortality and adverse events in patients with cardiovascular diseases and other diseases [29]. Recent studies have even evaluated the connection between GDF-15 levels and AECOPD, in which patients with AECOPD had higher baseline blood levels of GDF-15 and it is regarded as an independent predictor of the presence of AECOPD [37, 38]. Our data did not confirm that serum GDF-15 was an independent prognostic factor for short-time mortality in patients with AHRF who receive NPPV treatment, but suggested that it is dependent of IL-8 levels. To our knowledge no other study has addressed the role of GDF-15 in this clinical setting.

The predictive value of IL-8 on 28 days mortality was independent of the traditional biomarker CRP and it had a comparatively stronger association, although CRP levels also had an independent correlation to the endpoint. Our study does not allow any conclusions as to whether or not the relationship between IL-8 and short term mortality is causal, but in our opinion encourages further mechanistic studies to better understand this issue.

Our study has several limitations, the main one being the relatively small sample size, which also results in wide confidence intervals. Further studies are needed, which should include a larger group of patients with a larger spectrum of diagnoses and preferably even patients that are intubated if NPPV treatment is not successful. Another limitation is that only 85% of the patients did a chest radiography during the initial hours of the NPPV treatment. Nonetheless, the radiological results did not have any correlation to 28 days mortality.

The group of patients in this study had a high percentage of the "Do Not Resuscitate" order (72%), compared with an audit made by Roberts and al in UK (40%) [39]. A possible reason for this difference is that in the local guidelines, the admitting physician is obligated to make a resuscitation judgement if the patient is to be treated with NPPV. 28 days mortality was (28%) and can be regarded as more severely ill than groups of patients in some other studies in the field [8, 19], but similar to that reported in the UK audit (25% inhospital mortality) [39]. In this setting it is a challenge to recruit patients for research projects. Nonetheless, it is our opinion that more research in severely ill patients is necessary, to help clinicians make the choice between the use of demanding treatment such as NPPV or go directly to intubation. Our study did not include any patients that were later intubated so we cannot make any assumption as to how IL-8 values are effected by that. In our opinion it would be interesting to raise that question in further studies, and also evaluate the hypothesis that if IL-8 values do not become lower during noninvasive or invasive respiratory support, the prognosis would be poor in regards to short term mortality.

Another limitation of the study is the heterogeneity of the group. Subgroup analysis did not seem to influence the results though and the largest subgroup of patients, with AECOPD, have an even stronger association with the endpoint. Since the other two subgroups with AHF and AEOHS were so small in numbers, one should be careful to interpret the results in that clinical setting. The diagnosis of COPD and heart failure prior to admission came from the patients' medical records, but some data regarding spirometry and echocardiography was not present. Nonetheless, the primary discharge diagnosis was assessed by the same internist in all cases, and the probability of wrong diagnosis seems minimal because of the large amount of clinical data available during the admission. In our opinion, the heterogeneity of the group reflects the clinical setting in the ER where the underlying medical condition resulting in respiratory failure is commonly unknown, and the results can be applied in that context. Further studies of patients with AHRF in regards of clinically important prognostic factors are relevant because the treatment with NPPV can be costly and difficult for patients, and existing patient selection tools do not always help in treatment decision.

Conclusion

Our results show that IL-8 in serum is a target to explore further as a predictor of short-time mortality in patients with Acute Hypercapnic Respiratory Failure and Acute Exacerbation of COPD treated with Noninvasive Positive Pressure Ventilation. Its use in the initial assessment of this patient group should be addressed in studies with a larger number of patients but our result suggests a use of IL-8 as a tool to help physicians in treatment decisions.

Abbreviations
ABG: arterial blood gas; AECOPD: acute exacerbation of chronic obstructive pulmonary disease; AEOHS: acute exacerbation of obesity hypoventilation syndrome; AHF: acute heart failure; AHRF: acute hypercapnic respiratory failure; APACHE-II: acute physiology and chronic health evaluation ii; AVAPS: average volume assured pressure support; BMI: body mass index; CI: confidence interval; COPD: chronic obstructive pulmonary disease; CPAP: continuous positive airway pressure; CRP: C reactive protein; EPAP: expiratory positive airway pressure; ER: emergency room; FEV1: forced expiratory volume in 1 second; GDF-15: growth differentiation factor 15; HR: hazard ratio; ICU: intensive care unit; IL-8: interleukin-8; IPAP: inspiratory positive airway pressure; IQR: interquartile range; NPPV: noninvasive positive pressure ventilation; OHS: obesity hypoventilation syndrome; RLS: reaction level scale; SD: standard deviation

Acknowledgements
Not applicable.

Funding
Information about funding is available in the online article submission. The funding bodies had no roll in regards to design of the study, collection of data, analysis and interpretation of data or in writing the manuscript.

Authors' contributions
BJ had part in designing the study, thereafter collected, analyzed and interpreted the data, and was the main contributor to writing the manuscript. ÅJ participated in designing the study and in writing of the manuscript. CSM participated in the collection of data. OM had part in designing the study, was the main contributor to analysis and interpretation of data, and participated in writing the manuscript. All authors read and approved the final manuscript.

Competing interests
The authors declare that they have no competing interests.

Author details
[1]The Department of Clinical Sciences Malmo, Faculty of Medicine, Lund University, Lund, Sweden. [2]Department of Lung- and Allergy Medicine, Skåne University Hospital, Malmö, Sweden. [3]Department of Internal Medicine and Emergency Medicine, Skåne University Hospital, Malmö, Sweden.

References
1. Lopez AD, Shibuya K, Rao C, Mathers CD, Hansell AL, Held LS, Schmid V, Buist S. Chronic obstructive pulmonary disease: current burden and future projections. Eur Respir J. 2006;27(2):397–412.
2. Vestbo J, Hurd SS, Agusti AG, Jones PW, Vogelmeier C, Anzueto A, Barnes PJ, Fabbri LM, Martinez FJ, Nishimura M, Stockley RA, Sin DD, Rodriguez-Roisin R. Global strategy for the diagnosis, management, and prevention of chronic obstructive pulmonary disease: GOLD executive summary. Am J Respir Crit Care Med. 2013;187(4):347–65.
3. Brochard L, Mancebo J, Wysocki M, Lofaso F, Conti G, Rauss A, Simonneau G, Benito S, Gasparetto A, Lemaire F, et al. Noninvasive ventilation for acute exacerbations of chronic obstructive pulmonary disease. N Engl J Med. 1995;333(13):817–22.
4. Celikel T, Sungur M, Ceyhan B, Karakurt S. Comparison of noninvasive positive pressure ventilation with standard medical therapy in hypercapnic acute respiratory failure. Chest. 1998;114(6):1636–42.
5. Roberts CM, Brown JL, Reinhardt AK, Kaul S, Scales K, Mikelsons C, Reid K, Winter R, Young K, Restrick L, Plant PK. Non-invasive ventilation in chronic obstructive pulmonary disease: management of acute type 2 respiratory failure. Clin Med. 2008;8(5):517–21.
6. McCurdy BR. Noninvasive Positive Pressure Ventilation for Acute Respiratory Failure Patients With Chronic Obstructive Pulmonary Disease (COPD): An Evidence-Based Analysis. Ontario Health Technology Assessment Series. 2012;12(8):1–102.
7. Plant PK, Owen JL, Elliott MW. Early use of non-invasive ventilation for acute exacerbations of chronic obstructive pulmonary disease on general respiratory wards: a multicentre randomised controlled trial. Lancet. 2000; 355(9219):1931–5.
8. Cabrini L, Landoni G, Oriani A, Plumari VP, Nobile L, Greco M, Pasin L, Beretta L, Zangrillo A. Noninvasive ventilation and survival in acute care settings: a comprehensive systematic review and metaanalysis of randomized controlled trials. Crit Care Med. 2015;43(4):880–8.
9. Schnell D, Timsit JF, Darmon M, Vesin A, Goldgran-Toledano D, Dumenil AS, Garrouste-Orgeas M, Adrie C, Bouadma L, Planquette B, Cohen Y, Schwebel C, Soufir L, Jamali S, Souweine B, Azoulay E. Noninvasive mechanical ventilation in acute respiratory failure: trends in use and outcomes. Intensive Care Med. 2014;40(4):582–91.
10. Lightowler JV, Wedzicha JA, Elliott MW, Ram FS. Non-invasive positive pressure ventilation to treat respiratory failure resulting from exacerbations of chronic obstructive pulmonary disease: Cochrane systematic review and meta-analysis. BMJ. 2003;326(7382):185.
11. Plant PK, Owen JL, Elliott MW. Non-invasive ventilation in acute exacerbations of chronic obstructive pulmonary disease: long term survival and predictors of in-hospital outcome. Thorax. 2001;56(9):708–12.
12. Budweiser S, Jorres RA, Pfeifer M. Treatment of respiratory failure in COPD. Int J Chron Obstruct Pulmon Dis. 2008;3(4):605–18.
13. Ambrosino N, Vagheggini G. Non-invasive ventilation in exacerbations of COPD. Int J Chron Obstruct Pulmon Dis. 2007;2(4):471–6.
14. Confalonieri M, Garuti G, Cattaruzza MS, Osborn JF, Antonelli M, Conti G, Kodric M, Resta O, Marchese S, Gregoretti C, Rossi A. A chart of failure risk

for noninvasive ventilation in patients with COPD exacerbation. Eur Respir J. 2005;25(2):348–55.

15. Garpestad E, Brennan J, Hill NS. Noninvasive ventilation for critical care. Chest. 2007;132(2):711–20.

16. Confalonieri M, Potena A, Carbone G, Porta RD, Tolley EA, Umberto MG. Acute respiratory failure in patients with severe community-acquired pneumonia. A prospective randomized evaluation of noninvasive ventilation. Am J Respir Crit Care Med. 1999;160(5 Pt 1):1585–91.

17. Liesching T, Kwok H, Hill NS. Acute applications of noninvasive positive pressure ventilation. Chest. 2003;124(2):699–713.

18. Bello G, De Pascale G, Antonelli M. Noninvasive ventilation for the immunocompromised patient: always appropriate? Curr Opin Crit Care. 2012;18(1):54–60.

19. Mas A, Masip J. Noninvasive ventilation in acute respiratory failure. Int J Chron Obstruct Pulmon Dis. 2014;9:837–52.

20. Vital FM, Ladeira MT, Atallah AN. Non-invasive positive pressure ventilation (CPAP or bilevel NPPV) for cardiogenic pulmonary oedema. Cochrane Database Syst Rev. 2013;5:CD005351.

21. Berg KM, Clardy P, Donnino MW. Noninvasive ventilation for acute respiratory failure: a review of the literature and current guidelines. Intern Emerg Med. 2012;7(6):539–45.

22. Jones SF, Brito V, Ghamande S. Obesity hypoventilation syndrome in the critically ill. Crit Care Clin. 2015;31(3):419–34.

23. Carrillo A, Ferrer M, Gonzalez-Diaz G, Lopez-Martinez A, Llamas N, Alcazar M, Capilla L, Torres A. Noninvasive ventilation in acute hypercapnic respiratory failure caused by obesity hypoventilation syndrome and chronic obstructive pulmonary disease. Am J Respir Crit Care Med. 2012;186(12):1279–85.

24. Lemyze M, Taufour P, Duhamel A, Temime J, Nigeon O, Vangrunderbeeck N, Barrailler S, Gasan G, Pepy F, Thevenin D, Mallat J. Determinants of noninvasive ventilation success or failure in morbidly obese patients in acute respiratory failure. PLoS One. 2014;9(5):e97563.

25. Koutsokera A, Stolz D, Loukides S, Kostikas K. Systemic biomarkers in exacerbations of COPD: the evolving clinical challenge. Chest. 2012;141(2):396–405.

26. Shaw JG, Vaughan A, Dent AG, O'Hare PE, Goh F, Bowman RV, Fong KM, Yang IA. Biomarkers of progression of chronic obstructive pulmonary disease (COPD). J Thorac Dis. 2014;6(11):1532–47.

27. Wiklund K, Gransbo K, Lund N, Peyman M, Tegner L, Toni-Bengtsson M, Wieloch M, Melander O. Inflammatory biomarkers predicting prognosis in patients with acute dyspnea. Am J Emerg Med. 2016;34(3):370–4.

28. Bhowmik A, Seemungal TA, Sapsford RJ, Wedzicha JA. Relation of sputum inflammatory markers to symptoms and lung function changes in COPD exacerbations. Thorax. 2000;55(2):114–20.

29. Corre J, Hebraud B, Bourin P. Concise review: growth differentiation factor 15 in pathology: a clinical role? Stem Cells Transl Med. 2013;2(12):946–52.

30. Starmark JE, Stalhammar D, Holmgren E. The Reaction Level Scale (RLS85). Manual and guidelines. Acta Neurochir (Wien). 1988;91(1–2):12–20.

31. Lundberg M, Eriksson A, Tran B, Assarsson E, Fredriksson S. Homogeneous antibody-based proximity extension assays provide sensitive and specific detection of low-abundant proteins in human blood. Nucleic Acids Res. 2011;39(15):e102.

32. Proseek Multiplex. A Precision proteomics solution for targeted protein biomarker discovery. Uppsala: 2016. http://www.olink.com/products/proseek-multiplex/. Accessed 16 Aug 2016.

33. Plant PK, Owen JL, Parrott S, Elliott MW. Cost effectiveness of ward based non-invasive ventilation for acute exacerbations of chronic obstructive pulmonary disease: economic analysis of randomised controlled trial. BMJ. 2003;326(7396):956.

34. Koutsokera A, Kostikas K, Nicod LP, Fitting JW. Pulmonary biomarkers in COPD exacerbations: a systematic review. Respir Res. 2013;14:111.

35. Agusti A, Edwards LD, Rennard SI, MacNee W, Tal-Singer R, Miller BE, Vestbo J, Lomas DA, Calverley PM, Wouters E, Crim C, Yates JC, Silverman EK, Coxson HO, Bakke P, Mayer RJ, Celli B. Persistent systemic inflammation is associated with poor clinical outcomes in COPD: a novel phenotype. PLoS One. 2012;7(5):e37483.

36. Shafiek HA, Abd-Elwahab NH, Baddour MM, El-Hoffy MM, Degady AA, Khalil YM. Assessment of some inflammatory biomarkers as predictors of outcome of acute respiratory failure on top of chronic obstructive pulmonary disease and evaluation of the role of bacteria. ISRN Microbiol. 2012;2012:240841.

37. Freeman CM, Martinez CH, Todt JC, Martinez FJ, Han MK, Thompson DL, McCloskey L, Curtis JL. Acute exacerbations of chronic obstructive pulmonary disease are associated with decreased CD4+ & CD8+ T cells and increased growth & differentiation factor-15 (GDF-15) in peripheral blood. Respir Res. 2015;16:94.

38. Mutlu LC, Altintas N, Aydin M, Tulubas F, Oran M, Kucukyalin V, Kaplan G, Gurel A. Growth Differentiation Factor-15 Is a Novel Biomarker Predicting Acute Exacerbation of Chronic Obstructive Pulmonary Disease. Inflammation. 2015;38(5):1805–13.

39. Roberts CM, Stone RA, Buckingham RJ, Pursey NA, Lowe D. Acidosis, non-invasive ventilation and mortality in hospitalised COPD exacerbations. Thorax. 2011;66(1):43–8.

3

Unmet needs in the treatment of idiopathic pulmonary fibrosis—insights from patient chart review in five European countries

Toby M. Maher[1,8]*, Maria Molina-Molina[2], Anne-Marie Russell[1], Francesco Bonella[3], Stéphane Jouneau[4], Elena Ripamonti[5], Judit Axmann[6] and Carlo Vancheri[7]

Abstract

Background: Two antifibrotic drugs, pirfenidone and nintedanib, are approved by the European Medicines Agency and the US Food and Drug Administration for the treatment of idiopathic pulmonary fibrosis (IPF). In this analysis, treatment patterns of European patients with IPF were investigated to understand antifibrotic prescribing and identify unmet needs in IPF treatment practice.

Methods: Between February and March 2016, respiratory physicians from France, Germany, Italy, Spain, and the UK participated in an online questionnaire designed to collect information on IPF treatment patterns in patients under their care. Patients were categorized as treated (received approved antifibrotics) or untreated (did not receive approved antifibrotics, but may have received other unapproved therapies). Classification of IPF diagnosis (confirmed/suspected) and severity ('mild'/'moderate'/'severe') for each patient was based on the individual physician's report. Patients' perspectives were not recorded in this study.

Results: In total, 290 physicians responded to the questionnaire. Overall, 54% of patients with IPF did not receive treatment with an approved antifibrotic. More patients had a confirmed IPF diagnosis in the treated (84%) versus the untreated (51%) population. Of patients with a confirmed diagnosis, 40% did not receive treatment. The treated population was younger than the untreated population (67 vs 70 years, respectively; $p \leq 0.01$), with more frequent multidisciplinary team evaluation (83% vs 57%, respectively; $p \leq 0.01$). A higher proportion of untreated patients had forced vital capacity > 80% at diagnosis versus treated patients. Of patients with 'mild' IPF, 71% did not receive an approved antifibrotic versus 41% and 60% of patients with 'moderate' and 'severe' IPF, respectively.

Conclusions: Despite the availability of antifibrotic therapies, many European patients with confirmed IPF do not receive approved antifibrotic treatment. Importantly, there appears to be a reluctance to treat patients with 'mild' or 'stable' disease, and instead adopt a 'watch and wait' approach. More education is required to address diagnostic uncertainty, poor understanding of IPF and its treatments, and issues of treatment access. There is a need to increase physician awareness of the benefits associated with antifibrotic treatment across the spectrum of IPF severity.

Keywords: Antifibrotics, Idiopathic pulmonary fibrosis, Questionnaire, Treatment patterns, Unmet needs

* Correspondence: T.Maher@imperial.ac.uk
[1]NIHR Respiratory Biomedical Research Unit, Royal Brompton Hospital and Fibrosis Research Group, National Heart and Lung Institute, Imperial College London, London, UK
[8]Fibrosis Research Group, Inflammation, Repair and Development Section, NHLI, Sir Alexander Fleming Building, Imperial College London, London SW7 2AZ, UK
Full list of author information is available at the end of the article

Background

Idiopathic pulmonary fibrosis (IPF) is a chronic, debilitating, irreversible, and progressive lung disease characterized by exertional dyspnea and cough [1, 2]. Patients with IPF have a poor prognosis, with median survival following diagnosis previously reported as lower than that for many common types of cancer at between 2 and 5 years [1–8].

The reported incidence of IPF has been estimated to range from 2.8 to 9.3 cases per 100,000 population per year, in Europe and North America [9]. The prevalence of IPF in Europe is thought to range from 1.25 to 23.4 cases per 100,000 population [10]. There is evidence that the incidence, prevalence, and number of deaths from IPF may be increasing [9, 11–13].

Two antifibrotic drugs, pirfenidone and nintedanib, are approved by the European Medicines Agency and the US Food and Drug Administration for the treatment of IPF, and both are recommended in international treatment guidelines [14]. In the Phase III ASCEND and CAPACITY trials, pirfenidone significantly reduced the risk of disease progression or death compared with placebo [15, 16]. In the Phase III INPULSIS trials, nintedanib reduced the risk of disease progression versus placebo in patients with IPF [17].

Following the approval and recommendation of pirfenidone and nintedanib for the treatment of IPF, we conducted a patient chart audit using an online physician survey to investigate pharmacological treatment patterns, understand antifibrotic prescribing, and identify unmet needs in IPF treatment practice in Europe.

Methods

Study design and patients

This was a patient chart audit survey involving respiratory physicians from France, Germany, Italy, Spain, and the UK. Between February and March 2016, physicians participated in an online questionnaire (35–40 min) designed to collect information on IPF treatment patterns. The questionnaire was developed by Elma Research, an independent market research agency, on behalf of F. Hoffmann-La Roche Ltd. The questionnaire was available in English, French, German, Italian, and Spanish; all responses were precoded as numbers so translation was not required. Patients' perspectives were not recorded in this study.

Responses were collected from physicians who had consulted with at least six (France, Italy, Spain) or 10 (Germany, UK) patients with IPF within the previous 3 months. The number of patients with IPF required for each physician varied by country to account for inter-country differences in patient population size. Italian and British physicians were selected from a list of panelists held by Elma Research, which includes physicians

willing to take part in market research. In France, Germany, and Spain, external suppliers invited the physicians to participate on behalf of Elma Research. Physicians were asked to report on the last six patients (eight in the UK) with IPF they saw, regardless of any specific diagnostic or therapeutic features. No patient-identifiable data were collected and patients remained anonymous. All respondents received a cash incentive, which was awarded for participation in the research; i.e., this was not on a per-patient basis. Respondents agreed to complete the form personally, i.e., not to delegate the form completion to another staff member.

Patients were categorized as being in one of the following populations based on their last consultation:

- Treated population—those patients who had received approved antifibrotics for the treatment of IPF
- Untreated population—those patients who had not received approved antifibrotics.

In both the treated and untreated populations, patients may have been receiving concomitant therapies, such as N-acetylcysteine (NAC), steroids (prednisolone), immunosuppressants, and/or oxygen. Patients may also have received pharmacological therapies for the palliation of symptoms associated with IPF, and therapies for concomitant conditions. The retrospective nature of the survey meant that participation did not prompt any change in patient care; concomitant therapies may have been continuing or newly initiated at the last visit at the discretion of the treating physician. It is possible that continuing therapies may have been established in accordance with superseded clinical guidelines [2, 18].

Assessments

The questionnaire assessed a number of factors, including baseline demographics, IPF diagnosis, disease severity, treatments, and comorbidities (Additional files 1 and 2).

Pulmonary function and exercise capacity (6-min walk distance [6MWD]) were recorded from diagnosis and from the most recent consultation, where these data were available. Classification of IPF diagnosis (confirmed/suspected), severity ('mild'/'moderate'/'severe'), and evolution of severity (improvement/stable/worsening) for each patient was based on the individual physician's report, i.e., no pre-defined forced vital capacity (FVC) or carbon monoxide diffusing capacity (DLco) threshold was given to determine disease severity, and individual physicians may have applied different thresholds. Physicians were asked to report the number of acute exacerbations of IPF that resulted in hospitalization or an emergency room visit within the last year; acute exacerbations were defined according to clinical presentation and no standard criteria or adjudication were applied.

Statistical analysis

Statistical analyses were performed by a senior data analyst from Elma Research in April 2016 using Quantum v 5.8, once all questionnaires were completed and information on the number and percentage of respondents per answer were summarized. Comparisons between treated and untreated populations were performed using t-tests.

In the UK and Italy, expert centers were classified as those authorized to prescribe pirfenidone, while in France, Germany, and Spain, expert centers were defined as:

- General university hospital with > 60 patients in care and multidisciplinary team (MDT) available
- OR, office-based physicians who have an MDT available and care for > 60 patients
- OR, working in a lung clinic and have an MDT.

Centers not meeting these criteria, or who were not authorized to prescribe pirfenidone in the UK and Italy, were classed as non-expert centers. A subgroup analysis comparing expert and non-expert centers was performed for the following endpoints: IPF diagnosis, time until next consultation, goals with current treatment, and frequency of acute exacerbations. Comparisons between expert and non-expert subgroups were performed using t-tests.

Data for the number of physicians based at centers in the UK authorized to prescribe pirfenidone were weighted equally for prescribing and non-prescribing centers (50% each). In Italy, data were weighted 67% and 33% for prescribing and non-prescribing centers. To avoid duplication of data from patients treated with pirfenidone in Italy or in the UK, patients reported by non-prescribing centers as co-managed with an authorized prescribing center within the last 3 months were not included in the analysis.

Results

Physicians

Overall, there were 290 respondent physicians from Germany, France, Italy, the UK, and Spain reporting on 1838 patients. Out of 119 physicians from the UK and Italy, 80 (67.2%) were working in expert centers, which by definition were authorized to prescribe pirfenidone (Table 1). In France, Germany, and Spain, a total of 90/171 (52.6%) physicians were designated as being from expert centers. MDT evaluation, which alone did not confer status as an expert center, was available in the centers of 213 (73.4%) physicians (Table 1).

Patients

Of the 1838 patients, 55 patients in Italy and the UK were co-managed with a prescribing center and were therefore excluded from further analysis to avoid

Table 1 Physician characteristics

Factor, n (%)	Physicians N = 290
Country[a]	
Germany	60 (20.7)
France	51 (17.6)
Italy	70 (24.1)
United Kingdom (UK)	49 (16.9)
Spain	60 (20.7)
Type of practice	
General hospital	157 (54.1)
Centre specializing in lung diseases	120 (41.4)
Office-based practice	42 (14.5)
MDT available	213 (73.4)
MDT team members	
Respiratory specialist/pulmonologist	212 (99.5)
Radiologist	206 (96.7)
Pathologist	165 (77.5)
ILD/IPF Specialist Nurse	70 (32.9)
Other	44 (20.7)
Expert center (France, Germany, and Spain)[a]	90/171 (52.6)
General University Hospital with >60 patients and MDT[b]	40 (23.4)
Office-based physicians with >60 patients and MDT	5 (2.9)
Lung clinic with MDT available[b]	47 (27.5)
Expert center (UK and Italy)[a]	
Authorized to prescribe pirfenidone	80/119 (67.2)

For individual questions asked, please refer to Additional files 1 and 2
MDT multidisciplinary team, *ILD* interstitial lung disease, *IPF* idiopathic pulmonary fibrosis
[a]Unweighted data
[b]Two centers qualified under both criteria

double-counting. Of the remaining 1783 patients analyzed, 955 (53.6%) did not receive treatment with either approved antifibrotic drug (Fig. 1). The proportions of patients starting a new medication, switching to a different medication, or discontinuing a medication at their last consultation were 18.5, 6.8, and 1.2%, respectively.

Excluding patients who received palliative care only or palliative care only + oxygen therapy ($N = 46$), 828 patients (47.7%) received antifibrotic treatment and 909 patients (52.3%) did not receive antifibrotic treatment. More patients in the treated population had a confirmed diagnosis of IPF versus patients in the untreated population (Fig. 2a). Of 1158 patients with a confirmed IPF diagnosis, 462 (39.9%) did not receive treatment with an approved antifibrotic drug. More patients at expert centers had a confirmed diagnosis of IPF than at non-expert centers (70.1% vs 62.4%, respectively) (Fig. 2b); of patients with a confirmed diagnosis of IPF, antifibrotic

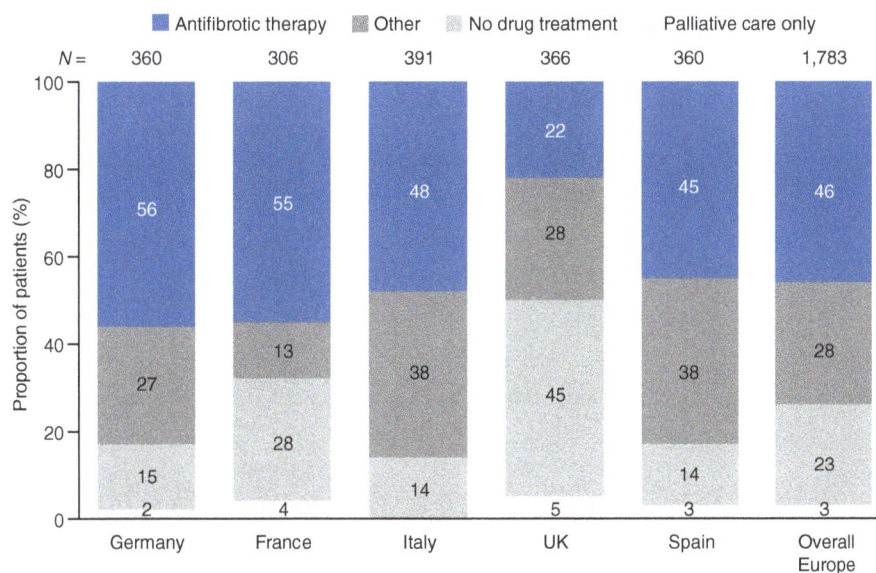

Fig. 1 Proportion of patients that are treated or untreated across European countries. Unweighted data. For individual questions asked, please refer to Additional files 1 and 2

treatment was received by 67.9% (461/679) of those at expert centers compared with 49.1% (235/479) of those at non-expert centers (Fig. 2b).

The treated population was younger than the untreated population and had more frequent MDT evaluation. Treated patients generally had a lower proportion of lung and cardiovascular comorbidities compared with untreated patients (Table 2). Significantly more treated patients were candidates for lung transplantation compared with untreated patients (Table 2).

A total of 1435 patients had data available regarding non-antifibrotic therapies that were being prescribed for IPF at the time of questionnaire completion (this information was not collected in France). Of 638 treated patients, the following patients also received another therapy: NAC = 88 (13.8%), steroids = 60 (9.4%), immunosuppressants = 11 (1.7%), palliative care = 3 (0.5%), oxygen = 172 (27.0%), and other pharmacological therapy = 164 (25.7%). In the untreated population (n = 797), the following patients received: NAC = 219 (27.5%), steroids = 251 (31.5%), immunosuppressants = 62 (7.8%), palliative care = 101 (12.7%), oxygen = 300 (37.6%), and other pharmacological therapy = 269 (33.8%).

Among untreated patients (including patients in France), 405 patients (45%) were reported as receiving 'no drug treatment'. Some of these patients were also reported as receiving oxygen therapy (61 [15.1%]), other therapy (pharmacological or non-pharmacological; 37 [9.1%]), or palliative care including morphine (13 [3.2%]). Untreated patients receiving palliative care only were older (mean age = 81 years) than those receiving no pharmacological treatment (71 years), oxygen therapy

(74 years), or other therapy (73 years). The most common reasons given for why the patient was not receiving any drug treatment were: lack of, or few, symptoms related to IPF (27%), stable disease (26%), old age (20%), and physician-reported good quality of life (20%).

The three most common treatment goals reported by physicians in both the treated and untreated populations were to prolong survival/reduce risk of mortality, improve quality of life, and stabilize disease (Table 3). To prolong survival/reduce risk of mortality was the most important treatment goal across all groups in the expert versus non-expert analyses, with the exception of the untreated non-expert population, where improvement in quality of life was the most important treatment goal (Table 3).

A larger proportion of the treated population (84.9%) had ≤ 3 months until their next consultation versus the untreated population (59.3%) (Additional file 3).

Disease severity and pulmonary function

Of 519 patients with 'mild' IPF, 71% (n = 370) did not receive treatment with an approved antifibrotic compared with 41% (n/N = 361/889) and 60% (n/N = 224/375) of patients with 'moderate' and 'severe' IPF, respectively (Fig. 3). The proportion of patients with 'mild' IPF who did not receive treatment with an approved antifibrotic was 40.4, 41.4, 37.5, 51.4, and 44.7% in Germany, France, Italy, the UK, and Spain, respectively.

In addition, a higher proportion of untreated versus treated patients had FVC > 80% or did not have their pulmonary function assessed at diagnosis (Table 4). At

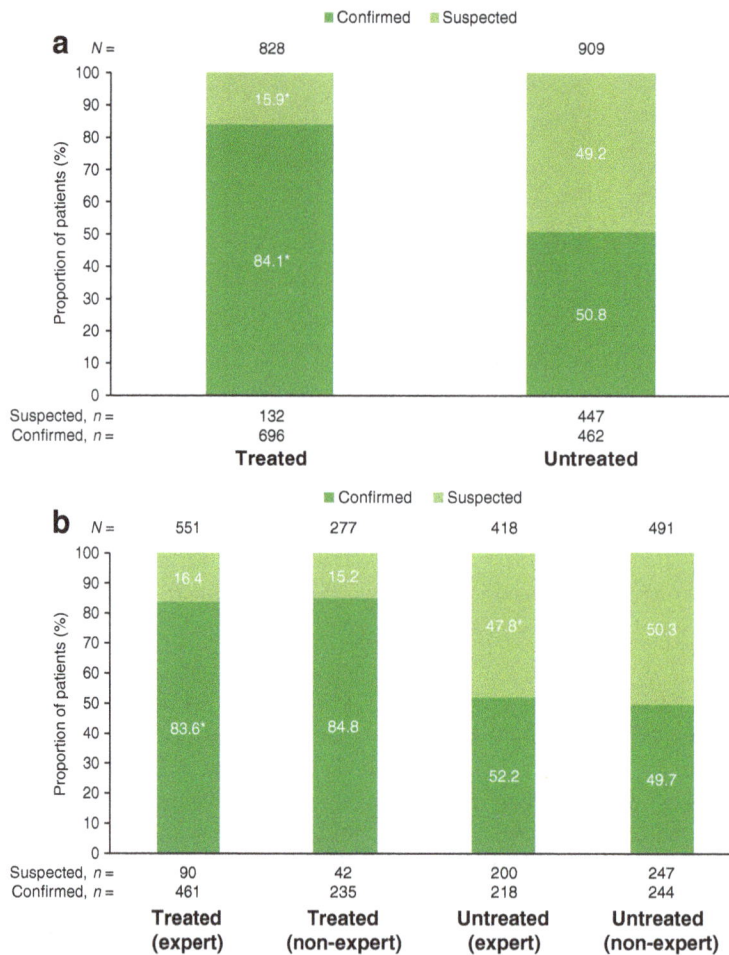

Fig. 2 Type of diagnosis, (**a**) pooled population (**b**) expert versus non-expert centers $^{*}p \leq 0.01$ for (**a**) treated population versus untreated population and (**b**) expert population versus non-expert population. Excluding patients receiving only palliative care. Number of patients with a confirmed diagnosis at expert (691/993, 69.6%) versus non-expert centers (494/790, 62.5%)—$p \leq 0.01$. Number of patients with confirmed IPF treated at expert (461/679, 67.9%) versus non-expert centers (235/479, 49.2%)—$p \leq 0.01$. For individual questions asked, please refer to Additional files 1 and 2. *IPF* idiopathic pulmonary fibrosis

the most recent consultation, significantly more untreated patients versus treated patients had 'mild' (40.7% vs 18.0%; $p \leq 0.01$) and/or stable (50.9% vs 31.3%; $p \leq 0.01$) IPF (Table 4). Likewise, more untreated patients had FVC > 80% at last check-up than treated patients; however, fewer untreated patients had an FVC measurement at their most recent check-up compared with treated patients (Table 4).

According to physician responses, a high proportion of patients had experienced an acute exacerbation of IPF in the year before completion of the survey, resulting in hospitalization or an emergency room visit (treated = 47.5% vs untreated = 39.6%) (Fig. 4a). A total of 16% of patients with 'mild' IPF had a physician-reported acute exacerbation compared with 38% and 32% of patients with 'moderate' and 'severe' IPF, respectively. Patients at non-expert centers had slightly

more acute exacerbations than patients at expert centers, whether they were treated or untreated (Fig. 4b).

Discussion

Our results show that approximately 40% of European patients with confirmed IPF do not receive antifibrotic treatment despite the regulatory approval of two antifibrotic therapies and the recommendation in international guidelines that the majority of individuals with IPF should be offered antifibrotic treatment. Indeed, at the time of the survey, antifibrotic therapy had been available for at least 2 years in all the countries surveyed, and it is therefore important to consider reasons for the observed treatment pattern.

Treatment requires a confident diagnosis of IPF, and it may be that a lack of awareness about IPF as a potential diagnosis and/or a lack of referral to specialist centers

Table 2 Patient characteristics

Factor, mean (SD) or n (%)	Treated (N = 828)	Untreated (N = 909)
Mean (SD) age, years	66.6 (9.3)	70.1 (11.4)[**]
Male	568 (68.6)	570 (62.7)[**]
MDT evaluation	687 (83.0)	520 (57.2)[**]
Confirmed IPF	696 (84.1)	462 (50.8)[**]
IPF severity at diagnosis		
Mild	213 (25.7)	395 (43.5)[**]
Moderate	530 (64.0)	367 (40.4)[**]
Severe	85 (10.3)	147 (16.2)[**]
Mean (SD) time from diagnosis to most recent consultation, months	15.8 (21.8)	15.9 (22.4)
Symptomatic at initiation of current treatment	746 (90.1)	430 (85.4)[a][**]
Candidate for lung transplantation	154 (18.6)	66 (7.3)[**]
Lung comorbidities	323 (39.0)	460 (50.6)[**]
Emphysema	187 (22.6)	299 (32.9)[**]
Lung cancer	20 (2.4)	46 (5.1)[**]
Pulmonary hypertension	184 (22.2)	229 (25.2)
CV comorbidities	320 (38.6)	406 (44.7)[*]
High risk of coronary artery disease	131 (15.8)	153 (16.8)
Coronary artery disease without history of MI or stroke	119 (14.4)	143 (15.7)
Coronary artery disease with history of MI	88 (10.6)	135 (14.9)[**]
Other comorbidities		
GERD	262 (31.6)	257 (28.3)
Depression	199 (24.0)	200 (22.0)
Obstructive sleep apnea syndrome	103 (12.4)	109 (12.0)
Increased risk of bleeding[b]	38 (4.6)	44 (4.8)
Other	111 (13.4)	149 (16.4)

p values represent treated population versus untreated population. [*]$p \leq 0.05$; [**]$p \leq 0.01$

[a]$N = 504$, patients who received no treatment were excluded

[b]e.g., due to use of anticoagulation therapy or concomitant diseases

For individual questions asked, please refer to Additional file 2

CV cardiovascular, GERD gastroesophageal reflux disease, IPF idiopathic pulmonary fibrosis, MDT multidisciplinary team, MI myocardial infarction, SD standard deviation

for MDT diagnostic assessment have an impact upon treatment practices. Our results show that a higher proportion of untreated patients had suspected IPF than treated patients and a lower proportion of untreated patients had an MDT evaluation at diagnosis. Uncertain diagnosis is also a key barrier to treatment in patients with suspected IPF, which will potentially be addressed by two clinical trials currently investigating the efficacy of antifibrotics in non-IPF interstitial lung diseases (NCT03099187 and NCT02999178).

In our analysis of treatment patterns in expert versus non-expert centers, more patients had a confirmed diagnosis of IPF at expert centers. In addition, a higher proportion of patients in the untreated population did not have an FVC (12% vs 8%), DLco (23% vs 15%), or 6MWD (57% vs 36%) measurement at baseline compared with the treated population. These differences

between the untreated and treated populations could reflect a number of issues, including difficulty with interpreting dynamic changes in pulmonary function or reduced monitoring in patients considered to be unsuitable for treatment by their physician.

Previous studies have shown that patients often visit several healthcare professionals before being diagnosed with IPF, with the process of obtaining a confirmed diagnosis taking in excess of 1 year in the majority of cases [19, 20]. Misdiagnosis and a lack of knowledge about IPF in primary care are cited as key reasons for delayed referral to specialist centers [20, 21]. Our data suggest that referral to a non-specialist pulmonologist may be another barrier to diagnosis and treatment access. Patients in several areas across the EU have reported limited access to a full MDT to facilitate diagnosis [21]. Once a diagnosis has been made, areas of unmet needs

Table 3 Most important treatment goals with current treatment

Goal, n (%)	Pooled population		Treated		Untreated	
	Treated N = 828	Untreated N = 405	Expert N = 551	Non-expert N = 277	Expert N = 176	Non-expert N = 229
Prolong survival/reduce risk of mortality	402 (48.6)	174 (43.0)	273 (49.5)	129 (46.6)	80 (45.5)	94 (41.0)
Improvement of quality of life	314 (37.9)	179 (44.2)*	194 (35.2)	120 (43.3)	75 (42.6)	104 (45.4)
Overall disease stabilization	334 (40.3)	152 (37.5)	234 (42.5)	100 (36.1)	64 (36.4)	88 (38.4)
Stabilization of predicted% FVC	279 (33.7)	56 (13.8)**	176 (32.0)	102 (36.8)	23 (13.1)	33 (14.4)
Stabilization of quality of life	248 (30.0)	135 (33.3)	164 (29.8)	83 (30.0)	70 (39.8)	65 (28.4)
Improvement of symptoms	236 (28.5)	142 (35.1)*	161 (29.2)	76 (27.4)	57 (32.4)	85 (37.1)
Stabilization of symptoms	215 (26.0)	143 (35.3)**	135 (24.5)	81 (29.2)	68 (38.6)	75 (32.8)
Decrease in number of exacerbations	208 (25.1)	94 (23.2)	153 (27.8)	55 (19.9)	40 (22.7)	53 (23.1)
Avoid pulmonary hospitalizations	156 (18.8)	122 (30.1)**	101 (18.3)	55 (19.9)	46 (26.1)	76 (33.2)
Stabilization of predicted% DLco	92 (11.1)	19 (4.7)**	61 (11.1)	31 (11.2)	3 (1.7)	15 (6.6)

DLco carbon monoxide diffusing capacity; FVC forced vital capacity
Respondents were asked to pick the three most important goals; for individual questions asked, please refer to Additional file 2
p values represent treated population versus untreated population. *$p \leq 0.05$; **$p \leq 0.01$

include a lack of awareness of available approved antifibrotic therapy and/or information and resources on pulmonary fibrosis from both a patient and a healthcare professional perspective [22–24]. Indeed, in our experience, informed patients with a good knowledge of their condition and the available treatments are more likely to request referral to specialist care and/or access to treatment than those with less knowledge about their condition. Similar factors were highlighted in the European IPF Patient Charter [21] and may contribute to the delayed diagnosis and treatment of IPF.

Our results indicate that many patients with IPF that is perceived to be 'mild' or 'stable' by their physician were not treated with an antifibrotic, suggesting physicians were adopting a 'watch and wait' approach. Indeed, a large group of patients who did not receive an antifibrotic received no treatment at all, with the most common reasons for this being lack of symptoms and/or lack of

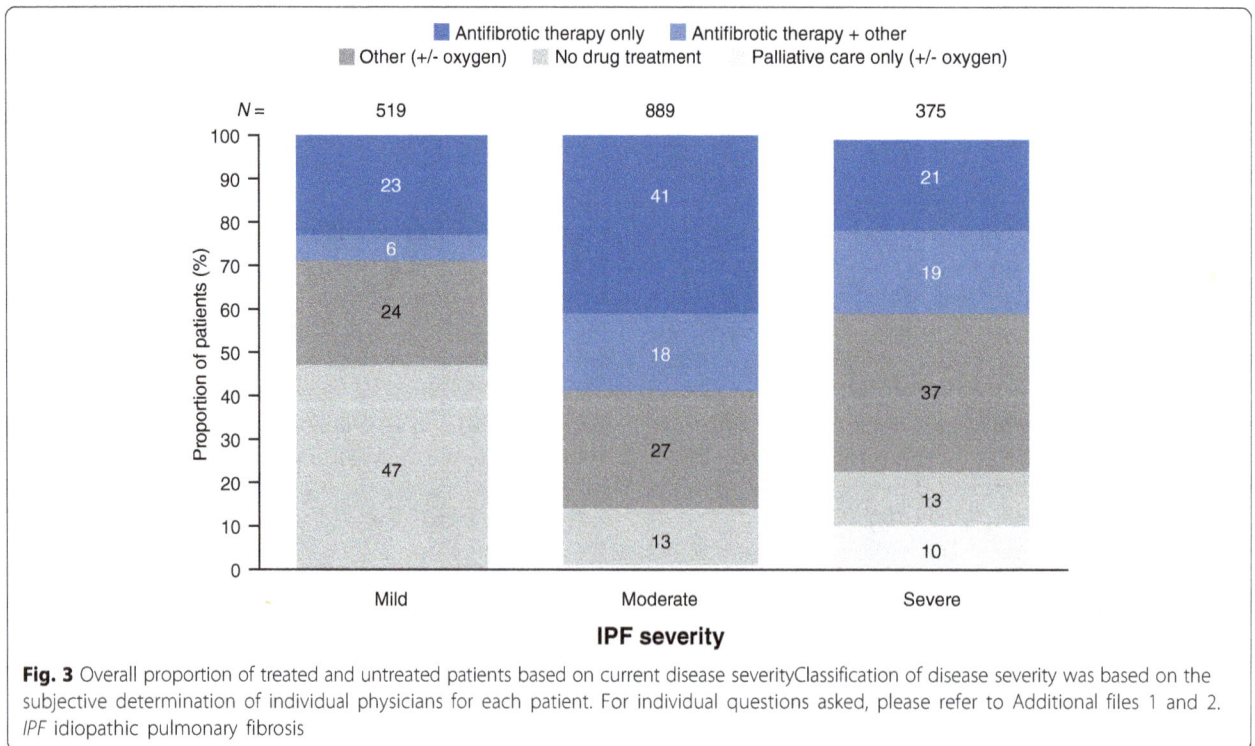

Fig. 3 Overall proportion of treated and untreated patients based on current disease severity Classification of disease severity was based on the subjective determination of individual physicians for each patient. For individual questions asked, please refer to Additional files 1 and 2. *IPF* idiopathic pulmonary fibrosis

Table 4 Disease characteristics

Factor, n (%)	Treated N = 828	Untreated N = 909
Diagnostic values		
FVC		
FVC > 80%	94 (11.4)	163 (17.9)**
FVC 71–80%	143 (17.3)	183 (20.1)
FVC 50–70%	425 (51.3)	335 (36.9)**
FVC < 50%	102 (12.3)	122 (13.4)
FVC not tested	64 (7.7)	106 (11.7)**
DLco		
DLco < 35%	74 (8.9)	85 (9.4)
DLco ≥ 35%	634 (76.6)	612 (67.3)**
DLco not tested	121 (14.6)	212 (23.3)**
6MWD		
6MWD < 150 m	71 (8.6)	71 (7.8)
6MWD ≥ 150 m	460 (55.6)	323 (35.5)**
Not tested	297 (35.9)	516 (56.8)**
Last visit		
Mild IPF (current level)	149 (18.0)	370 (40.7)**
FVC		
FVC > 80%	39 (4.7)	119 (13.1)**
FVC 71–80%	116 (14.0)	134 (14.7)
FVC 50–70%	427 (51.6)	279 (30.7)**
FVC < 50%	148 (17.9)	141 (15.5)
FVC not tested	98 (11.8)	236 (26.0)**
Evolution in severity level[a] from diagnosis to last check-up		
Improvement	38 (4.6)	36 (4.0)
Stable	637 (76.9)	782 (86.0)**
Worsening	154 (18.6)	92 (10.1)**
Type of progression		
Stable IPF	259 (31.3)	463 (50.9)**
Slow progressing	383 (46.3)	291 (32.0)**
Progressive	159 (19.2)	114 (12.5)**
Fast progressing	27 (3.3)	41 (4.5)

For individual questions asked, please refer to Additional file 2

6MWD 6-min walk distance, *DLco* carbon monoxide diffusing capacity, *FVC* forced vital capacity, *IPF* idiopathic pulmonary fibrosis

[a]Evolution in severity levels was defined as follows: Improvement = from Moderate to Mild/from Severe to Moderate or Mild; Stable = unchanged level of severity at diagnosis to last check-up; Worsening = from Mild to Moderate or Severe/from Moderate to Severe

p values represent treated population versus untreated population.

*$p \leq 0.05$; **$p \leq 0.01$

disease progression. The data gathered in this survey suggest that treated patients had more severe disease than untreated patients: they were more likely to have an FVC < 70% at diagnosis and follow-up, they were more likely to have disease rated as 'moderate' by their physician, they

tended to have more acute exacerbations than untreated patients, and they were more likely to be candidates for lung transplantation (although it should be acknowledged that this may have been because they were younger and/or had fewer comorbidities than untreated patients, rather than reflecting more severe disease).

One possible explanation for patients with 'mild' or 'stable' IPF remaining untreated is a lack of physician confidence in the evidence base. The limitations of our survey design prevented further investigation of this possibility; however, a survey of respiratory physicians has previously reported that physicians who waited for disease progression before initiating antifibrotic therapy were less likely to agree that antifibrotics can significantly slow disease progression compared with physicians who treated within 4 months of diagnosis [25]. However, the available evidence increasingly points toward early intervention in this progressive, unpredictable, irreversible, and fatal disease [1, 26–31], especially as experience from other lung diseases suggests that physicians tend to underestimate the severity of disease [32, 33]. Antifibrotic treatment in patients with limited lung function impairment has been demonstrated to reduce FVC decline compared with placebo [28, 30, 31], and patients who progress on antifibrotic therapy still appear to benefit from continued therapy [34]. Furthermore, in a post-hoc analysis of data from the pooled ASCEND and CAPACITY population, pirfenidone showed similar efficacy in patients with more-preserved and less-preserved baseline lung function [27], a finding that has also been reported with nintedanib in a post-hoc subgroup analysis of data from the INPULSIS trials [29]. These data suggest that earlier treatment with antifibrotics may help to preserve lung function at higher levels if started in the early stages of the disease.

Goals for patient care may also have influenced treatment decisions. Overall, the three most important goals given by physicians were to prolong survival or reduce the risk of mortality, improve quality of life, and stabilize disease. However, the importance placed on these goals differed in treated and untreated patients, with improvement and/or stabilization in quality of life being more frequent for untreated patients (78%) than treated patients (68%). There may be a perception among physicians that antifibrotic treatment might have a detrimental effect on quality of life, possibly via the common side effects associated with treatment, and that the potential risks outweigh the benefit of treatment, particularly in patients with preserved lung function. Validating IPF-specific quality-of-life endpoints is still a work in progress and, so far, findings have been inconsistent with the treatment response (as measured with clinical endpoints) [35]. However, the available evidence from clinical trials suggests antifibrotic treatment results in

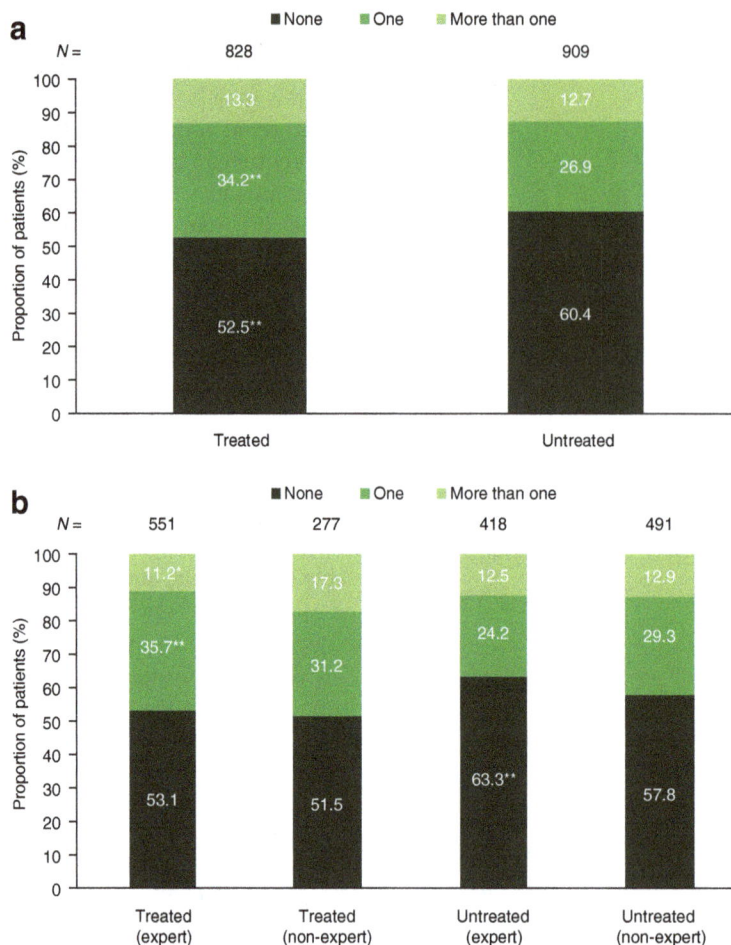

Fig. 4 Exacerbations in the last year, (**a**) pooled population (**b**) expert versus non-expert centers. *$p \leq 0.05$; **$p \leq 0.01$ for (**a**) treated population versus untreated population and (**b**) expert population versus non-expert population. Excluding patients receiving only palliative care. For individual questions asked, please refer to Additional file 1 and Fig. 2

statistically non-significant improvements in quality-of-life endpoints or has no net effect on these endpoints [15, 17, 36].

Access to IPF treatment differs in each country, for example because of reimbursement restrictions, and this may also have resulted in some differences in treatment practices. In Italy, patients must have a DLco > 35% and be < 80 years of age to be eligible for treatment reimbursement, while patients in the UK and in several regions in Spain must have an FVC < 80%. Interpretation of our data is limited because the survey did not specifically ask about access restrictions; however, the proportion of patients in the UK with 'mild' disease who were untreated was higher (51.4%) compared with countries without an upper FVC limit, such as France and Germany (41.1 and 40.4%, respectively). Overall, a greater proportion of the untreated population had an FVC > 80% compared with treated patients, both at diagnosis (17.9% vs 11.4%) and at last check up (13.1% vs 4.7%).

Both pirfenidone and nintedanib are associated with a number of adverse events, which may limit tolerability or result in treatment discontinuation due to potentially harmful events, e.g., rare elevations in liver enzymes [37, 38]. Patients may occasionally be prevented from taking specific antifibrotics due to contraindications [37, 38]. Although emphysema and lung cancer are not direct contraindications to antifibrotic treatment, untreated patients in our analysis were more likely to have these comorbidities. The results suggest that physicians are reluctant to treat patients with other lung diseases, perhaps due to a perception that these individuals may be more susceptible to adverse effects from treatment, or concerns about the benefit of treating fibrosis in individuals who may have other life-limiting disease. It should be noted, however, that patients with some degree of emphysema were included in the CAPACITY and INPULSIS trials [15, 17].

In Europe, pirfenidone is indicated for the treatment of 'mild to moderate' IPF [37], thereby excluding patients with 'severe' disease, often considered to be those with FVC < 50%. In fact, a minority of treated patients in our analysis had an FVC < 50%, and this proportion was similar in the untreated population. Other reasons for non-treatment could include patient choice, particularly in those with 'mild disease,' or lack of adherence to treatment due to social or personal circumstances.

The focus of the current analysis was to investigate antifibrotic treatment patterns; however, in general, many patients in our analysis appeared to receive inadequate additional symptom management measures. Treatment guidelines recommend oxygen supplementation and other therapies for symptom control and management of comorbidities [2]; however, oxygen therapy and supportive treatments, such as anti-cough treatments, vaccines, etc., were used in only half of patients overall and in approximately a quarter of patients in the treated population. Supportive treatments for comorbidities, symptom control, or side-effect management may help with adherence to antifibrotic therapy and also improve patients' perceptions of treatment. Furthermore, only 59/1783 patients (3%) overall received palliative care (46 patients were reported as having received palliative care only ± oxygen and a further 13 were reported as receiving no drug treatment and palliative care only ± oxygen). Amongst patients with IPF considered 'severe' by their doctor, only 10% were receiving palliative care. This is similar to previous findings, which highlighted poor or variable access and ineffective utilization of palliative care services, despite increasing evidence that access to palliative care services or having end-of-life discussions early in the course of IPF is desired by patients and can also improve quality of life, symptom control, and mood [21, 39–41]. Variable information regarding the disease and treatment, and access to other aspects of IPF management, such as supplementary oxygen, comorbidities, and palliative care, have been identified as unmet needs in the IPF Patient Charter; our observations support the findings of the Charter and suggest improvements in IPF awareness are still needed [21].

The conclusions from this study are limited by the nature of questionnaire-based research, which may have introduced bias. Furthermore, the quality of the data collected in this survey was reliant upon case notes recorded by physicians during patient consultations prior to their awareness of the survey. Physicians might not have reported on consecutive patients as directed, and may instead have selected cases that they considered representative of their medical decision making. The number of acute exacerbations resulting in hospitalization or an emergency room visit in the previous year (40–47%) was much higher than expected when compared with an annual acute exacerbation rate of 5–10% in the published literature [42–44], suggesting that these data are limited by the subjective acute exacerbation diagnoses made by individual physicians and the lack of specific criteria defining acute exacerbations in the survey. There is also no consensus on how to categorize disease severity or disease progression in IPF, and our analysis is limited by the subjective determination made by individual physicians as to whether disease was 'mild,' 'moderate,' or 'severe,' or whether the patient had stable or worsening disease. We recognize that there is an unmet need for an objective severity staging system to capture the nature and progression of IPF. In particular, 'mild' is an inadequate description of a disease that can impair quality of life and undergo periods of acute exacerbation even in its early stages, and other classifications including 'subclinical IPF' may become more appropriate in the future. Finally, this analysis focused on five European countries (France, Germany, Italy, Spain, and the UK); therefore, the results may not be comparable in the rest of the world.

Treatment patterns in IPF will require further evaluation in future studies as more evidence is presented regarding available pharmacological treatments. The impact of early intervention and the potential for combining antifibrotics need further investigation [45, 46].

Conclusion

In summary, this study highlights the high proportion of patients who are diagnosed with IPF, but do not receive antifibrotic treatment. The factors affecting treatment prescription in this analysis appear to involve diagnostic uncertainty and a lack of understanding around important features of both the disease and treatment as well as issues relating to treatment access. We acknowledge that a small proportion of patients will make an informed decision to not proceed with treatment. However, the adoption by physicians of a 'watch and wait' approach is of particular concern when evidence suggests immediate intervention can improve outcomes for patients with IPF. Increased education about IPF, in line with the European IPF Patient Charter, may help to empower patients to become more actively involved in treatment decisions and may improve treatment patterns in patients with IPF.

Endnotes

[1]Became a wholly owned Roche subsidiary in 2014.

Abbreviations

6MWD: 6-min walk distance; CV: Cardiovascular; DLco: Carbon monoxide diffusing capacity of the lungs; FVC: Forced vital capacity; GERD: Gastroesophageal reflux disease; ILD: Interstitial lung disease;

IPF: Idiopathic pulmonary fibrosis; MDT: Multidisciplinary team; MI: Myocardial infarction; NAC: N-acetylcysteine; SD: Standard deviation

Acknowledgments

The authors would like to thank the staff at Elma Research for their support with data analysis. Medical writing support was provided by Catherine Stanton on behalf of Complete Medical Communications Ltd., funded by F. Hoffmann-La Roche Ltd.

Funding

This study was sponsored by F. Hoffmann-La Roche Ltd.

Authors' contributions

All authors were involved in the design of this study and/or the interpretation of study results. ER coordinated a team of researchers from Elma Research S.R.L in preparing the online questionnaire and summarizing outcomes. All authors contributed to the manuscript from the outset and read and approved the final draft.

Competing interests

TMM has received grants, consulting fees, and speaker fees from GSK and UCB, and grants from Novartis. He has also received consulting fees and speaker fees from AstraZeneca, Bayer, Biogen Idec, Boehringer Ingelheim, Cipla, Lanthio, InterMune International AG,[1] F. Hoffmann-La Roche Ltd., Sanofi-Aventis, and Takeda. TMM is supported by a National Institute for Health Research Clinician Scientist Fellowship (NIHR Ref: CS:-2013-13-017). MM-M has received grants and consulting fees from GSK, Boehringer Ingelheim, AstraZeneca, Chiesi, InterMune International AG,[1] Esteve-Teijin, and F. Hoffmann-La Roche Ltd. AMR has received educational grants, speaker fees, and consultancy fees from InterMune International AG[1] and F. Hoffmann-La Roche Ltd.; and a research grant from the Pulmonary Fibrosis Trust (UK). She has received travel scholarships from Action for Pulmonary Fibrosis UK, Boehringer Ingelheim, and the British Lung Foundation. AMR is a director of the ILD Interdisciplinary Network. She is supported by a National Institute for Health Research Clinical Doctoral Fellowship. FB has received speaker fees, advisory board honoraria, or grants from InterMune International AG,[1] Boehringer Ingelheim, Serendex, Centocor, and F. Hoffmann-La Roche Ltd. SJ has received grants, advisory board honoraria, consulting fees, and/or speaker fees from Actelion, Association pour les Insuffisants Respiratoire de Bretagne (AIRB), AstraZeneca, Bristol-Myers Squibb, Boehringer Ingelheim, Chiesi, GSK, Mundipharma, Novartis, Pfizer Inc., and F. Hoffmann-La Roche Ltd., and research project funding from AIRB, Boehringer Ingelheim, Novartis, and F. Hoffmann-La Roche Ltd. ER has no conflicts of interest to declare. JA is an employee of F. Hoffmann-La Roche Ltd. CV was previously part of the InterMune International AG[1] scientific board. He is now part of the F. Hoffmann-La Roche Ltd. scientific board. He has received consulting fees and/or speaker fees from AstraZeneca, Boehringer Ingelheim, Chiesi, F. Hoffmann-La Roche Ltd., and Menarini.

Author details

[1]NIHR Respiratory Biomedical Research Unit, Royal Brompton Hospital and Fibrosis Research Group, National Heart and Lung Institute, Imperial College London, London, UK. [2]University Hospital of Bellvitge, Institut d'Investigacions Biomèdiques de Bellvitge (IDIBELL), Barcelona, and Centro de Investigación Biomédica en Red Enfermedades Respiratorias (CIBERES), Barcelona, Spain. [3]Ruhrlandklinik, University Hospital Essen, Essen, Germany. [4]Hôpital Pontchaillou, IRSET UMR 1085, Université de Rennes 1, Rennes, France. [5]Elma Research S.R.L., Milan, Italy. [6]F. Hoffmann-La Roche Ltd., Basel, Switzerland. [7]Regional Referral Centre for Rare Lung Diseases, University of Catania, Catania, Italy. [8]Fibrosis Research Group, Inflammation, Repair and Development Section, NHLI, Sir Alexander Fleming Building, Imperial College London, London SW7 2AZ, UK.

References

1. Ley B, Collard HR, King TE Jr. Clinical course and prediction of survival in idiopathic pulmonary fibrosis. Am J Respir Crit Care Med. 2011;183:431–40.
2. Raghu G, Collard HR, Egan JJ, Martinez FJ, Behr J, Brown KK, et al. An official ATS/ERS/JRS/ALAT statement: idiopathic pulmonary fibrosis: evidence-based guidelines for diagnosis and management. Am J Respir Crit Care Med. 2011;183:788–824.
3. American Cancer Society. Cancer Facts and Figures 2016 2016. http://www.cancer.org/acs/groups/content/@research/documents/document/acspc-047079.pdf. Accessed 4 Dec 2016.
4. Meltzer EB, Noble PW. Idiopathic pulmonary fibrosis. Orphanet J Rare Dis. 2008;3:8.
5. Nathan SD, Shlobin OA, Weir N, Ahmad S, Kaldjob JM, Battle E, et al. Long-term course and prognosis of idiopathic pulmonary fibrosis in the new millennium. Chest. 2011;140:221–9.
6. Siegel RL, Miller KD, Jemal A. Cancer statistics, 2016. CA Cancer J Clin. 2016;66:7–30.
7. Strand MJ, Sprunger D, Cosgrove GP, Fernandez-Perez ER, Frankel SK, Huie TJ, et al. Pulmonary function and survival in idiopathic vs secondary usual interstitial pneumonia. Chest. 2014;146:775–85.
8. Vancheri C, Failla M, Crimi N, Raghu G. Idiopathic pulmonary fibrosis: a disease with similarities and links to cancer biology. Eur Respir J. 2010;35:496–504.
9. Hutchinson J, Fogarty A, Hubbard R, McKeever T. Global incidence and mortality of idiopathic pulmonary fibrosis: a systematic review. Eur Respir J. 2015;46:795–806.
10. Nalysnyk L, Cid-Ruzafa J, Rotella P, Esser D. Incidence and prevalence of idiopathic pulmonary fibrosis: review of the literature. Eur Respir Rev. 2012;21:355–61.
11. Navaratnam V, Fleming KM, West J, Smith CJ, Jenkins RG, Fogarty A, et al. The rising incidence of idiopathic pulmonary fibrosis in the U.K. Thorax. 2011;66:462–7.
12. Navaratnam V, Fogarty AW, McKeever T, Thompson N, Jenkins G, Johnson SR, et al. Presence of a prothrombotic state in people with idiopathic pulmonary fibrosis: a population-based case-control study. Thorax. 2014;69:207–15.
13. Raimundo K, Chang E, Broder MS, Alexander K, Zazzali J, Swigris JJ. Clinical and economic burden of idiopathic pulmonary fibrosis: a retrospective cohort study. BMC Pulm Med. 2016;16:2.
14. Raghu G, Rochwerg B, Zhang Y, Garcia CA, Azuma A, Behr J, et al. An official ATS/ERS/JRS/ALAT clinical practice guideline: treatment of idiopathic pulmonary fibrosis. An update of the 2011 clinical practice guideline. Am J Respir Crit Care Med. 2015;192:e3–19.
15. King TE Jr, Bradford WZ, Castro-Bernardini S, Fagan EA, Glaspole I, Glassberg MK, et al. A phase 3 trial of pirfenidone in patients with idiopathic pulmonary fibrosis. N Engl J Med. 2014;370:2083–92.
16. Noble PW, Albera C, Bradford WZ, Costabel U, Glassberg MK, Kardatzke D, et al. Pirfenidone in patients with idiopathic pulmonary fibrosis (CAPACITY): two randomised trials. Lancet. 2011;377:1760–9.
17. Richeldi L, du Bois RM, Raghu G, Azuma A, Brown KK, Costabel U, et al. Efficacy and safety of nintedanib in idiopathic pulmonary fibrosis. N Engl J Med. 2014;370:2071–82.
18. American Thoracic Society. Idiopathic pulmonary fibrosis: diagnosis and treatment. International consensus statement. American Thoracic Society (ATS), and the European Respiratory Society (ERS). Am J Respir Crit Care Med. 2000;161:646–64.
19. Russell AM, Ripamonti E, Vancheri C. Qualitative European survey of patients with idiopathic pulmonary fibrosis: patients' perspectives of the disease and treatment. BMC Pulm Med. 2016;16:10.
20. Sampson C, Gill BH, Harrison NK, Nelson A, Byrne A. The care needs of patients with idiopathic pulmonary fibrosis and their carers (CaNoPy): results of a qualitative study. BMC Pulm Med. 2015;15:155.
21. Bonella F, Wijsenbeek M, Molina-Molina M, Duck A, Mele R, Geissler K, et al. European IPF patient charter: unmet needs and a call to action for healthcare policymakers. Eur Respir J. 2016;47:597–606.
22. Schoenheit G, Becattelli I, Cohen AH. Living with idiopathic pulmonary fibrosis: an in-depth qualitative survey of European patients. Chron Respir Dis. 2011;8:225–31.
23. Collard HR, Tino G, Noble PW, Shreve MA, Michaels M, Carlson B, et al. Patient experiences with pulmonary fibrosis. Respir Med. 2007;101:1350–4.
24. Wuyts WA, Peccatori FA, Russell AM. Patient-centred management in idiopathic pulmonary fibrosis: similar themes in three communication models. Eur Respir Rev. 2014;23:231–8.
25. Maher T, Swigris J, Kreuter M, Wijsenbeek M, Axmann J, Ireland L, et al. Differences in patient and physician viewpoints of the management of idiopathic pulmonary fibrosis (IPF). Poster presented at the ATS. 2017
26. Antoniou KM, Wuyts W, Wijsenbeek M, Wells AU. Medical therapy in idiopathic pulmonary fibrosis. Semin Respir Crit Care Med. 2016;37:368–77.

27. Albera C, Costabel U, Fagan EA, Glassberg MK, Gorina E, Lancaster L, et al. Efficacy of pirfenidone in patients with idiopathic pulmonary fibrosis with more preserved lung function. Eur Respir J. 2016;48:843–51.

28. Costabel U, Inoue Y, Richeldi L, Collard HR, Tschoepe I, Stowasser S, et al. Efficacy of Nintedanib in idiopathic pulmonary fibrosis across Prespecified subgroups in INPULSIS. Am J Respir Crit Care Med. 2016;193:178–85.

29. Kolb M, Richeldi L, Behr J, Maher TM, Tang W, Stowasser S, et al. Nintedanib in patients with idiopathic pulmonary fibrosis and preserved lung volume. Thorax. 2017;72:340–6.

30. Noble PW, Albera C, Kirchgaessler KU, Gilberg F, Petzinger U, Costabel U. Benefit of treatment with pirfenidone (PFD) persists over time in patients with idiopathic pulmonary fibrosis (IPF) with limited lung function impairment [abstract]. Eur Respir J. 2016;48(suppl 60):OA1809.

31. Noble PW, Albera C, Bradford WZ, Costabel U, du Bois RM, Fagan EA, et al. Pirfenidone for idiopathic pulmonary fibrosis: analysis of pooled data from three multinational phase 3 trials. Eur Respir J. 2016;47:243–53.

32. Mapel DW, Dalal AA, Johnson P, Becker L, Hunter AG. A clinical study of COPD severity assessment by primary care physicians and their patients compared with spirometry. Am J Med. 2015;128:629–37.

33. Vennera Mdel C, Picado C, Herráez L, Galera J, Casafont J. Factors associated with severe uncontrolled asthma and the perception of control by physicians and patients. Arch Bronconeumol. 2014;50:384–91.

34. Nathan SD, Albera C, Bradford WZ, Costabel U, du Bois RM, Fagan EA, et al. Effect of continued treatment with pirfenidone following clinically meaningful declines in forced vital capacity: analysis of data from three phase 3 trials in patients with idiopathic pulmonary fibrosis. Thorax. 2016;71:429–35.

35. Wijsenbeek M, van Manen M, Bonella F. New insights on patient-reported outcome measures in idiopathic pulmonary fibrosis: only PROMises? Curr Opin Pulm Med. 2016;22:434–41.

36. Kreuter M, Wirtz H, Prasse A, Pittrow D, Koschel D, Klotsche J, et al. Symptoms and quality-of-life in relation to lung function and comorbidities in patients with idiopathic pulmonary fibrosis: INSIGHTS-IPF registry [abstract]. Eur Res J. 2016;48:OA4570.

37. European Medicines Agency. Summary of Product Characteristics - Esbriet (pirfenidone) 2015. http://www.ema.europa.eu/docs/en_GB/document_library/EPAR_-_Product_Information/human/002154/WC500103049.pdf. Accessed 15 Mar 2017.

38. European Medicines Agency. Summary of Product Characteristics - OFEV (nintedanib) 2016. http://www.ema.europa.eu/docs/en_GB/document_library/EPAR_-_Product_Information/human/003821/WC500182474.pdf. Accessed 13 Mar 2017.

39. Bajwah S, Higginson IJ, Ross JR, Wells AU, Birring SS, Patel A, et al. Specialist palliative care is more than drugs: a retrospective study of ILD patients. Lung. 2012;190:215–20.

40. Bajwah S, Koffman J, Higginson IJ, Ross JR, Wells AU, Birring SS, et al. 'I wish I knew more ...' the end-of-life planning and information needs for end-stage fibrotic interstitial lung disease: views of patients, carers and health professionals. BMJ Support Palliat Care. 2013;3:84–90.

41. Ravaglia C, Tomassetti S, Gurioli C, Buccioli M, Tantalocco P, Derni S, et al. Palliative medicine and end-of-life care in idiopathic pulmonary fibrosis. J Palliat Med. 2013;16:339.

42. Kim DS. Acute exacerbations in patients with idiopathic pulmonary fibrosis. Respir Res. 2013;14:86.

43. Antoniou KM, Wells AU. Acute exacerbations of idiopathic pulmonary fibrosis. Respiration. 2013;86:265–74.

44. Johannson K, Collard HR. Acute exacerbation of idiopathic pulmonary fibrosis: a proposal. Curr Respir Care Rep. 2013;2

45. Kreuter M, Bonella F, Wijsenbeek M, Maher TM, Spagnolo P. Pharmacological treatment of idiopathic pulmonary fibrosis: current approaches, unsolved issues, and future perspectives. Biomed Res Int. 2015;2015:329481.

46. Wuyts WA, Antoniou KM, Borensztajn K, Costabel U, Cottin V, Crestani B, et al. Combination therapy: the future of management for idiopathic pulmonary fibrosis? Lancet Respir Med. 2014;2:933–42.

4

An implantable pump Lenus pro® in the treatment of pulmonary arterial hypertension with intravenous treprostinil

Marcin Kurzyna[1*], Katarzyna Małaczyńska-Rajpold[2] (ID), Andrzej Koteja[3], Agnieszka Pawlak[4], Łukasz Chrzanowski[5], Michał Furdal[6], Zbigniew Gąsior[7], Wojciech Jacheć[8], Bożena Sobkowicz[9], Justyna Norwa[1], Tatiana Mularek-Kubzdela[2] and Adam Torbicki[1]

Abstract

Background: Subcutaneous treprostinil is a prostacyclin analogue used to treat pulmonary arterial hypertension (PAH). Due to local pain it can cause a deterioration of heart related quality of life (HRQoL) or even abandonment of treatment. The aim of this paper was to assess the feasibility of treatment with intravenous treprostinil administered by means of the Lenus Pro® implantable pump.

Methods: This was a retrospective, multi-center study involving 12 patients (8 females) with PAH treated with a subcutaneous infusion of treprostinil with intolerable pain at the infusion site. Clinical evaluation, including HRQoL assessment with SF-36 questionnaire was performed, before pump implantation and 2–9 months after. The median time of follow-up time was 14 months (4–29 months).

Results: After implantation of the Lenus Pro® pump, no statistically significant changes were observed in the 6-min walking distance and NT-proBNP. After implantation 50% of patients were in II WHO functional class (33% before, $p = 0,59$). There was a significant improvement in HRQoL within the Physical Component Score (28 ± 7 vs 38 ± 8 pts., $p < 0,001$) and in specific domains of SF-36 form: physical role (31 ± 7 pts. vs. 41 ± 12 pts., $p = 0,03$), bodily pain (31 ± 12 vs. 50 ± 14 pts., $p = 0,02$), and vitality (37 ± 8 pts. vs. 50 ± 14 pts., $p = 0,03$). During the periprocedural period, one patient developed a recurrent haematoma at the implantation site. During follow-up in one patient, the drug delivering cannula slipped out of the subclavian vein, what required repositioning repeated twice, and in another patient an unexpected increase in the drug administration rate was observed.

Conclusions: In patients with PAH who do not tolerate subcutaneous infusion of treprostinil, the use of the Lenus Pro® implantable pump results in significant subjective improvement of vitality and physical aspect of the HRQoL with acceptable safety profile.

Keywords: Pulmonary arterial hypertension, Treprostinil, Implantable pump, Quality of life, SF-36 form

Background

Treprostinil, a prostacyclin analogue, is a drug that is widely used to treat pulmonary arterial hypertension (PAH) [1–3]. Its efficacy was confirmed in studies that compared it to placebo [1, 4] and to epoprostenol [4]. Due to the stability of treprostinil sodium solution and its relatively long half-life compared to prostacyclin [5, 6], the drug enabled PAH patients to receive safe long-term treatment. Treprostinil is administered as a continuous subcutaneous infusion using an insulin-like pump. In the case of this route of administration, its half-life is about 3 h [6]. Unfortunately, due to reaction at the infusion site many patients report significant deterioration of quality of life, and some of them (about 5–10%) even abandon treatment [1, 7]. There are trials in progress to find a more convenient method of administration for this drug. The efficacy of oral administration has been uncertain –

* Correspondence: marcin.kurzyna@ecz-otwock.pl
[1]Department of Pulmonary Circulation, Thromboembolic Diseases and Cardiology, Centre of Postgraduate Medical Education, European Health Centre Otwock, Borowa 14/18, 05-400 Otwock, Poland
Full list of author information is available at the end of the article

reports are contradictory [8–12], while inhalation remains a valid alternative for patients in a less advanced stage of the disease [13]. Therefore, for patients whose illness is more severe, only continuous parenteral administration of the drug remains an option.

The Lenus Pro® implantable pump appears to be a promising alternative to an external pump. By means of this method, treprostinil sodium is administered as a continuous intravenous infusion, and the drug reservoir is refilled every 28 days. Thermal stability of treprostinil at body temperature was confirmed during a 60-day observation [5]; concentrations of the drug administered intravenously are comparable to subcutaneous administration, and the only differing parameter is a shorter half-life of less than 1 h [14]. The first experiences with implantable pumps originate in Austria [15, 16] and Germany [17] and present this method of treatment as a milestone in PAH therapy. In Poland, the first implantation of a Lenus Pro® pump took place in 2013 [18]. Functionally similar pump, was tested in US with comparable results in efficacy and safety [19].

The aim of this paper was to assess the feasibility of treatment with intravenous treprostinil administered by means of the Lenus Pro® implantable pump and its impact at quality of life.

Methods

During the years from 2013 to 2016 the number of patients with PAH treated with subcutaneous infusion of treprostinil sodium (Remodulin®, PubChem CID: 23663413) in Poland ranged from 52 to 98. Among them 12 patients (8 males/4 females, aged 42 ± 13 yrs) treated with subcutaneous treprostinil infusion were qualified for implantable pump because they did not tolerate the therapy due to local inflammatory reactions, pain at the infusion site and infection-related complications. Additional inclusion criteria were good clinical response for sc treprostinil infusion guarantying improvement during further therapy. We retrospectively reviewed their clinical data and HRQoL (Short Form 36, SF36) [20, 21] questionnaires obtained before and during 2–9 months after Lenus Pro® pump implantation. Non-invasive clinical evaluation was made, including: WHO functional class (WHO FC), 6-min walking test (6MWT), and concentration of NT-proBNP. All patients gave informed consent for pump implantation. Local Bioethics Committee at Poznan University of Medical Sciences was notified about the study and decided this retrospective analysis does not require formal approval (KB 576/17).

Lenus pro implantable pump

Lenus Pro® pump (Tricumed Medizintechnik GmbH, Kiel, Germany) is a metal device of diameter of 8 cm and a thickness of 2 cm with two compartments inside (Fig. 1).

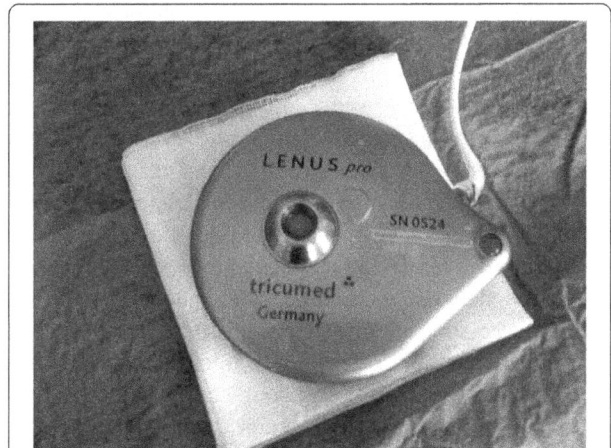

Fig. 1 Photography of the Lenus Pro® pump prepared for implantation

One with capacity of 40 ml is the drug reservoir and latter is filled with noble gas. Both compartments are divided by movable membrane and filling the pump with drug effects in gas compression and causes drug flow toward the patients. The special chip with thin capillary created inside of piece of glass causes constant drug flow (about 1,3 ml/day) irrespectively of gas pressure (high after filling and low close to next refill). As the flow of the drug solution is constant for specific device the dose of the drug is adjusted by changing its concentration. Pump should be refilled every about 28 days by percutaneous puncture of silicone port located on the top of the devices. The second smaller port is designed for pump flushing. No mechanical parts requiring powering are installed inside causing no need for periodic replacement like in case of pacemaker. The pump is usually located in subcostal area and connected with tunnelized catheter inserted via subclavian vein into superior caval vein. The Lenus Pro pump was approved in EU for use in humans according to the Medical Devices Act and is MRI compatible up to 3 Tesla machines.

Pump implantation procedure

Prior to pump implantation the subcutaneous dose of treprostinil was escalated up to the highest dose tolerated by a particular patient. The procedure of pump implantation was carried out in European Health Center Otwock under general anesthesia (n = 11) or shallow analgosedation (fentanyl and propofol) combined with local anesthesia with lidocaine 2% (n = 1) in Zabrze. At first, a silicone catheter with a diameter of 6F was introduced via the subclavian vein into the superior vena cava using Seldinger's technique. The tip of the catheter was placed in the superior vena cava, 1–2 cm above its ostium into the right atrium. Subsequently, the Lenus Pro® pump was implanted either in the right or left subcostal area suprafascially, and in one patient, subfascially due to very scarce subcutaneous adipose tissue. A catheter was then tunneled from the implanted pump under the skin of the abdomen and chest to the subclavian area where it was connected to the tip of the catheter introduced into the subclavian vein by means of a special connector. The pump was filled with treprostinil prior to its implantation, without changing the dose of the drug administered by subcutaneous infusion. The external pump delivering the drug subcutaneously was detached after about 3 h, when treprostinil administered by mean of the Lenus Pro® pump filled its catheter and reached the patient's bloodstream. During this period patient stayed in intensive care unit.

Statistical analysis

Data are presented as means and standard deviations (SD) or medians and interquartile range (IQR). The Wilcoxon signed rank test was used for statistical analysis of data obtained prior to and following implantation. A p value <0.05 was considered significant.

Results

At the time of starting therapy with subcutaneous treprostinil, all patients exhibited symptoms of advanced PAH – mean pulmonary artery pressure was 64 ± 17 mmHg, cardiac index was 2.56 ± 1.1 L/min*m2, mean right atrial pressure 10 ± 4 mmHg, and pulmonary vascular resistance was 14.8 ± 7.1 Wood Units. 75% of patients were WHO functional class III, while the remaining ones were WHO functional class IV. The median time of subcutaneous therapy prior to Lenus Pro® pump implantation was 8 months (from 1 to 51 months, IQR 6–18).

The clinical characteristics of patients who had a Lenus Pro® pump implanted are presented in Table 1.

Efficacy of switch from sc to iv infusion with Lenus pro® pump

Immediately before Lenus Pro® pump implantation, 4 (33%) patients were functional class II and 8 (67%) were functional class III. After implantation, 6 (50%) patients were functional class II, and 5 (42%) and 1 (8%) were functional class III and IV, respectively (p = 0,59; Fig. 2). The treprostinil dose used was increased significantly after implantation of the Lenus Pro® pump – 33.9 ± 12.5 vs. 41.3 ± 14.0 ng/kg/min (p = 0.003). The blood concentration of NT-pro-BNP decreased from 1771 ± 1772 pg/ml to 1320 ± 929 pg/ml. However, this trend did not prove to be statistically significant (p = 0.24). Six-minute walking distance did not change – 398 ± 140 m vs. 402 ± 105 m (p = 0.59) (Fig. 3).

Safety of implantable pump

During implantation, no complications associated with surgical anesthesia were observed. During the postoperative period, in 4 cases small hematoma in the pump implantation bed was diagnosed that required a single evacuation by puncture. In one patient (pt. #11), puncturing of the pump bed area was required 3 times due to recurrence of the hematoma. This patient presented coagulopathy because of splenomegaly associated with liver cirrhosis resulting in thrombocytopenia.

During the follow-up with the median time of 14 months (from 4 to 29 months, IQR 11–20), one patient (#5) died of lung cancer, while others survived and were treated further with treprostinil.

In one patient, the drug delivery cannula slipped out of the subclavian vein during stretching gymnastics. It required the repositioning catheter twice [22]. In two cases, there was a reduction in the drug administration rate that required the flushing procedure to be carried out (pts #8 and #11) resulted in restoration of the original flow ratio. Those patients reported more aggravated fatigue without signs of right ventricular decompensation. Flushing was performed through service point with heparinized saline after complete emptying of the pump. In one patient (pt #3), an unexpected increase in the drug administration rate was observed – from 1.3 mL/day to 1.7 mL/day, which resulted in total emptying of the pump 1 day before refill visit with symptoms of deterioration of exercise capacity and fatigue, but without hemodynamic collapse. The flow acceleration required adjustment of the dose and frequency of follow-up visits. Other problems with the implantable pumps were of local nature and did not require any additional interventions. No clinically significant complications were observed during pump refill procedures, which were performed in authors' centers.

Health related quality of life

With regard to quality of life evaluated by means of the SF36 form, there was a significant improvement within the Physical Component Score – 28 ± 7 vs. 38 ± 8 points. (p < 0.001) and in specific domains: Physical Role – 31 ± 7 vs. 41 ± 12 points, (p = 0.03), Bodily Pain – 31 ± 12 vs. 50 ± 14 points (p = 0.02), and Vitality – 37 ± 8 vs. 50 ± 14 points (p = 0.03; Fig. 3). At general question "How would you rate your health in general compared to period before pump implantation?" 10 patients (83%) answered "Much better now" and 2 patients answered "Somewhat better now" and "About the same", respectively.

Discussion

The most important finding emerging from this study is the confirmation of positive effect at patients' HRQoL and relative safety of treating PAH with treprostinil by means of the Lenus Pro® subcutaneous implantable pump.

Table 1 Clinical characteristics of patients treated with subcutaneous treprostinil referred for the pump implantation and the postimplantation parameters

Pt	Age range [yrs.]	PAH etiology	Duration of sc. therapy [months]	Dose sc. [ng/kg/min]	Dose iv. [ng/kg/min]	WHO FC before implantation	WHO FC after implantation	FU [months]	Complications
1	42	Corrected CHD	6	38,0	40,0	II	II	29	None
2	28	Corrected CHD	50	62,5	80,0	III	III	24	None
3	37	Idiopathic PAH	6	20,0	30,5	III	III	21	Unexpected acceleration in drug delivery
4	40	Idiopathic PAH	8	22,5	22,5	II	II	19	Slight dislocation of pump without clinical implications
5	68	Connective tissue disease	8	27,0	30,0	II	III	12	Died because of lung cancer, no problems with the pump
6	54	Eisenmenger	6	25,5	43,5	III	II	16	None
7	25	Eisenmenger	9	41,3	42,0	III	III	15	None
8	38	Idiopathic PAH	27	40,2	41,3	III	III	13	Dislocation of the catheter, decrease in delivery rate
9	57	Connective tissue disease	10	33,9	35,4	II	II	11	None
10	53	Idiopathic PAH	29	40,4	44,0	II	II	10	None
11	30	Corrected CHD	7	17,0	40,0	III	IV	4	Recurrent hematoma at implantation site, decrease in delivery rate
12	32	Connective tissue disease	2	39,0	46,0	III	II	4	None

PAH – pulmonary arterial hypertension, CHD – congenital heart disease, WHO FC – WHO functional class, FU – follow-up [months]

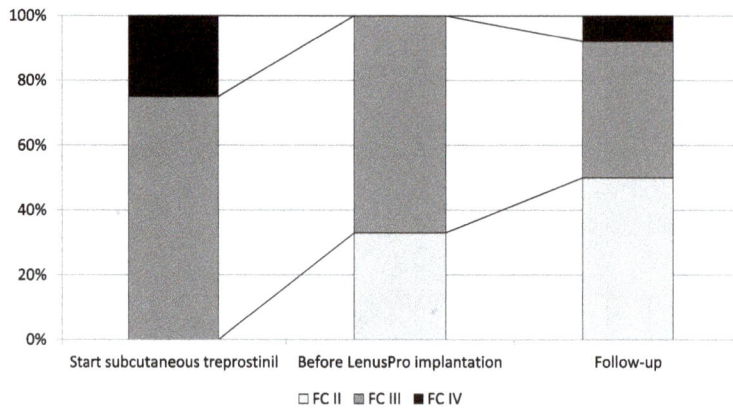

Fig. 2 Changes in WHO functional class assessed at the time of starting subcutaneous treprostinil infusion, before Lenus Pro® pump implantation and in follow-up

Patients evaluated in the study benefited after implantation of the implantable pump despite the fact it was no change in active substance but only the route of administration. It may partially result from the fact that it was possible to increase the medication dose after pump implantation thanks to elimination of the infusion site pain. Although the concentration of NT-proBNP did not change significantly and the 6-min walking distance did not increase, patients reported better physical performance, which was consistent with functional class evaluation made by a physician. However, assessment of functional class was not blinded and was based on patients' report, so placebo effect cannot be completely excluded. An increase in the 6MWT distance was noticeable in some patients – particularly in those, in whom this distance at the baseline was very short (about 150 m) (Fig. 3b). Improvement in treatment outcomes may also have been caused by elimination of activities related to external pump handling, which had resulted in unintentional errors. Moreover, better outcomes could also be caused by improvement of patient compliance in terms of continuous drug administration and maintenance of a fixed or increasing dose. It seems that due to implantation of a subcutaneous pump, the therapeutic

effect of treprostinil has taken advantage to the fullest extent – without limitations associated with the previous method of administration.

From the SF-36 questionnaire, it was found that improvement in HRQoL resulting from pump implantation was related first and foremost to reduction of experienced pain and the physical limitations associated both with the disease and the presence of an external pump. Bourge et al. also found improvement in activity scale of CAMPHOR questionnaire after switch from external system for delivery of treprostinil to implantable pump of different type [19]. Pain at the infusion site results from the topical effect of treprostinil that dilates the vessels in the subcutaneous tissue, leading to its hyperemia and pain fibers irritation [13] . Administrating the drug directly into the central vein allows the patient to avoid that bothersome side effect. Additionally, the presence of an external pump is associated with limitations to physical activity resulting from the patient being afraid of damaging the delicate infusion set construction and the drug-delivering catheter attached to it, and the necessity to detach the pump e.g. when bathing. Additionally, an external pump requires the drug to be replenished every 2–4 days, and in the case of some patients this

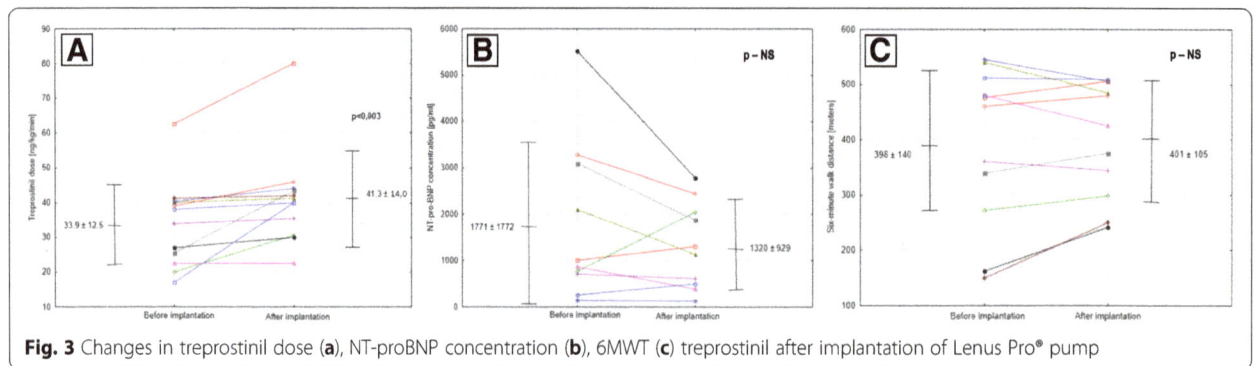

Fig. 3 Changes in treprostinil dose (**a**), NT-proBNP concentration (**b**), 6MWT (**c**) treprostinil after implantation of Lenus Pro® pump

requires assistance of a third person due to manual or language limitations. The complexity of treprostinil therapy by an external pump is therefore much higher than in the case of an implantable pump. Although the procedure of pump implantation itself bears a certain risk, the subsequent handling, which requires only a monthly refilling in the treating center, is much more patient-friendly. In this study, this directly translated into an improvement of the physical aspect of the quality of life (PCS – physical component score) (Fig. 4). Interestingly, patients demonstrated an increase in vitality after implantation of the Lenus Pro® pump, as reported in appropriate domain of the SF-36 questionnaire. However, due to a lack of objective indicators of clinical improvement in the form of 6MWT and NT-proBNP, it can be assumed that the increase in vitality results from "rebuilding" the energy that patients lost due to the use of an external pump and due to the feeling of stigmatization associated with it. Additional factor leading to improve in the vitality might be withdrawal some analgesics taken previously because of pain at infusion site.

This study showed safety of surgical procedure of pump implantation with general anesthesia in severely ill PAH patients. In Poland treatment with treprostinil is the second line anti-PAH therapy, restricted for patients deteriorating on oral therapies or being in functional class IV at diagnosis. In periprocedural period only minor complications were observed including hematoma in the pump implantation bed that required an evacuation by a puncture. In one case recurrent hematoma was found in patient with coagulopathy but it was also managed without surgical intervention. Richter et al. in series of 51 patients who were implanted with Lenus Pro pump reported two deaths because of right heart failure during hospital stay. Three patients suffered from atrial fibrillation related to catheter irritation, and in one case

hematoma and one case of seroma with catheter dislocation occurred [23].

Major complications during follow-up included an unexpected increase in the drug flow rate in the pump that required a change in the drug concentration and frequency of refilling, and dislocation of the drug-delivering catheter that required two repositioning procedures. The issue of drug flow changes requires further in-depth analysis and verification of the filling protocol, as it might be potentially life threatening complications related to stop of drug delivery for several hours. In few available publications, the that complications have not been described [15, 16]. However, in 2013 producer of Lenus Pro pump issued safety note informing that more than 10% acceleration in drug delivery might happen, especially when pumps are used for longer periods of time (2 to 4 years). It was postulated that the treprostinil would cauterize the glass surface within the capillary increasing its diameter. The corrective action was introduced by the new development of a chip canal with a more resistant glass [24]. As the pumps implanted in our patients came from upgraded series it should not be responsible for delivery acceleration. The fever or direct exposition of abdomen for sun which may increase the gas pressure inside pump and accelerate delivery rate were either excluded in this case. The issue of instability of flow delivery was also reported by Bourge et al. with different type of implantable pump [19].

The catheter dislocation was the next important complication during follow-up. In observed patient, it was clearly dependent on excessive physical activity including stretching and rap dancing. After reposition and cessation of above mentioned activities the catheter's position was stable. Thus, it seems sensible to carry out periodic follow-ups of the catheter location using an imaging technique (e.g. chest X-ray or fluoroscopy).

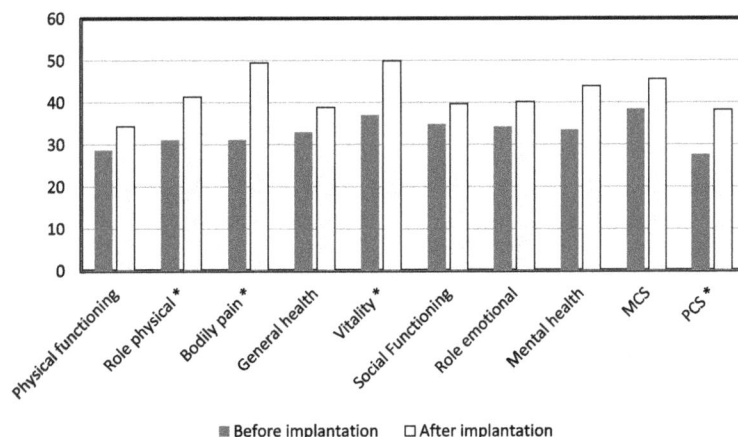

Fig. 4 Changes in quality of life measured with the SF-36 ver2 form. Norm based scores provided for 9 patients who completed the SF36 form. MCS – mental component score PCS – physical component score, * - $p < 0.05$

Our study confirmed safety of refiling process as well. Hohenforst-Schmidt et al. described one case, where erroneous administration of a monthly dose of treprostinil outside of the lumen of the pump while refilling resulted in circulatory collapse that was managed within a day using supportive therapy [25].

Limitations of the study

The main limitation of the study was a small number of patients and a lack of the control group. When considering the number of pumps implanted in relation to the number of patients treated with subcutaneous treprostinil, it seems that only 5–10% of patients will require changing of the subcutaneous therapy. It is consisted with percentage of patients withdrawing from sc therapy observed in previous trials [1, 2]. The lack of the control group may make it difficult to evaluate the impact of the placebo effect on improvement of the HRQoL. However, we found no negative effect on NT-pro-BNP, an objective indicator of heart failure. Moreover, this study presents only short-term and mid-term effects of changing the way of treprostinil administration. In order to carry out long-term evaluation, it would be necessary to prolong the observation period.

Conclusions

In patients with PAH who do not tolerate subcutaneous treprostinil infusion, the use of the Lenus Pro® implantable pump eliminates pain at infusion site and results in significant subjective improvement of vitality and physical aspect of the HRQoL. Therapy with the use of the Lenus Pro® pump is characterized by efficacy comparable to that of subcutaneous administration of treprostinil and acceptable safety profile, which however requires further observation.

Abbreviations
6MWT: 6-mintute walking test; CHD: congenital heart disease; FU: follow-up [months]; HRQoL: health-related quality of life; NT-proBNP: N-terminated brain natriuretic propeptide; PAH: pulmonary arterial hypertension; PCS: physical component score; WHO FC: World Health Organization functional class

Acknowledgements
We would like express our gratitude to Mrs. Małgorzata Suder (certified nurse) for her excellent assistance during pump implantation procedures.

Funding
This research did not receive any specific grant from funding agencies in the public, commercial, or not-for-profit sectors. The publication costs were covered by Pulmonary Hypertension Foundation, Warsaw, Poland.

Chemical compounds studied in this article
Treprostinil sodium (PubChem CID: 23663413)

Authors' contributions
All authors come from different centers, in which they treat patients with pulmonary arterial hypertension. They had referred the patients for pump implantation and continue with the follow-up and refiling procedures (KMR, AP, ŁC, MF, ZG, WJ, BS, TMK, AT). MK and KMR were the major contributors in writing the manuscript. MK and AK were the only implantators of the Lenus Pro® pump. JN performed the quality of life questionnaires. All authors have read and revised the manuscript and they agree for its publication in BMC Pulmonary Medicine.

Author information
AT is a member of the European Society of Cardiology (ESC) Working Group on Pulmonary Hypertension and is one of the authors of the most recent ESC guidelines for the management of patients with pulmonary hypertension.
MK was a reviewer of the above mentioned guidelines as a delegate of National Society.

Competing interests
The authors declare that they have no competing interests.

Author details
[1]Department of Pulmonary Circulation, Thromboembolic Diseases and Cardiology, Centre of Postgraduate Medical Education, European Health Centre Otwock, Borowa 14/18, 05-400 Otwock, Poland. [2]1st Department of Cardiology, University of Medical Sciences, Poznan, Poland. [3]Department of Anesthesiology and Intensive Care, European Health Centre Otwock, Otwock, Poland. [4]Department of Invasive Cardiology, Central Clinical Hospital of the Ministry of the Interior and Administration, Warsaw, Poland. [5]Department of Cardiology, Medical University of Lodz, Lodz, Poland. [6]Department of Cardiology, Provincial Specialist Hospital in Wroclaw, Research and Development Centre, Wrocław, Poland. [7]Department of Cardiology, SHS, Medical University of Silesia, Katowice, Poland. [8]2nd Department of Cardiology, School of Medicine with Dentistry Division, Medical University of Silesia, Zabrze, Poland. [9]Department of Cardiology, Medical University of Bialystok, Białystok, Poland.

References
1. Simonneau G, Barst RJ, Galie N, Naeije R, Rich S, Bourge RC, et al. Continuous subcutaneous infusion of treprostinil, a prostacyclin analogue, in patients with pulmonary arterial hypertension: a double-blind, randomized, placebo-controlled trial. Am J Respir Crit Care Med. 2002;165:800–4.
2. Lang I, Gomez-Sanchez M, Kneussl M, Naeije R, Escribano P, Skoro-Sajer N, et al. Efficacy of long-term subcutaneous treprostinil sodium therapy in pulmonary hypertension. Chest. 2006;129:1636–43. doi:10.1378/chest.129.6.1636.
3. Galiè N, Humbert M, Vachiery J-L, Gibbs S, Lang I, Torbicki A, et al. 2015 ESC/ERS guidelines for the diagnosis and treatment of pulmonary hypertension. Eur Heart J. 2016;37:67–119.
4. McLaughlin VV, Gaine SP, Barst RJ, Oudiz RJ, Bourge RC, Frost A, et al. Efficacy and safety of treprostinil: an epoprostenol analog for primary pulmonary hypertension. J Cardiovasc Pharmacol. 2003;41:293–9.
5. Xu QA, Trissel LA, Pham L. Physical and chemical stability of Treprostinil sodium injection packaged in plastic syringe pump reservoirs. Int J Pharm Compd. 8:228–30.
cutaneous treprostinil for severe pulmonary hypertension. J Heart Lung Transplant. 2012;31:735–43. doi: 10.1016/j.healun.2012.02.025.
8. Jing Z-C, Parikh K, Pulido T, Jerjes-Sanchez C, White RJ, Allen R, et al. Efficacy and safety of oral treprostinil monotherapy for the treatment of pulmonary arterial hypertension: a randomized, controlled trial. Circulation. 2013;127:624–33. doi: 10.1161/CIRCULATIONAHA.112.124388.
9. Skoro-Sajer N, Lang I. Extended-release oral treprostinil for the treatment of pulmonary arterial hypertension. Expert Rev Cardiovasc Ther. 2014;12:1391–9. doi: 10.1586/14779072.2014.975209.
10. Hellawell JL, Bhattacharya S, Farber HW. Pharmacokinetic evaluation of treprostinil (oral) for the treatment of pulmonary arterial hypertension. Expert Opin Drug Metab Toxicol. 2014;10:1445–53. doi: 10.1517/17425255.2014.958466.

11. Pugliese SC, Bull TM. Clinical use of extended-release oral treprostinil in the treatment of pulmonary arterial hypertension. Integr Blood Press Control. 2016;9:1–7.

12. Chin KM, Ruggiero R, Bartolome S, Velez-Martinez M, Darsaklis K, Kingman M, et al. Long-term therapy with oral treprostinil in pulmonary arterial hypertension failed to lead to improvement in important physiologic measures: results from a single center. Pulm Circ. 2015;5:513–20.

13. Skoro-Sajer N. Optimal use of treprostinil in pulmonary arterial hypertension: a guide to the correct use of different formulations. Drugs. 2012;72:2351–63. doi: 10.2165/11638260-000000000-00000.

14. Wade M, Baker FJ, Roscigno R, DellaMaestra W, Hunt TL, Lai AA. Absolute bioavailability and pharmacokinetics of treprostinil sodium administered by acute subcutaneous infusion. J Clin Pharmacol. 2004;44:83–8.

15. Steringer-Mascherbauer R, Eder V, Ebner C, Niel J, Fuegger R, Wittrich S, et al. First experiences with intravenous Treprostinil delivered by an implantable pump (Lenus pro®) with filling intervals of 28 days in patients with pulmonary arterial hypertension (PAH) - a series of five cases. CHEST J. 2011;140:904A.

16. Steringer-Mascherbauer R, Eder V, Huber C, Wittrich S, Marecek I, Nesser HJ. Intravenous treprostinil delivered by the implantable pump Lenus pro®: a innovative "surgical" approach to management of PAH. J Hear Lung Transplant. 2013;37:S64.

17. Desole S, Velik-Salchner C, Fraedrich G, Ewert R, Kähler CM. Subcutaneous implantation of a new intravenous pump system for prostacyclin treatment in patients with pulmonary arterial hypertension. Heart Lung. 2012;41:599–605.

18. Pawlak A, Koteja A, Starska A, Kurzyna M, Gil RJ. The first LENUS pro® pump implantation in Poland in patient with pulmonary hypertension. Kardiol Pol. 2016;74:300. doi: 10.5603/KP.2016.0030.

19. Bourge RC, Waxman AB, Gomberg-Maitland M, Shapiro SM, Tarver JH, Zwicke DL, et al. Treprostinil administered to treat pulmonary artery hypertension using a fully implantable programmable intravascular delivery system: results of the DelIVery for PAH trial. Chest. 2016;150:27–34.

20. Ware JE, Sherbourne CD. The MOS 36-item short-form health survey (SF-36). I. Conceptual framework and item selection. Med Care. 1992;30:473–83.

21. Tylka J, Piotrowicz R. Quality of life assessment questionnaire (SF-36) - polish version. Kardiol Pol. 2009;67:1166–9.

22. Malaczynska-Rajpold K, Kurzyna M, Koteja A, Torbicki A, Mularek-Kubzdela T. The "bouncing" catheter. Cardiol J. 2016;23:552–3.

23. Richter MJ, Ewert R, Warnke C, Gall H, Classen S, Grimminger F, et al. Procedural safety of a fully implantable intravenous prostanoid pump for pulmonary hypertension. Clin Res Cardiol. 2016:1–9.

24. Bülow M, Otto K-H. Tricumed. Urgent Safety Information 2013. https://www.swissmedic.ch/recalllists_dl/08938/Vk_20131223_02-e1.pdf.

25. Hohenforst-Schmidt W, Hornig J, Friedel N, Zarogoulidis P, Zarogoulidis K, Brachmann J. Successful management of an inadvertent excessive treprostinil overdose. Drug Des Devel Ther. 2013;7:161–5.

5

Case report: continued treatment with alectinib is possible for patients with lung adenocarcinoma with drug-induced interstitial lung disease

Tatsuya Nitawaki* ⓘ, Yoshihiko Sakata, Kodai Kawamura and Kazuya Ichikado

Abstract

Background: Alectinib, a second-generation anaplastic lymphoma kinase (ALK) inhibitor, is a key drug for ALK rearranged lung adenocarcinoma. Interstitial lung disease (ILD) is an important adverse effect of alectinib, which generally requires termination of treatment. However, we treated two patients with drug-induced ILD who continued to receive alectinib.

Case presentation: Patient 1 was a 57-year-old male with an *ALK*-rearranged Stage IV lung adenocarcinoma who was administered alectinib as first-line therapy. Computed tomography (CT) detected asymptomatic ground-glass opacity (GGO) on day 33 of treatment. Alectinib therapy was therefore discontinued for 7 days and then restarted. GGO disappeared, and the progression of ILD ceased. Patient 2 was a 64-year-old woman with an *ALK*-positive lung adenocarcinoma who was administered alectinib as third-line therapy. One year later, CT detected GGO; and she had a slight, nonproductive cough. Alectinib therapy was continued in the absence of other symptoms, and GGO slightly diminished after 7 days. Two months later, CT detected increased GGO, and alectinib therapy was continued. GGO diminished again after 7 days. The patient has taken alectinib for more than 2 years without progression of ILD.

Conclusions: Certain patients with alectinib-induced ILD Grade 2 or less may continue alectinib therapy if they are closely managed.

Keywords: Lung cancer, Non-small cell lung cancer, ALK, Alectinib, Interstitial lung disease, GGO

Background

Alectinib is one of the key drugs for treating patients with ALK-positive non-small cell lung cancer (NSCLC), because it is effective and is well tolerated [1]. Interstitial lung disease (ILD) is an important adverse effect associated with alectinib treatment as well as with all tyrosine kinase inhibitors (TKI) [2]. Generally, when ILD occurs, TKI therapy should be terminated, although treatment with certain molecular targeting inhibitors such as those specific for mammalian target of rapamycin (mTOR) can be continued [3]. It is unclear whether the physician should continue alectinib when ILD is diagnosed. Here we report two patients with alectinib-induced ILD who were able to continue alectinib therapy.

Case presentation

Patient 1

A 57-year-old male smoker with lung adenocarcinoma of his right lower lobe was positive for *EML4-ALK* and positive for ALK. Metastases were present at the third left rib and bilateral adrenal glands, leading to a diagnosis of Stage IV disease. Alectinib (300 mg twice daily) was administered as first-line treatment as per standard of care. CT revealed that the sizes of the primary lesion and other metastases were much smaller compared with baseline. However, 33 days after alectinib administration, CT revealed patchy ground glass opacity (GGO) of the

* Correspondence: tatsuya-nitawaki@saiseikaikumamoto.jp
Division of Respiratory Medicine, Saiseikai Kumamoto Hospital, 5-3-1 Chikami, Kumamoto 861-4193, Japan

left lower lobe (Fig. 1a). We suspected alectinib-induced ILD, and discontinued treatment. Laboratory data did not detect significant inflammation. Bronchoalveolar lavage fluid (BALF) analysis of the left B9 revealed to be lymphocyte-predominant for 54%. The results of blood tests and microbial culture of the BALF did not indicate any infection (Table 1), so we diagnosed alectinib-induced ILD. But we did not use corticosteroid because he had no symptom of ILD.Alectinib was therefore reintroduced on day 40with careful observation. The GGO in the left lower lobe disappeared on day 61 (Fig. 1b). The patient did not show any symptoms after a 7-month course of alectinib.

Patient 2

A 64-year-old woman nonsmoker had experienced relapsing adenocarcinoma 19 months after undergoing lung surgery and postoperative chemotherapy. She was positive for *EML4-ALK*. Crizotinib therapy was started as first-line treatment. However, multiple lung and brain metastases and carcinomatous lymphagitis developed after 5 months. Whole brain radiotherapy and two cycles of pemetrexed, bevacizumab maintenance therapy after 4 cycles of carboplatin-pemetrexed-bevacizumab therapy were administered. However, 6 months later, brain MRI revealed tumor dissemination to the meninges. Therefore, she received 300-mg alectinib twice daily. Twelve months later, a chest CT revealed GGO in the left lower lobe (Fig. 2a). She presented with a slight, nonproductive cough, no fever or dyspnea, and her blood values were within their normal ranges. Alectinib-induced ILD Grade 2 (Common Terminology Critera for Adverse Events version 4.0) was suspected. Since her symptom was only cough and very slight, we had continued alectinib with careful observation, not using corticosteroid. After 7 days, her cough and the GGO had been improved spontaneously (Fig. 2b), so alectinib treatment was continued. But it became more pronounced 2 months later (Fig. 2c). Then she did not present cough and any other symptoms or abnormal laboratory values. Blood tests and microbial culture of BALF did not detect any infection and cell count of BALF was normal (Table 1). There was no other cause of the GGO, so we diagnosed alectinib-induced ILD. But she was not considered to have significant symptom caused by ILD, we therefore continued alectinib treatment and found that the GGO diminished after 1 week. (Fig. 2d). She has taken alectinib for 2 years without progression of ILD.

Discussion and conclusions

Alectinib is a key drug for treating patients with *EML4-ALK*-positive NSCLC. In particular, alectinib is highly effective and well tolerated [1], although some patients may experience severe acute ILD [4]. In the ALEX trial and the J-ALEX trial, the incidence of alectinib-induced ILD was reported 1% and 8%, respectively [5, 6]. Physicians

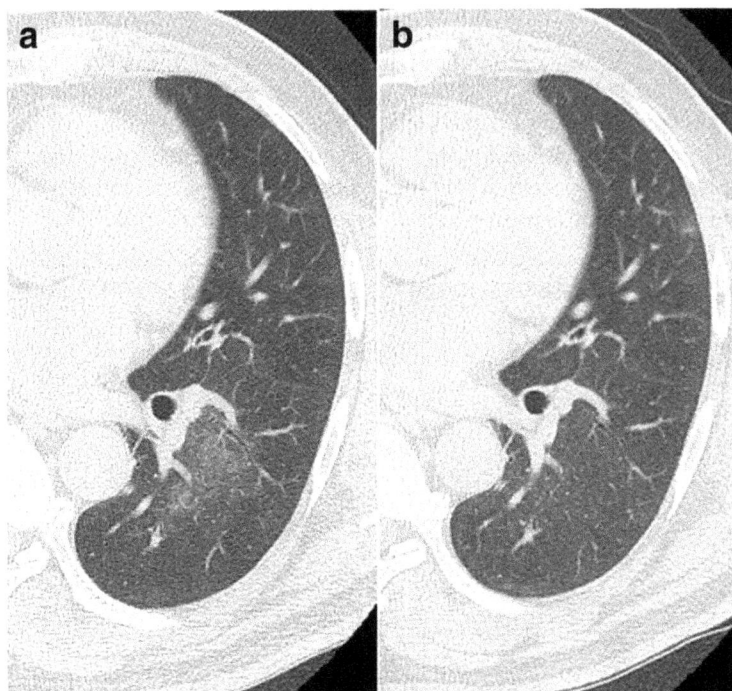

Fig. 1 GGO, Case 1. **a** On day 33 of alectinib therapy, a GGO was detected in the left lower lobe. Alectinib was discontinued. **b** On day 61, the GGO disappeared after reintroducing alectinib on day 40

Table 1 The results of laboratory test of the blood and the bronchoalveolar lavage fluid (BALF)

	Case1	Case2
Blood examination		
WBC (/μL)	6,800	4,500
CRP (mg/dL)	0.02	0.03
LDH (IU/L)	222	202
SP-D (ng/mL)	37	19.3
KL-6 (IU/mL)	299	211
β-D-glucan (pg/mL)	negative	negative
CMV antigen pp65 C7-HRP (antigenemia)	negative	negative
BALF		
Fluid (mL)	17/100	23/150
cell count (/mL)	4×10^5	1×10^5
Lymphocyte (%)	54.5	17
Neutrophil (%)	1	25
Eosinophil (%)	5	1
Basophil (%)	0	0
Histiocyte (%)	39.5	57
CD4/CD8 rate	1.2	0.65
culture	negative	negative
Arterial blood gas		
pH	7.396	NA
PaO$_2$ (mmHg)	36.0	NA
PaCO$_2$ (mmHg)	82.5	NA
HCO$_3^-$ (mmol/L)	21.6	NA
BE	−2.2	NA

generally must discontinue alectinib in such cases, although we believe that certain patients can continue therapy.

In general, drug-induced ILD is suspected when the following criteria are met:(1) history of exposure to the suspected drug, (2) report of suspected previous drug-induced ILD, (3) exclusion of other causes, (4) improvement after discontinuation of a suspected drug, and (5) recurrence of symptoms on rechallenge [7]. Patient 1 did not meet criteria 5 and patient 2 did not meet criteria 4 and 5.; however, there was no evidence of infection and other etiologies of ILD. Furthermore, *Ikeda* et al. reported a patient with alectinib-induced ILD who had GGO and no clinical symptoms, similar to our patients [8]. We conclude therefore that our patients had alectinib-induced ILD.

Generally, drug-induced ILD is characterized by lymphocyte-predominant BALF, while bacterial pneumonia may be associated with neutrophil-predominant BALF. *Ait-Tahar* et al. reported higher immune responses of B and cytotoxic T cells in ALK-positive patients with anaplastic large cell lymphoma than in ALK-negative patients [9]. It is suggested that having ALK fusion gene may lead to higher immune response. Analysis of the BALF of Patient 1 revealed lymphocyte-predominant disease, which might reflect "ALK fusion gene-related drug hypersensitivity". This "hypersensivity" may lead to the risk of ILD. Otherwise the BALF of Patient 2 was neutrophil-predominant, which may be influenced by the low recovery rate from BALF. Additionally, since there was no evidence of other etiology of the GGO, the absence of lymphocyte-predominant BALF did not exclude drug-induced ILD.

We continued alectinib despite the suspicion of ILD, because patient1 did not have any symptoms, patient 2 had only very sligh cough. *Créquit P* et al. reported that six of 29 patients with ILD who were treated with crizotinib, the first available ALK inhibitor for treating NSCLC, had few clinical symptoms [10]. Moreover, they reported that patients with crizotinib-induced ILD had longer median progression-free survival compared with those without crizotinib-ILD (19.9 vs 6.2 months, $p = 0.04$).

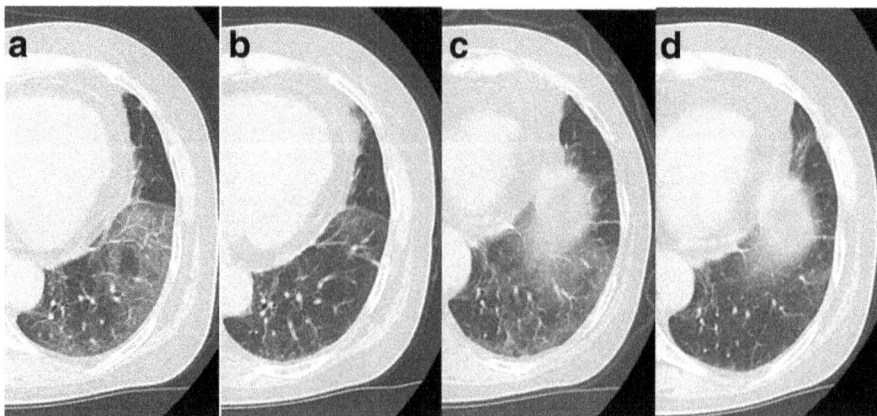

Fig. 2 GGO, Case 2. **a** GGO in the left lower lobe 1 year after administration of alectinib. **b** The GGO disappeared after 1 week. **c** Relapse of the GGO after 2 months. **d** The GGO disappeared again after 8 days

Therefore, these findings suggest that a patient with ALK inhibitor-induced ILD may exhibit a higher response compared with those without ALK inhibitor-induced ILD. To our knowledge, this is the first report that patients with ILD Grade 2 or less were able to continue alectinib therapy.

Alectinib may induce severe ILD. For example, CT detected bilateral GGO in a patient with progressive dyspnea [4]. According to *Créquit P* et al., a patient with crizotinib-induced ILD died from acute respiratory distress syndrome on day 28 after the initiation of crizotinib therapy, and this patient previously experienced reversible erlotinib-induced ILD [10]. Therefore, if physicians want to continue alectinib treatment for a patient with alectinib-ILD Grade2 or less, the very careful observation is needed.

There are some limitations to the present study. First, we retrospectively studied two patients who were treated at a single center, and more patients must be studied, or a multicenter prospective study will be required. Second, the recovery rate of BALF was insufficient, so BALF analysis may not have reflected the effect of alectinib for the lungs accurately. Third, it is not clear if our patients responded longer to therapy compared with those without alectinib-induced ILD.

We conclude that certain patients with alectinib-induced ILD Grade2 or less may continue alectinib therapy if they are closely managed, because they may therefore achieve a prolonged response to therapy that leads to longer survival.

Abbreviations
ALK: Anaplastic lymphoma kinase; BALF: Bronchoalveolar lavage fluid; CT: Computed tomography; GGO: Ground-glass opacity; ILD: Interstitial lung disease; mTOR: Mammalian target of rapamycin; NSCLC: Non-small cell lung cancer; TKI: Tyrosine kinase inhibitor

Acknowledgments
I am deeply grateful to all the people who were associated with our medical practice.

Funding
This research did not receive any specific grant from funding agencies in the public, commercial, or not-for-profit sectors.

Authors' contributions
TN wrote the initial draft of the manuscript. YS contributed to collect data, and assisted in the preparation of the manuscript. All other authors have contributed to review the manuscript. All authors approved the final version of the manuscript, and agree to be accountable for all aspects of the work in ensuring that questions related to the accuracy or integrity of any part of the work are appropriately investigated and resolved.

Competing interests
The authors declare that they have no competing interests.

References
1. Seto T, Kiura K, Nishio M, Nakagawa K, Maemondo M, Inoue A, Hida T, Yamamoto N, Yoshioka H, Harada M, Ohe Y, Nogami N, Takeuchi K, Shimada T, Tanaka T, Tamura T. CH5424802 (RO5424802) for patients with ALK-rearranged advanced non-small-cell lung cancer (AF-001JP study): a single-arm, open-label, phase 1-2 study. Lancet Oncol. 2013;14:590–8.
2. Cohen MH, Williams GA, Sridhara R, Chen G, Pazdur R. FDA drug approval summary: Gefitinib (ZD1839) (Iressa®) tablets. Oncologist. 2003;8:303–6.
3. White D, Camus P, Endo M, Escudier B, Calvo E, Akaza H, Uemura H, Kpamegan E, Kay A, Robson M, Ravaud A, Motzer RJ. Noninfectious Pneumonitis after Everolimus therapy for advanced renal cell carcinoma. Am J Respir Crit Care Med. 2010;182:396–403.
4. Yamamoto Y, Okamoto I, Otsubo K, Iwama E, Hamada N, Harada T, Takayama K, Nakanishi Y. Severe acute interstitial lung disease in a patient with anaplastic lymphoma kinase rearrangement-positive non-small cell lung cancer treated with alectinib. Investig New Drugs. 2015;33:1148–50.
5. Peters S, Camidge DR, Shaw AT, Gadgeel S, Ahn JS, Kim DW, Ou SHI, Pérol M, Dziadziuszko R, Rosell R, Zeaiter A, Mitry E, Golding S, Balas B, Noe J, Morcos PN, Mok T. Alectinib versus Crizotinib in untreated ALK-positive non. Small-cell lung cancer. N Engl J Med. 2017;(6) 10.1056/NEJMoa1704795.
6. Hida T, Nokihara H, Kondo M, Kim YH, Azuma K, Seto T, Takiguchi Y, Nishio M, Yoshioka H, Imamura F, Hotta K, Watanabe S, Goto K, Satouchi M, Kozuki T, Shukuya T, Nakagawa K, Mitsudomi T, Yamamoto N, Asakawa T, Asabe R, Tanaka T, Tamura T. Alectinib versus crizotinib in patients with ALK-positive non-small-cell lung cancer (J-ALEX): an open-label, randomised phase 3 trial. Lancet. 2017;390:29–39.
7. Schwaiblmair M, Behr W, Haeckel T, Markl B, Foerg W, Berghaus T. Drug induced interstitial lung disease. Open Respir Med J. 2012;6:63–74.
8. Ikeda S, Yoshioka H, Arita M, Sakai T, Sone N, Nishiyama A, Niwa T, Hotta M, Tanaka T, Ishida T. Interstitial lung disease induced by alectinib (CH5424802 /RO5424802). Jpn J Clin Oncol. 2015;45:221–4.
9. Ait-Tahar K, Cerundolo V, Banham AH, Hatton C, Blanchard T, Kusec R, Becker M, Smith GL, Pulford K. B and CTL responses to the ALK protein in patients with ALK-positive ALCL. Int J Cancer. 2006;118:688–95.
10. P. Créquit, M. Wislez, J. Fleury Feith, N. Rozensztajn, L. Jabot, S. Friard S, A. Lavole, V. Gounant, J. Fillon, M. Antoine, J. Cadranel J. Crizotinib associated with ground-glass opacity predominant pattern interstitial lung disease. A retrospective observational cohort study with a systematic literature review. J Thorac Oncol. 10 (2015) 1148-1155.

6

The impacts of baseline ventilator parameters on hospital mortality in acute respiratory distress syndrome treated with venovenous extracorporeal membrane oxygenation

Meng-Yu Wu[1,2]*[iD], Yu-Sheng Chang[1], Chung-Chi Huang[3], Tzu-I Wu[4,5] and Pyng-Jing Lin[1]

Abstract

Background: Venovenous extracorporeal membrane oxygenation (VV-ECMO) is a valuable life support in acute respiratory distress syndrome (ARDS) in adult patients. However, the success of VV-ECMO is known to be influenced by the baseline settings of mechanical ventilation (MV) before its institution. This study was aimed at identifying the baseline ventilator parameters which were independently associated with hospital mortality in non-trauma patients receiving VV-ECMO for severe ARDS.

Methods: This retrospective study included 106 non-trauma patients (mean age: 53 years) who received VV-ECMO for ARDS in a single medical center from 2007 to 2016. The indication of VV-ECMO was severe hypoxemia ($P_aO_2/$ FiO_2 ratio < 70 mmHg) under pressure-controlled MV with peak inspiratory pressure (PIP) > 35 cmH_2O, positive end-expiratory pressure (PEEP) > 5 cmH_2O, and F_iO_2 > 0.8. Important demographic and clinical data before and during VV-ECMO were collected for analysis of hospital mortality.

Results: The causes of ARDS were bacterial pneumonia ($n = 41$), viral pneumonia ($n = 24$), aspiration pneumonitis ($n = 3$), and others ($n = 38$). The median duration of MV before ECMO institution was 3 days and the overall hospital mortality was 53% ($n = 56$). The medians of $PaO_2/$ FiO_2 ratio, PIP, PEEP, and dynamic pulmonary compliance (PC_{dyn}) at the beginning of MV were 84 mmHg, 32 cmH_2O, 10 cmH_2O, and 21 mL/cmH_2O, respectively. However, before the beginning of VV-ECMO, the medians of $PaO_2/$ FiO_2 ratio, PIP, PEEP, and PC_{dyn} became 69 mmHg, 36 cmH_2O, 14 cmH_2O, and 19 mL/cmH_2O, respectively. The escalation of PIP and the declines in $PaO_2/$ FiO_2 ratio and PC_{dyn} were significantly correlated with the duration of MV before ECMO institution. Finally, the duration of MV (OR: 1.184, 95% CI: 1.079–1.565, $p < 0.001$) was found to be the only baseline ventilator parameter that independently affected the hospital mortality in these ECMO-treated patients.

Conclusion: Since the duration of MV before ECMO institution was strongly correlated to the outcome of adult respiratory ECMO, medical centers are suggested to find a suitable prognosticating tool to determine the starting point of respiratory ECMO among their candidates with different duration of MV.

(Continued on next page)

* Correspondence: david3627@gmail.com
[1]Department of Cardiovascular Surgery, Chang Gung Memorial Hospital and Chang Gung University, Taoyuan, Taiwan
[2]School of Traditional Chinese Medicine, Chang Gung University, Taoyuan, Taiwan
Full list of author information is available at the end of the article

(Continued from previous page)

Keywords: Venovenous extracorporeal membrane oxygenation, Adult respiratory distress syndrome, Lung recruitment, Lung-protective mechanical ventilation

Background

Extracorporeal Membrane Oxygenation (ECMO) is currently an important life support for acute respiratory distress syndrome (ARDS) in adult patients [1, 2]. According to the 2016 international report of the Extracorporeal Life Support Organization (ELSO) Registry, 58% of the adult patients receiving ECMO for severe respiratory failure can be saved and discharged from hospital [3]. This report also reveals that about 90% of the 9812 ECMO runs for adult respiratory failure are in venovenous (VV)-associated configurations [3]. The niche of VV-ECMO in the management of ARDS is to provide a pre-pulmonary blood gas exchange to the venous blood and reduce the patient's dependence on pulmonary ventilation [2].While the patient's dependence on pulmonary ventilation is reduced, the risk and the severity of ventilator-induced lung injury (VILI) can theoretically be mitigated. Although the popularity of adult respiratory ECMO is continuously increasing, the applications of ECMO are still limited in large medical centers and reserved for the most advanced diseases [1]. The discrepancy in user experience leads to considerable controversies about the timing of respiratory ECMO among experts worldwide. Currently, the timing of respiratory ECMO is mostly determined by the severity of hypoxemia which is represented by the ratio of arterial oxygen tension (PaO_2) to the fraction of inspired oxygen (FiO_2) under mechanical ventilation (MV). In the ELSO Guidelines for Adult Respiratory Failure, the suggested threshold value of PaO_2/FiO_2 (PF) ratio for ECMO institution is 100 mmHg or less [4]. However, under the inclusion criteria based on PF ratio, patients with a relatively slow-progressive disease may experience a significant escalation in the driving force of MV before their PF ratio can finally meet the threshold value for ECMO [5]. Since the therapeutic goal of respiratory ECMO is to reduce the negative influence of MV on the success of adult respiratory ECMO, the starting point of respiratory ECMO should also take the determinant ventilator parameters into consideration. Therefore, the study was aimed at identifying the baseline ventilator parameters which were independently associated with hospital mortality in patients receiving VV-ECMO for severe ARDS.

Methods

Settings and patients

From March 2007 to March 2016, a total of 151 adult patients received VV-ECMO for advanced respiratory support at Chang Gung Memorial Hospital Linko Branch. The university-affiliated hospital is a tertiary referral center with 3400 beds. To avoid the influences of trauma or surgery on blood coagulation and compliance of the respiratory system, we only enrolled 106 adult non-trauma patients who had a single run of VV-ECMO and survived on VV-ECMO >24 h in this retrospective study. This study was conducted in accordance with the amended Declaration of Helsinki. The ethics committee of the Chang Gung Medical Foundation approved this protocol (CGMF IRB no. 201601483B0) and waived the necessity of individual patient consent.

Managements of adult VV-ECMO

Our techniques of applying MV and ECMO to improve hypoxemia in patients with ARDS were described previously [5–9]. Before ECMO is considered, patients with ARDS were treated with the lung-protective MV and paralyzed with neuromuscular blockers. Our lung-protective MV is pressure-controlled ventilation which uses a peak airway pressure (PIP) less than 35 mmHg to drive a tidal volume (V_T) no more than 6 ml/ kg. To prevent carbon dioxide (CO_2) retention and oxygen toxicity, the respiratory rate, the positive end-expiratory pressure (PEEP), and the F_iO_2 of MV are set at 20 to 25/ min, 10 to 18 cmH_2O, and less than 0.8, respectively. VV-ECMO would be delivered to suitable candidates if they required a higher PIP and FiO_2 for maintaining a PF not less than 70 mmHg. Nevertheless, VV-ECMO was contraindicated in candidates showing (1) uncontrolled hemorrhages, (2) major brain damages, and (3) significant hemodynamic instability. The definition of significant hemodynamic instability here was circulatory shock (systolic arterial blood pressure < 90 mmHg) that required a high-dosed inotrope/vasopressor therapy (dopamine >15 mcg/kg/min, epinephrine >0.1 mcg/kg/min, or norepinephrine >0.1 mcg/kg/min). Our ECMO devices include a centrifugal pump [Capiox emergent bypass system (Terumo, Tokyo, Japan) or Bio-console 560 system (Medtronic, Minneapolis, MN, USA)], an oxygenator with silicone membrane (Medtronic, Minneapolis, MN, USA) or polymethylpentene membrane (Terumo Capiox-SX or Medos Hilite 7000), and two vascular cannulae (DLP Medtronic, Minneapolis, MN, USA). We conduct VV-ECMO via percutaneous cannulation of the common femoral vein (inflow, with a cannula of 19–23 French) and the right internal jugular vein (outflow, with a cannula of 17–21 French). After implantation of VV-ECMO, we initially maximize the sweep gas flow (10 L/min, pure oxygen) to rapidly remove CO_2, and gradually increase the ECMO pump flow to achieve a steady flow that carries the best pulse oximetry-detected oxyhemoglobin saturation (SpO_2). To rest the injured lungs, we gradually downgrade the original MV settings to a non-injurious level (PIP ≤ 30 cmH_2O and MV FiO_2 ≤ 0.4). According to the data of arterial and post-oxygenator blood gas samplings, we dynamically adjust the flows of ECMO to provide an optimal SpO_2 (> 90%) and arterial oxyhemoglobin saturation (SaO_2; > 85%). A modest anticoagulation (activated partial thromboplastin time between 40 and 55 s) is achieved with systemic heparinization except in hemorrhagic patients. We would try to wean the improved patients from VV-ECMO as long as the arterial oxygenation could be maintained with small V_T and ventilator FiO_2 no more than 0.6.

Data collection

We retrospectively reviewed the electronic medical records of every patient and collected their relevant demographic and clinical data before and during ECMO run. Since sequential organ failure assessment (SOFA) score [10] and respiratory extracorporeal membrane oxygenation survival prediction (RESP) score [11] have become our major prognosticating tools for adult respiratory ECMO now, we collected the essential data to calculate the two scores in each patient. Therefore the following variables were collected: age, gender, body weight and height, acute respiratory diagnosis (viral pneumonia, bacterial pneumonia, asthma, trauma/burn, aspiration, and others), immunocompromised status (malignancy, organ transplantation, liver cirrhosis Child B or C, or autoimmune diseases requiring long-term immunosuppressive therapy), non-pulmonary infection, duration of MV before institution of VV-ECMO, MV settings [measured ventilation volume, PIP, mean airway pressure (MAP), PEEP, dynamic driving pressure, dynamic pulmonary compliance (PC_{dyn}), and oxygen index (OI)] soon (1 to 2 h) after institution of MV and just (1–2 h) before institution of VV-ECMO, special medications (neuromuscular blockers, bicarbonate or vasopressors) before institution of VV-ECMO, the latest results of blood tests (arterial blood gas sampling, blood cell counts, creatinine, and total bilirubin) before institution of VV-ECMO, durations of hospital and ECMO stay, and outcomes (survived or died in hospital). In the survivors, we also collected the MV settings just before and after 24 h of ECMO removal. The V_T was defined as the measured ventilation volume dividing by the ideal body weight. The dynamic driving pressure was defined as the difference of PIP and PEEP. PC_{dyn} was defined as the measured ventilation volume dividing by the difference of PIP and PEEP. The OI was defined as the product of MAP and FiO_2 dividing by PaO_2. The baseline value of a given variable was the value obtained just before institution of VV-ECMO. For our practical purposes, we made some modifications of the definitions in the original RESP score. First, we assigned the patients with fungal pneumonia to the category of bacterial pneumonia, because fungal pneumonia was not a category of diagnosis in RESP score and the number of fungal pneumonia in our patient cohort was small. Second, we excluded the item of nitric oxide inhalation because this information was often missing in our patient cohort. Third, we assigned a SOFA neurological assessment score to each patient according to his/her neurological status before sedation [12].

Outcome measures

The endpoint of this study was to identify the predictors of hospital mortality in adult respiratory ECMO among the baseline ventilator parameters.

Statistical analyses

Statistical analyses were performed with SPSS for Windows (Version 21, IBM, Inc., NY, USA). For all analyses, the statistical significance was set at $p < 0.05$. The independent T-test or the Mann-Whitney U test was used for univariate comparison of numerical variables. The Chi-square or Fisher's exact test was used for univariate comparison of categorical variables. The data were presented as mean (± standard deviation) for numerical variables with normal distribution or median (interquartile range; IQR) for numerical variables without normal distribution. The categorical data were presented as number (percentage). The multivariate logistic regression method was used to identify the independent predictors of hospital mortality and to build up the mortality risk prediction model. All variables with a $p < 0.05$ in univariate tests were firstly processed by the logistic regression method with a backward stepwise selection procedure. The variables showed a $p < 0.05$ in the logistic regression process were re-tested by the logistic regression method with a forward stepwise selection procedure to build the final prediction model. The final model was evaluated by the Hosmer-Lemeshow test and the receiver operating characteristic curve analysis for its goodness-of-fit and the predictive power for hospital mortality.

Results

Patient characteristics

Our therapeutic protocol and associated patient distribution are presented in fig. 1. The results of univariate comparisons of important demographic and clinical data between the survivors and the non-survivors are presented in Table 1. The causes of ARDS were categorized into 4 groups: bacterial pneumonia ($n = 41$; three were fungal pneumonia, and the top three found bacteria were *Staphylococcus aureus, Pseudomonas aeruginosa,* and *Acinetobacter baumannii*), viral pneumonia ($n = 24$; all influenza type A), aspiration pneumonitis ($n = 3$), and

others ($n = 38$). The "others" group included (1) pneumonia without identifiable pathogens ($n = 24$); (2) pulmonary hemorrhage caused by autoimmune vasculitis ($n = 2$); (3) pneumonia after near-drowning ($n = 1$); and (4) pulmonary edema due to acute on chronic renal failure ($n = 4$), acute pancreatitis ($n = 3$), or after percutaneous interventions ($n = 4$; 3 for cardiac lesions and 1 for cerebral aneurysm). All patients received VV-ECMO in our institution. Three patients received MV support before they were transferred to our hospital, and the duration of MV support before their ER admission were 10 h, 18 h, and 4 days. Diagnoses in the 37

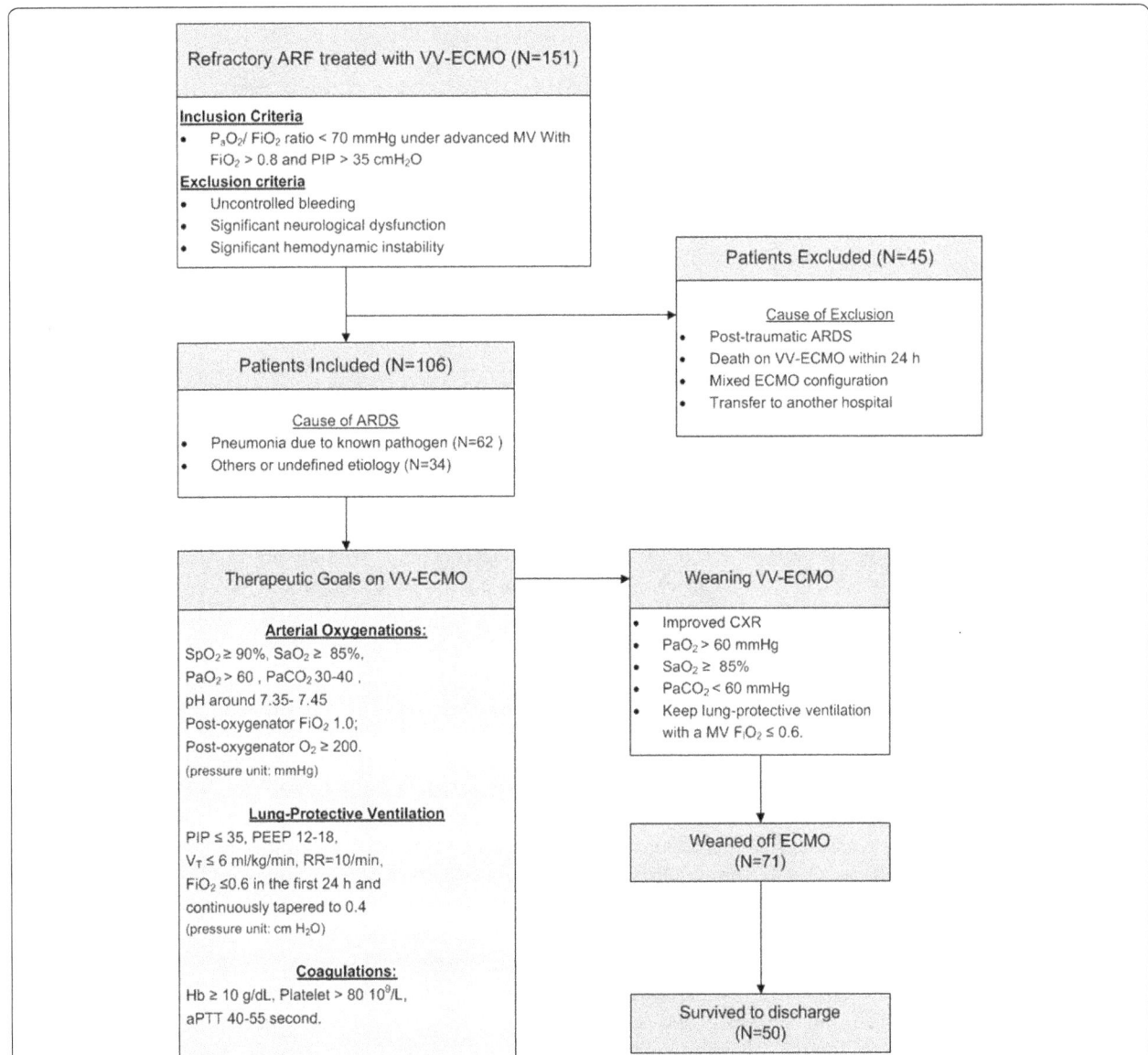

Fig. 1 Flow chart of patient distribution and managements during venovenous extracorporeal membrane oxygenation. ARF: Acute respiratory failure. FiO2: The fraction of inspired oxygen. PaO2: Arterial oxygen tension. PEEP: Positive end-expiratory pressure. PIP: Peak inspiratory pressure. RR: Respiratory rate. SaO2: Arterial oxygen saturation; SpO2: Oxyhemoglobin saturation by pulse oximetry. V_T: Tidal volume. VV-ECMO: Venovenous extracorporeal membrane oxygenation

Table 1 Patient characteristics before venovenous extracorporeal membrane oxygenation

	All (n = 106)	Survivor (n = 50)	Non-survivor (n = 56)	P
Age (year)	53 ± 15	51 ± 15	55 ± 15	0.11
Male	71 (67)	35 (70)	36 (64)	0.53
Predicted body weight[a] (kg)	55 ± 14	55 ± 16	55 ± 11	0.89
Hospital day before ECMO	6 (1–14)	2(1–9)	11(4–20)	<0.001*
Mechanical ventilation before ECMO (day)	3 (1–9)	1(0–4)	6(1–12)	<0.001*
Cause of ARDS				
Viral pneumonia	24 (21)	11 (22)	13 (23)	0.88
Bacterial pneumonia	38 (37)	16 (32)	22 (39)	0.54
Fungal pneumonia	3 (3)	0	3 (6)	0.25
Aspiration pneumonitis	3 (3)	3 (6)	0	0.10
Other acute respiratory diagnoses	38 (36)	20 (40)	18 (32)	0.40
Acute associated infection	24 (21)	11 (22)	13 (23)	0.88
Immunocompromised status[b]	37 (35)	11 (22)	26 (46)	0.008*
Renal failure requiring dialysis	28 (26)	13 (26)	15 (27)	0.93
Creatinine (mg/dL)	1.6 (0.8–3.4)	2.8 ± 3.3	2.3 ± 2.3	0.36
Total bilirubin (mg/dL)	1.5 ± 2.5	1.1 ± b1.2	1.9 ± 3.2	0.14
Platelet count (10^9/L)	137 (83–218)	172 (113–237)	106 (60–161)	0.002*
Hemoglobin (g)	10 (9–12)	11 (9–12)	10 (9–11)	0.08
SOFA score	10 (8–11)	9 (7–10)	10 (9–12)	0.002*
RESP score	2 ± 3	2 ± 3	1 ± 3	0.05*

Data were presented as mean ± standard deviation in normal-distributed numerical variables, median (interquartile range) in numerical variables not normal-distributed, and n (%) in categorical variables. ECMO Extracorporeal membrane oxygenation, SOFA sequential organ failure assessment, RESP score Respiratory extracorporeal membrane oxygenation survival prediction score, ARDS Acute respiratory distress syndrome. [a] Ideal body weight is calculated by the ARDSnet formulas. [b]Immunocompromised status includes hematologic malignancy, solid tumor, solid organ transplantation, liver cirrhosis Child B or C, or autoimmune diseases requiring long-term immunosuppressive therapy
*p < 0.05. (in the comparisons between survivors and non-survivors)

immunocompromised patients were malignancies (n = 16; 15 solid tumor and 1 lymphoma), autoimmune diseases (n = 10; 2 dermatomyositis, 2 idiopathic thrombocytopenia, 2 granulomatosis with polyangiitis, 1 psoriatic arthritis, 1 rheumatoid arthritis, 1 systemic lupus erythematosus, and 1 Graves'disease), immunosuppressive therapy in solid organ transplantation (n = 8; 6 liver transplantation and 2 renal transplantation), advanced liver cirrhosis (n = 2), and steroid therapy in asthma (n = 1). Fifty-six patients died in hospital and 35 of them died on VV-ECMO. Six patients died on VV-ECMO due to hemorrhagic complications including intracranial hemorrhages (n = 2), intra-abdominal or retroperitoneal hemorrhages (n = 1), and gastrointestinal tract hemorrhages (n = 4). The multiple-organ failure syndrome with sepsis was the cause of death for the other non-survivors. The results of univariate comparisons of ventilator parameters between the survivors and non-survivors are also presented in Table 2. These parameters were obtained soon after the beginning of MV and just before the beginning of VV-ECMO. The 3 patients receiving MV support in other hospital were excluded from the analysis of ventilator parameters just after the beginning of

MV. Differences between the pre-ECMO and the early MV data of a given ventilator parameter were also calculated to present the deterioration of pulmonary function and the corresponding escalation of ventilation pressures before ECMO institution.

Multivariate prediction model of hospital death

According to the results of multivariate analysis, the pre-ECMO duration of MV [Odd ratio (OR): 1.184; 95% confident interval (CI): 1.079–1.565, p < 0.001] and the pre-ECMO SOFA score (OR: 1.299; 95% CI: 1.077–1.302; p = 0.006) were identified to be the independent predictors of hospital mortality in adult non-trauma patients who received VV-ECMO for severe ARDS. The mortality prediction model built with these factors was presented as follows: Predicted mortality $(y) = e^X / (1 + e^X)$. $X = -3.218 + 0.169 \times$ (days of MV before institution of VV-ECMO) $+ 0.262 \times$ (SOFA score before institution of VV-ECMO). The model explained 30% (Nagelkerke R^2) of the variance in hospital mortality and correctly classified 68.9% of the cases (sensitivity: 66.1%; specificity: 72%). This predictive model also

Table 2 Ventilator parameters before venovenous extracorporeal membrane oxygenation

	All (n = 106)	Survivor (n = 50)	Non-survivor (n = 56)	P
Just after intubation				
P_aO_2/F_iO_2 (mmHg)	112 ± 76	90 ± 55	129 ± 85	0.009*
Peak inspiratory pressure (cmH$_2$O)	33 ± 6	32 ± 5	33 ± 6	0.86
Mean airway pressure (cmH$_2$O)	18 ± 4	18 ± 4	18 ± 5	0.85
PEEP (cmH$_2$O)	12 ± 3	12 ± 3	12 ± 3	0.56
Dynamic driving pressure[a] (cmH$_2$O)	21 ± 5	21 ± 5	22 ± 5	0.86
Measured tidal volume (ml/kg)	7.7 ± 2.3	7.7 ± 2.3	7.8 ± 2.3	0.73
Dynamic compliance[b] (ml/cmH$_2$O)	22 ± 9	23 ± 10	21 ± 8	0.15
Oxygen index[c]	25 ± 19	29 ± 22	21 ± 15	0.11
Just before ECMO				
P_aO_2/F_iO_2 (mmHg)	72 ± 17	72 ± 19	72 ± 16	0.93
Peak inspiratory pressure (cmH$_2$O)	36 ± 6	35 ± 5	37 ± 6	0.16
Mean airway pressure (cmH$_2$O)	21 ± 4	21 ± 4	22 ± 4	0.13
PEEP (cmH$_2$O)	14 ± 3	14 ± 3	14 ± 3	0.79
Dynamic driving pressure[a] (cmH$_2$O)	22 ± 6	21 ± 5	23 ± 6	0.22
Measured tidal volume (ml/kg)	6.7 (6–7.8)	6.8 (6.1–8.7)	6.7 (5.8–7.7)	0.22
Dynamic compliance[b] (ml/cmH$_2$O)	19 (15–23)	21 (15–25)	17 (12–21)	0.01*
Oxygen index[c]	39 ± 13	39 ± 14	38 ± 13	0.66
Difference				
Δ P_aO_2/F_iO_2 (mmHg)	−16 (−71–9)	0 (−51–21)	−31 (−95–5)	0.009*
Δ Peak inspiratory pressure (cmH$_2$O)	4 ± 6	4 ± 6	4 ± 7	0.18
Δ PEEP (cmH$_2$O)	3 ± 4	3 ± 3	3 ± 4	0.92
Δ Dynamic driving pressure[a] (cmH$_2$O)	1 ± 6	1 ± 6	1 ± 7	0.33
Δ Measured tidal volume (ml/kg)	−0.3 (−1.9–0.8)	0 (−1.5–1.2)	−0.8 (−1.9–0.2)	0.05*
Δ Dynamic compliance[b] (ml/cmH$_2$O)	−2 ± 11	−1 ± 11	−3 ± 11	0.72
Δ Oxygen index[c]	14 ± 2	10 ± 21	17 ± 19	0.35

Data were presented as mean ± standard deviation in normal-distributed numerical variables, median (interquartile range) in numerical variables not normal-distributed, and n (%) in categorical variables. *ECMO* Extracorporeal membrane oxygenation, *PEEP* Positive end expiratory pressure. [a]Driving pressure = (Peak inspiratory pressure – Positive end-expiratory pressure)
[b]Dynamic pulmonary compliance = Measured tidal volume/ Driving pressure
[c]Oxygen index = [(Mean airway pressure□x□FiO$_2$□x 100)/ arterial oxygen tension]
*$p < 0.05$. Δ: The data obtained before ECMO - the data obtained after intubation

fitted the dataset well (Hosmer-Lemeshow test: $\chi^2 = 7.526$, $p = 0.376$) and showed a fair predictive power of hospital mortality (c-index: 0.763, $p < 0.001$, 95% CI: 0.674–0.851). Figure 2 demonstrates the observed hospital mortality rates among patients grouped by their baseline SOFA score.

Serial changes of arterial oxygenation during the course of treatment

To get a deeper understanding of the influences of VV-ECMO combining lung-protective MV on arterial oxygenation during the course of treatment, we collected the ventilator parameters at several time points (T0: 1 to 2 h after intubation for MV, T1: 1 to 2 h before ECMO cannulation, T2:24 h after ECMO institution, T3: 1 to

2 h before ECMO decannulation, and T4: 24 h after ECMO removal) for analysis and the results are demonstrated in Table 3. It is notable that only the survivors could go through the whole treatment and show data in all of the 5 points. The survivors' trends of PF ratio and dynamic driving pressure are also illustrated in fig. 3.

Discussion

This study revealed that the duration of MV before ECMO institution was the only baseline ventilator parameter which was independently associated with hospital mortality in non-trauma patients receiving VV-ECMO for severe ARDS, although the mechanism of how a prolonged duration of MV could jeopardize the survival in these ECMO-treated patients was still

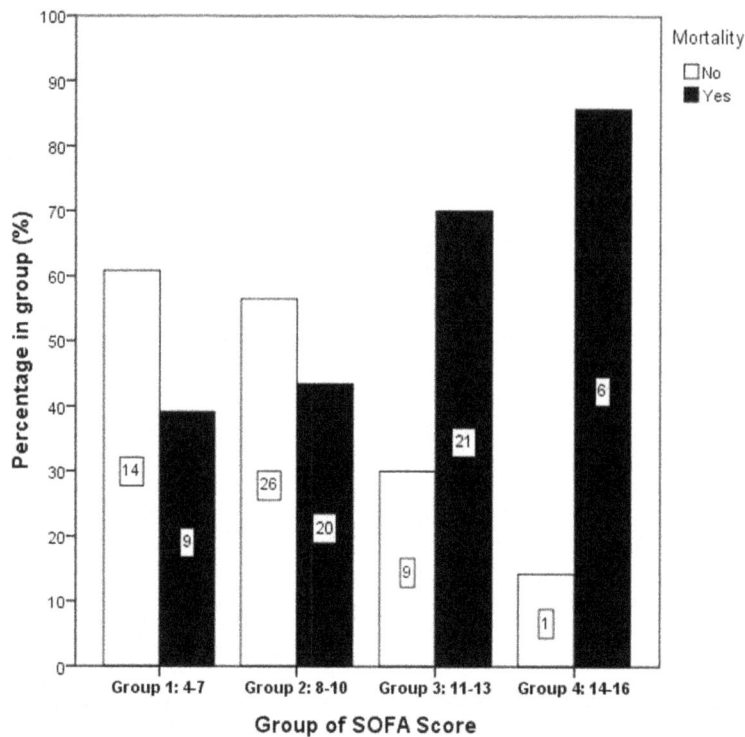

Fig. 2 Observed mortality rates among patients categorized by the baseline sequential organ failure assessment (SOFA) score. The case number in each group is also presented

unclear. In fact, this duration is a reciprocal measure of the declining rate of PF ratio from the value obtained at the beginning of MV to the given threshold value for ECMO. Clinically, this declining rate of PF ratio is significantly affected by the etiology of ARDS, patient characteristics, and the institutional experience on advanced modes of MV, as the conclusion of CESAR trial [11, 13]. These uncertainties make the suitable duration of MV before ECMO individualized among institutions. Nevertheless, limitation of this duration should still be important to adult candidates of respiratory ECMO. According to Table 2, regardless of the value of initial PF ratio, most of our patients were found to have severely non-compliant lungs at the beginning of MV. The mean PC_{dyn} measured at the beginning of MV was 22 cm H_2O in all of the patients, which was only accounted for 10% or less of the normal value [14]. This finding implied that these patients were very sensitive and vulnerable to the cyclic pulmonary manipulation of MV [15–17]. When the disease progresses and involves more pulmonary segments, clinicians often need to open the collapsed segments with an increased driving pressure of MV to maintain an acceptable blood-gas exchange. This attempt of lung recruitment may considerably increase the amount of dead space ventilation rather than effectively improve the blood-gas exchange, since the local perfusion of the distended segments may

drop, as demonstrated by Gattinoni et al. [18]. The over-distended lungs may also increase the intrathoracic pressure and compromise the cardiac output [19]. Therefore, if available and not contraindicated, VV-ECMO combining lung-protective MV is a valuable strategy to reduce pulmonary manipulation and reverse some of the pulmonary segments performing dead space ventilation under high-pressure MV to the segments performing effective blood-gas exchange under a reduced inspiratory pressure. However, the benefit of VV-ECMO is often small in patients with prolonged ventilation (often >7 days) or severe multiple organ dysfunctions [2]. From this viewpoint, it should be important for ECMO centers to have a practical tool to determine the starting point of respiratory ECMO among candidates with different duration of MV. Technically, there are three common ways to reduce the risk of a prolonged MV before ECMO institution. The first is choosing an arbitrary deadline which is set according to general experiences, such as a 7-day period [20]. The second is loosening the threshold value of PF ratio for ECMO from 100 mmHg to 150 mmHg, as per the suggestion of ELSO Guidelines. The third is creating a risk assessment model for a multi-axial evaluation, as is our choice here.

What interested us was that the baseline PIP could not be identified as a prognostic predictor of adult respiratory

Table 3 The serial changes of pressure settings of mechanical ventilation and index of arterial oxygenation during and after removal of venovenous extracorporeal membrane oxygenation

	24 h after ECMO institution (T2)	Just before ECMO removal. (T3)	24 h after ECMO removal (T4)
Survivors (n = 50)			
P_aO_2/F_iO_2 (mmHg)	226 ± 85*	206 ± 89	216 ± 94
Peak inspiratory pressure (cmH$_2$O)	30 ± 5	30 ± 5	24 ± 13
Mean airway pressure (cmH$_2$O)	17 ± 3	17 ± 4	17 ± 4
PEEP (cmH2O)	12 (10–14)	10 (10–12)	12 (10–12)
Dynamic driving pressure[a] (cmH2O)	18 ± 6	19 ± 5	19 ± 6
Measured tidal volume (ml/kg)	7 ± 1	8 ± 2	7 ± 4
Dynamic compliance[b] (ml/cmH$_2$O)	24 ± 9*	28 ± 12	22 ± 15
Oxygen index[c]	8 ± 4*	10 ± 6	10 ± 6
ECMO outflow PaO$_2$ (mmHg)	391 (338–449)	50 (38–133)	–
ECMO outflow PaCO$_2$ (mmHg)	35 (28–40)	40 (36–59)	–
ECMO outflow O$_2$ saturation (%)	100	100	–
Non-Survivors (n = 56)			–
P_aO_2/F_iO_2 (mmHg)	164 ± 84*	–	–
Peak inspiratory pressure (cmH$_2$O)	32 ± 5	–	–
Mean airway pressure (cmH$_2$O)	18 ± 4	–	–
PEEP (cmH2O)	13 ± 3	–	–
Dynamic driving pressure[a] (cmH2O)	19 ± 6	–	–
Measured tidal volume (ml/kg)	6 ± 3	–	–
Dynamic compliance[b] (ml/cmH$_2$O)	19 ± 10*	–	–
Oxygen index[c]	14 ± 7*	–	–
ECMO outflow PaO$_2$ (mmHg)	408 ± 79	–	–
ECMO outflow PaCO$_2$ (mmHg)	36 ± 6	–	–
ECMO outflow O$_2$ saturation (%)	100	–	–

Only the survivors showed data recorded just before and 24 h after ECMO removal

Data were presented as mean ± standard deviation in normal-distributed numerical variables, median (interquartile range) in numerical variables not normal-distributed, and n (%) in categorical variables. *ECMO* Extracorporeal membrane oxygenation, *PEEP* Positive end expiratory pressure

*The mean values of a specific variable in the T2 column are significant different between the survivors and non-survivors while analyzed by independent T-test ($p < 0.05$)

[a]Driving pressure = (Peak inspiratory pressure – Positive end-expiratory pressure)

[b]Dynamic pulmonary compliance = Measured tidal volume/ Driving pressure

[c]Oxygen index = [(Mean airway pressure □x□FiO$_2$□x 100)/ arterial oxygen tension]

ECMO in the current study, which was different from the suggestion of RESP score. The RESP score is derived from a retrospective analysis of 2355 adult patients in ELSO's registry and reveals that the baseline PIP, with a threshold value of 42 cmH$_2$O, is a predictive factor for hospital mortality in adult patients receiving respiratory ECMO [11]. However, in the current study including 106 patients, the patients with a baseline PIP > 42 cm H$_2$O (n = 14) showed a significantly lower hospital mortality rate than the patients with a baseline PIP ≤ 42 cm H$_2$O (21% vs. 58%, $p = 0.02$). We thought that the discrepancy in sample size between the two studies should have some connection to this unexplained result. In the original study of RESP score [11], the odds ratio of baseline PIP for hospital survival is close to 1.0 (0.992). Furthermore, the medians

of baseline PIP were surprisingly both the same (36 cmH$_2$O) in the survivors (n = 1338) and non-survivors (n = 1017). Therefore, the baseline PIP might not be a very suitable criterion to initiate respiratory ECMO. Some researchers suggest that the baseline plateau pressure (P_{plat}) is also a valuable indicator used for this purpose [21]. Although P_{plat} is a better airway pressure than PIP for measuring the pressure applied to lung itself during MV, we were unable to reproduce the above-mentioned result because the data of P_{plat} were severely incomplete in this retrospective study due to unknown reason.

Although the impact of the baseline pressure settings of MV remains equivocal on the outcomes of adult respiratory ECMO, an unreduced static or dynamic driving

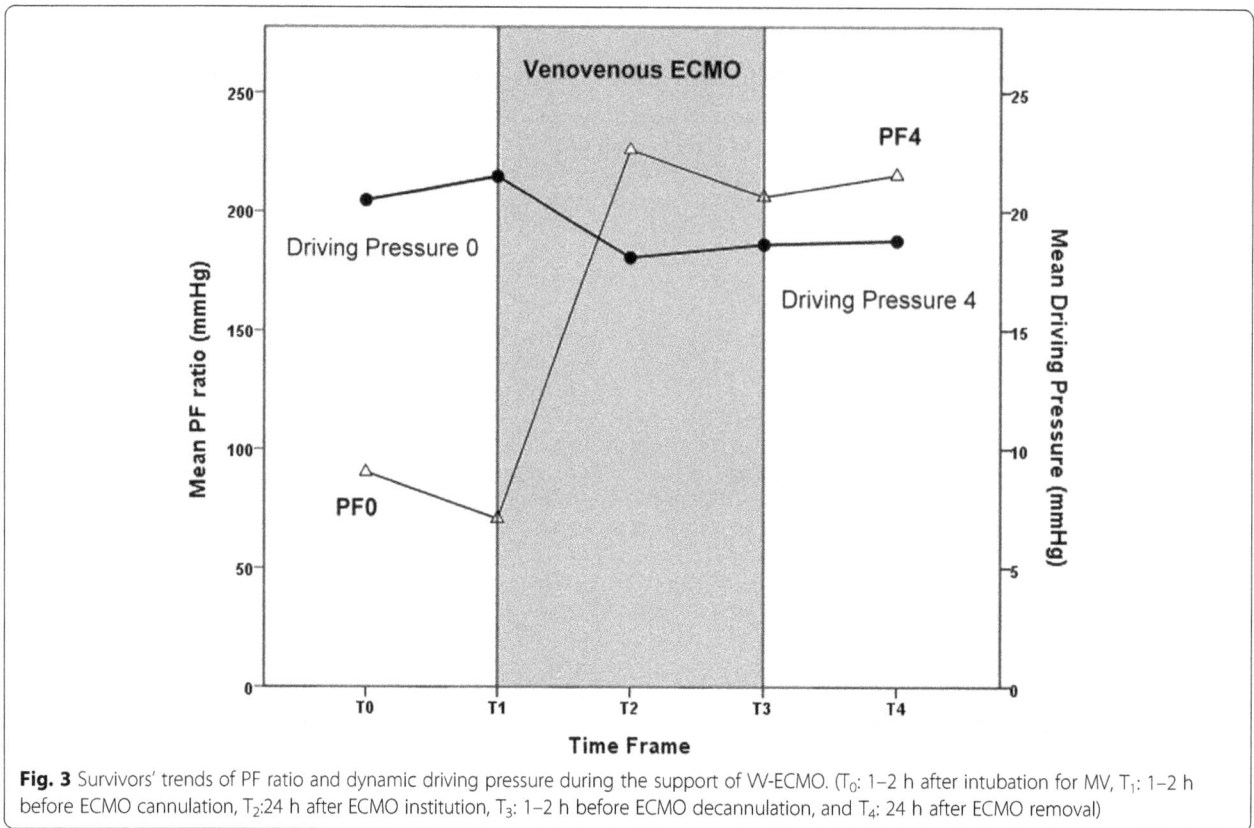

Fig. 3 Survivors' trends of PF ratio and dynamic driving pressure during the support of VV-ECMO. (T_0: 1–2 h after intubation for MV, T_1: 1–2 h before ECMO cannulation, T_2:24 h after ECMO institution, T_3: 1–2 h before ECMO decannulation, and T_4: 24 h after ECMO removal)

pressure of MV during the first three days of adult respiratory ECMO is recently reported to be a predictor of hospital mortality in these ECMO-treated patients [22, 23]. When the results of these updated investigations on adult respiratory ECMO are reviewed together, researchers may find that there seem to be some links among the duration of MV before ECMO institution, the driving pressure of MV during ECMO, and the outcomes of ECMO. According to Tables 2 and 3, all of the patients showed an improvement in arterial oxygenation and a downgrade of driving pressure of MV during the first 24 h of ECMO institution. Since the collapsed alveoli should be difficult to be re-opened by a decreased driving pressure, we could assume that the improvement in arterial oxygenation should depend on the oxygenator and the non-collapsed alveoli. However, as shown in fig. 3, only patients maintaining the trend of improvement in arterial oxygenation throughout the ECMO support could eventually wean ECMO and survive. It is notably that the pulmonary compliance remained impaired in the survivors after a successful rescue of ECMO. These findings implied that the size of the non-collapsed pulmonary segments before ECMO should be one of the key contributors to the patient's progression on ECMO and the outcome. To keep the non-collapsed pulmonary segments opened under a reduced driving pressure during ECMO, the decrease in the

driving pressure during the early support of ECMO was achieved by a reduction in PIP rather than in PEEP. Actually, choosing a moderate high PEEP is also an important issue in patients treated with lung-protective MV [17]. Despite not used in this study, an esophageal balloon is considered to be a useful tool to measure the serial changes of transpulmonary pressure and suggested an appropriate level of PEEP and driving pressure in this scenario [24]. In general, ventilating the patients with an unreduced driving pressure is not an effective solution to improve hypoxemia on VV-ECMO, since this behavior means that the clinicians still want to recruit the collapsed segments. In cases with a refractory hypoxemia during VV-ECMO, the circuit of ECMO should be rearranged to a hybrid configuration which may promptly correct the arterial hypoxemia and allow a decrease in driving pressure [25]. However, significant hypoxemia may recur during the weaning process of ECMO in any configuration if the pulmonary parenchyma is extensively damaged and the residual reservoir is below the requirement for surviving without ECMO.

The major limitations of this study are its retrospective design and moderate sample size. This study did not provide a comprehensive discussion of adult respiratory ECMO since only non-trauma patients treated with pressure-controlled ventilation and VV-

ECMO in a single center were included. Further collaborative and prospective studies that adopt new techniques to obtain novel respiratory parameters in a large cohort of ECMO-treated ARDS patients are necessary to validate our hypothesis and determine the influences of baseline ventilator parameters on outcomes of adult respiratory ECMO.

Conclusion

Among the baseline ventilator parameters included in this study, duration of MV was the only parameter independently associated with hospital mortality in adult non-trauma patients treated with VV-ECMO. The benefit of VV-ECMO was small in patients with prolonged ventilation or severe multiple organ dysfunctions. Therefore, medical centers were suggested to find a suitable prognosticating tool to determine the starting point of respiratory ECMO among their candidates with different duration of MV.

Abbreviations
AaDO2: Alveolar-arterial oxygen difference; APTT: Activated partial thromboplastin time; ARDS: Acute respiratory failure; ECMO: Extracorporeal membrane oxygenation; FiO_2: Fraction of inspiratory oxygen; LPV: Lung-protective ventilation; MV: Mechanical ventilation; OI: Oxygen Index; $PaCO_2$: Arterial carbon dioxide tension; PaO_2: Arterial oxygen tension; PEEP: Positive end-expiratory pressure; PIP: Peak inspiratory pressure; PT: Prothrombin time; RV: Right ventricle; SaO_2: Arterial oxygen saturation; SOFA: Sequential organ failure assessment; SpO_2: Oxyhemoglobin saturation by pulse oximetry; VA: Venoarterial; VILI: Ventilator induced lung injury; VV: Venovenous

Acknowledgements
We are grateful to all of the members in the ECMO Team and the Respiratory Support Group in Chang Gung Memorial Hospital for their feedback on the patient survey.

Funding
This study was supported by no funding.

Authors' contributions
WMY contributed to the conception and design of the study, acquisition and interpretation of data, and revision of the manuscript. Y-SC also contributed to the revision of the manuscript. Both WMY and YSC had equal contribution to the final version of the manuscript (Co-first authors). HCC and LPJ contributed to the literature review and the formation of therapeutic protocol. WTI performed statistical analysis. WMY also contributed to manuscript composition and was responsible for the final product. All authors read and approved the final manuscript.

Competing interests
None of the authors have a conflict of interest to declare in relation to this work.

Author details
[1]Department of Cardiovascular Surgery, Chang Gung Memorial Hospital and Chang Gung University, Taoyuan, Taiwan. [2]School of Traditional Chinese Medicine, Chang Gung University, Taoyuan, Taiwan. Department of Thoracic Medicine, Chang Gung Memorial Hospital and Chang Gung University, Taoyuan, Taiwan. [4]Department of Obstetrics and Gynecology, School of Medicine, College of Medicine, Taipei Medical University, Taipei, Taiwan. [5]Department of Obstetrics and Gynecology, Wan Fang Hospital, Taipei Medical University, Taipei, Taiwan.

References
1. Combes A, Brodie D, Bartlett R, Brochard L, Brower R, Conrad S, et al. Position paper for the organization of extracorporeal membrane oxygenation programs for acute respiratory failure in adult patients. Am J Respir Crit Care Med. 2014;190:488–96.
2. Fan E, Gattinoni L, Combes A, Schmidt M, Peek G, Brodie D, et al. Venovenous extracorporeal membrane oxygenation for acute respiratory failure : a clinical review from an international group of experts. Intensive Care Med. 2016;42:712–24.
3. Thiagarajan RR, Barbaro RP, Rycus PT, Mcmullan DM, Conrad SA, Fortenberry JD, et al. Extracorporeal life support organization registry international report 2016. ASAIO J. 2017;63:60–7.
4. Extracorporeal Life Support Organization (ELSO) Guidelines for Adult Respiratory Failure V1.3. 2013. https://www.elso.org/resources/guidelines.aspx. Accessed 1 Jan 2017.
5. MY W, Huang CC, TI W, Wang CL, Lin PJ. Venovenous extracorporeal membrane oxygenation for acute respiratory distress syndrome in adults: prognostic factors for outcomes. Medicine (Baltimore). 2016;95:e2870.
6. Tsai HC, Chang CH, Tsai FC, Fan PC, Juan KC, Lin CY, et al. Acute respiratory distress syndrome with and without extracorporeal membrane oxygenation: a score matched study. Ann Thorac Surg. 2015;100:458–64.
7. Cheng YT, MY W, Chang YS, Huang CC, Lin PJ. Developing a simple preinterventional score to predict hospital mortality in adult venovenous extracorporeal membrane oxygenation: a pilot study. Medicine (Baltimore). 2016;95:e4380.
8. Chiu LC, Tsai FC, HC H, Chang CH, Hung CY, Lee CS, et al. Survival predictors in acute respiratory distress syndrome with extracorporeal membrane oxygenation. Ann Thorac Surg. 2015;99:243–50.
9. MY W, Lin PJ, Tseng YH, Kao KC, Hsiao HL, Huang CC. Venovenous extracorporeal life support for posttraumatic respiratory distress syndrome in adults: the risk of major hemorrhages. Scand J Trauma Resusc Emerg Med. 2014;22:56.
10. Vincent JL, Moreno R, Takala J, Willatts S, De Mendonça A, Bruining H, et al. The SOFA (sepsis-related organ failure assessment) score to describe organ dysfunction/failure. Intensive Care Med. 1996;22:707–10.
11. Schmidt M, Bailey M, Sheldrake J, Hodgson C, Aubron C, Rycus PT, et al. Predicting survival after extracorporeal membrane oxygenation for severe acute respiratory failure. The respiratory extracorporeal membrane oxygenation survival prediction (RESP) score. Am J Respir Crit Care Med. 2014;189:1374–82.
12. Livingston BM, Mackenzie SJ, MacKirdy FN, Howie JC. Should the pre-sedation Glasgow coma scale value be used when calculating acute physiology and chronic health evaluation scores for sedated patients? Scottish Intensive Care Society audit group. Crit Care Med. 2000;28:389–94.
13. Peek GJ, Mugford M, Tiruvoipati R, Wilson A, Allen E, Thalanany MM, et al. Efficacy and economic assessment of conventional ventilatory support versus extracorporeal membrane oxygenation for severe adult respiratory failure (CESAR): a multicentre randomised controlled trial. Lancet. 2009; 374:1351–63.
14. Galetke W, Feier C, Muth T, Ruehle KH, Borsch-Galetke E, Randerath W. Reference values for dynamic and static pulmonary compliance in men. Respir Med. 2007;101:1783–9.
15. Carney D, DiRocco J, Nieman G. Dynamic alveolar mechanics and ventilator-induced lung injury. Crit Care Med. 2005;33:S122–S8.
16. Barbas CS, de Matos GF, Pincelli MP, da Rosa Borges E, Antunes T, de Barros JM, et al. Mechanical ventilation in acute respiratory failure: recruitment and high positive end-expiratory pressure are necessary. Curr Opin Crit Care. 2005;11:18–28.
17. Rouby JJ, Liu Q, Goldstein I. Selecting the right level of positive end-expiratory pressure in patients with acute respiratory distress syndrome. Am J Respir Crit Care Med. 2002;165:1182–6.

18. Gattinoni L, Caironi P, Cressoni M, Chiumello D, Ranieri VM, Quintel M, et al. Lung recruitment in patients with the acute respiratory distress syndrome. N Engl J Med. 2006;354:1175–86.

19. Boissier F, Katsahian S, Razazi K, Thille AW, Roche-Campo F, Leon R, et al. Prevalence and prognosis of cor pulmonale during protective ventilation for acute respiratory distress syndrome. Intensive Care Med. 2013;39:1725–33.

20. Bohman JK, Vogt MN, Hyder JA. Retrospective report of contraindications to extracorporeal membrane oxygenation (ECMO) among adults with acute respiratory distress syndrome (ARDS). Heart Lung. 2016;45:227–31.

21. Schmidt M, Zogheib E, Roze H, Repesse X, Lebreton G, Luyt CE, et al. The PRESERVE mortality risk score and analysis of long-term outcomes after extracorporeal membrane oxygenation for severe acute respiratory distress syndrome. Intensive Care Med. 2013;39:1704–13.

22. Serpa Neto A, Schmidt M, Azevedo LC, Bein T, Brochard L, Beutel G, et al. Associations between ventilator settings during extracorporeal membrane oxygenation for refractory hypoxemia and outcome in patients with acute respiratory distress syndrome: a pooled individual patient data analysis : mechanical ventilation during ECMO. Intensive Care Med. 2016;42:1672–84.

23. Chiu LC, HC H, Hung CY, Chang CH, Tsai FC, Yang CT, et al. Dynamic driving pressure associated mortality in acute respiratory distress syndrome with extracorporeal membrane oxygenation. Ann Intensive Care. 2017;7:12.

24. Talmor D, Sarge T, Malhotra A, O'Donnell CR, Ritz R, Lisbon A, et al. Mechanical ventilation guided by esophageal pressure in acute lung injury. N Engl J Med. 2008;359:2095–104.

25. Montisci A, Maj G, Zangrillo A, Winterton D, Pappalardo F. Management of refractory hypoxemia during venovenous extracorporeal membrane oxygenation for ARDS. ASAIO J. 2015;61:227–36.

7

Potential benefit of bosentan therapy in borderline or less severe pulmonary hypertension secondary to idiopathic pulmonary fibrosis—an interim analysis of results from a prospective, single-center, randomized, parallel-group study

Yosuke Tanaka[1*], Mitsunori Hino[1] and Akihiko Gemma[2]

Abstract

Background: No drugs have been approved for the treatment of patients with pulmonary hypertension (PH) secondary to idiopathic pulmonary fibrosis (IPF), particularly those with idiopathic honeycomb lung. This study was conducted to investigate the long-term efficacy and safety of bosentan for PH based on changes in prognosis and respiratory failure.

Methods: IPF patients with borderline or less severe PH and completely organized honeycomb lung were randomized (1:1) to bosentan or no treatment for PH for 2 years and assessed at baseline and every 6 months for respiratory failure, activities of daily living (ADL), lung and heart functions by right cardiac catheterization, and other parameters. An interim analysis was performed, however, following detection of a significant survival benefit favoring bosentan therapy.

Results: Significant differences were noted for the bosentan-treated ($n = 12$) vs. untreated ($n = 12$) groups in hospital-free survival (603.44 ± 50.074 days vs. 358.87 ± 68.65 days; hazard ratio [HR], 0.19; $P = 0.017$) and overall survival (671 days vs. 433.78 ± 66.98 days; HR, 0.10; $P = 0.0082$). Again, significant improvements were noted for the bosentan-treated group from baseline to month 6 or 12 in several indices in ADL, pulmonary circulation, and %DLCO. Without requiring O_2 inhalation, bosentan was associated with no increase but a trend toward a decrease in adverse events and an improvement in respiratory status.

Conclusions: Bosentan tended to improve prognosis and ADL without worsening respiratory failure in IPF patients with borderline or less severe PH and completely organized honeycomb lung alone.

Keywords: Pulmonary hypertension, Idiopathic pulmonary fibrosis, Right heart catheterization, Echocardiography, Endothelin receptor antagonists

* Correspondence: yosuke-t@nms.ac.jp
[1]Department of Respiratory Medicine, Nippon Medical School, Chiba Hokusoh Hospital, 1715 Kamagari, Inzai, Chiba 270-1694, Japan
Full list of author information is available at the end of the article

Background

Idiopathic pulmonary fibrosis (IPF) is a disorder associated with poor prognosis. Pulmonary arterial hypertension (PAH), which is likely to lead to right heart overload, is also associated with poor prognosis. Patients with IPF are at risk of developing pulmonary hypertension (PH) as the underlying condition worsens or becomes severer, thus further compromising their prognosis [1–8]. However, it remains unclear how long it may typically take for patients with IPF to start developing PH or for its associated influence on cardiac function to become manifest [1]. Given that, once elevated, pulmonary arterial pressure (PAP) becomes irreversible because of established vascular remodeling [1, 9], it appears that efficacious treatment should be started before its onset. Furthermore, it is assumed that cardiac overload starts even before the onset of PH. However, to date, no drugs have been approved for the treatment of PH secondary to respiratory diseases, such as IPF [1].

Drugs specific for PAH, such as bosentan (Tracleer Tablets®), have been reported in some studies to effectively improve PH in patients with respiratory diseases, such as COPD and IPF [1, 10–13].

While the results of randomized controlled studies conducted to date, such as BUILD-1 and BUILD-3 studies [11], appear to argue against the use of bosentan in patients with pulmonary hypertension (PH), these studies involved a wide range of patients from those with fibrotic idiopathic interstitial pneumonia (f-IIP) and fibrotic nonspecific interstitial pneumonia (f-NSIP) to those with highly elevated pulmonary arterial pressure (PAP) and decreased cardiac index (CI), where the presence of multiple risk factors for IPF in these patients may have additively or synergistically contributed to the therapeutic outcomes reported in these studies. Again, the benefit of early intervention with bosentan may not have been sufficiently explored in those with mildly elevated PAP in these trials, while bosentan was indeed shown to be efficacious against IP in a subset of patients in the BUILD-1 study, despite the observation that many patients with IPF are associated with rapidly elevated PAP as well as progression of IPF and that elevated PAP is associated with poor prognosis [7].

Against this background, the present bosentan study focused on IPF patients with completely organized honeycomb lung without any pulmonary (including IP) lesions who chiefly complained of symptoms suggestive of progressive respiratory failure, i.e., progressive dyspnea with minimal IPF activity.

Thus, the IPF patients with completely organized honeycomb lung alone were enrolled in this study to ensure that the subjects in this study had pathologically stable IPF and required regular hospital visits for treatment. An interim analysis was performed, however, in patients with borderline or less severe PH (25 mmHg ≤ mean pulmonary arterial pressure [mPAP] at rest <35 mmHg and/or mPAP on effort [mPAPOE] ≥ 30 mmHg), following detection of a greater-than-expected significant survival benefit in patients with borderline or less severe PH treated with bosentan at an early phase of the trial when the number of patients enrolled was still small.

Methods

Study design and methods

This was a prospective, single-center, interventional, parallel, randomized, open-label study.

Target patient population

This study was conducted in patients with IPF (WHO functional class II, III or IV) who showed no signs of hypoxia during 6-min walk test (6MWT) and therefore had enough functional capacity for ADL and who gave written informed consent to participate in the study.

Eligibility criteria

To be included in this study, patients had to fulfill all of the following inclusion criteria but none of the following exclusion criteria:

Inclusion criteria

1) Patients aged 20 years old or older (both sexes)
2) Patients diagnosed at this hospital as having IPF (WHO functional class II, III or IV) without hypoxia at rest or during 6MWT (to exclude those with decreased ADL and dyspnea in daily living associated with hypoxia and to minimize the influence of hypoxic pulmonary vasoconstriction [HPV] as a potential cause of PH associated with decreased partial pressure of oxygen in arterial blood [PaO_2]) ($PaO_2 < 60$ mmHg)*.
   *Including those whose hypoxia ($PaO_2 < 60$ mmHg) had been corrected with long-term oxygen therapy (LTOT)
3) Patients with stable IPF who had not required any change of treatment within 3 months prior to study entry, i.e., those confirmed to have completely organized honeycomb lung and no active inflammatory lesion, such as grand glass opacity (GGO) (chronic IIP based on high-resolution computed tomography (CT) findings for which no effective therapy exists); and who presented to our hospital for the first time with symptoms of progressive respiratory failure and had not received any medical treatment for IPF within 3 months prior to their visit.
   *Excluding those whose progressive respiratory failure required no treatment for IPF itself and those who had an increased LTOT dose as a minimum requirement for progressive respiratory failure.

4) Inpatients and outpatients
5) Patients who provided written informed consent to participate in this study

Exclusion criteria

1) Patients who had received bosentan or any other drug specific for PAH (e.g., phosphodiestetrase type 5 [PDE-5] inhibitors, endothelin receptor antagonists, or prostaglandin analogs) prior to their enrollment
2) Patients with any disease that could cause right heart overload
3) Patients with hypoxia during 6MWT (PaO_2 < 60 mmHg)*.
   a. Excluded were those whose hypoxia (PaO_2 < 60 mmHg) had been corrected with LTOT (i.e., those in whom LTOT is in place to ensure PaO_2 > 60 mmHg both at rest and during 6MWT, who were deemed equivalent to IPF patients receiving routine therapy in clinical practice to allow them to be monitored for changes in their condition, prognosis and functional capacity for ADL).
4) Women who were pregnant or might have been pregnant, and who were lactating
5) Patients with moderate or severe liver disorder
6) Patients receiving treatment with cyclosporine, tacrolimus, or glibenclamide
7) Other patients judged by the investigator to be ineligible for this study (e.g., those with any disease or condition other than IPF that might affect their ADL, such as arrhythmia, LV failure, pulmonary thromboembolism, connective tissue diseases, intervertebral disc herniation, as they were confirmed by history taking, physical examination, chest x-ray, echocardiography [ECG], lung perfusion scintigraphy, and measurements of various parameters conducted during the run-in period).

Grouping of patients

In order to include those with minimal IPF activity alone, of all patients first diagnosed with IPF at our hospital based on the presence of chronic f-IIP as confirmed by high-resolution CT findings, those whose chief complaints suggested progressive respiratory failure and who were suffering from progressive dyspnea were evaluated for PAP by right heart catheterization (RHC) and ECG, as well as for right heart function by ECG.

According to the current diagnostic criteria, if mPAP at rest is <25 mmHg, the patient is not diagnosed as having PH even if the mPAPOE is ≥30 mmHg. In our study, however, this state was defined as borderline PH representing a very mild form of PH; and besides, 25 mmHg ≤ mPAP at rest <35 mmHg was defined as less severe PH. Since the aim of this study was to evaluate the efficacy

and safety of early therapeutic intervention with bosentan in PH, borderline PH or PH was diagnosed if mPAP at rest was ≥25 mmHg and/or mPAPOE was ≥30 mmHg and mPAWP was ≤15 mmHg. Moreover, borderline PH or less severe PH was defined as mPAP <25 mmHg and mPAPOE ≥30 mmHg or 25 mmHg ≤ mPAP <35 mmHg; severe PH was defined as mPAP ≥35 mmHg; and non-borderline PH or PH was defined as non-PH (mPAP <25 mmHg and mPAPOE <30 mmHg).

Drug-treated and untreated patients

All patients who met the eligibility criteria and gave informed consent to participate in this study were evaluated for PAP and right heart function and those with mPAP at rest ≥25 mmHg and/or mPAPOE ≥30 mmHg were stratified by mPAP: mPAP at rest <35 mmHg vs. ≥ 35 mmHg. Patients in each subgroup were randomly allocated to either bosentan (drug-treated group) or no treatment (untreated group) by the envelope method. Patients diagnosed with non-PH (mPAP at rest <25 mmHg with mPAPOE <30 mmHg) were assigned to the untreated group.

The drug-treated group comprised those who were diagnosed at this hospital as having IPF without hypoxia (PaO_2 > 60 mmHg) and who gave informed consent to participate in this study after PAP and right heart function assessments.

The untreated group comprised those diagnosed at this hospital as having IPF without hypoxia (PaO_2 > 60 mmHg) and who gave their informed consent to participate in this study after PAP and right heart function assessments. This group included those with severe PH (mPAP at rest ≥35 mmHg), borderline or less severe PH (25 mmHg ≤ mPAP at rest <35 mmHg and/or mPAPOE ≥30 mmHg), and non-PH (without borderline PH or PH). (Fig. 1; see also Additional file 1).

An interim analysis was performed, however, in patients with borderline or less severe PH (25 mmHg ≤ mPAP at rest <35 mmHg and/or mPAPOE ≥30 mmHg), following detection of a greater-than-expected significant survival benefit in patients with borderline or less severe PH treated with bosentan, at an early phase of the trial when the number of patients enrolled was still small.

The study required that IPF patients be randomized to drug-treated and untreated groups to investigate their clinical course in real-world settings, with no change of treatment allowed including bosentan for 2 years or until their death as a rule, except for minimal symptomatic therapy (including oxygen volume adjustments required to ensure similar oxygen conditions among the patients), which met none of the exclusion criteria.

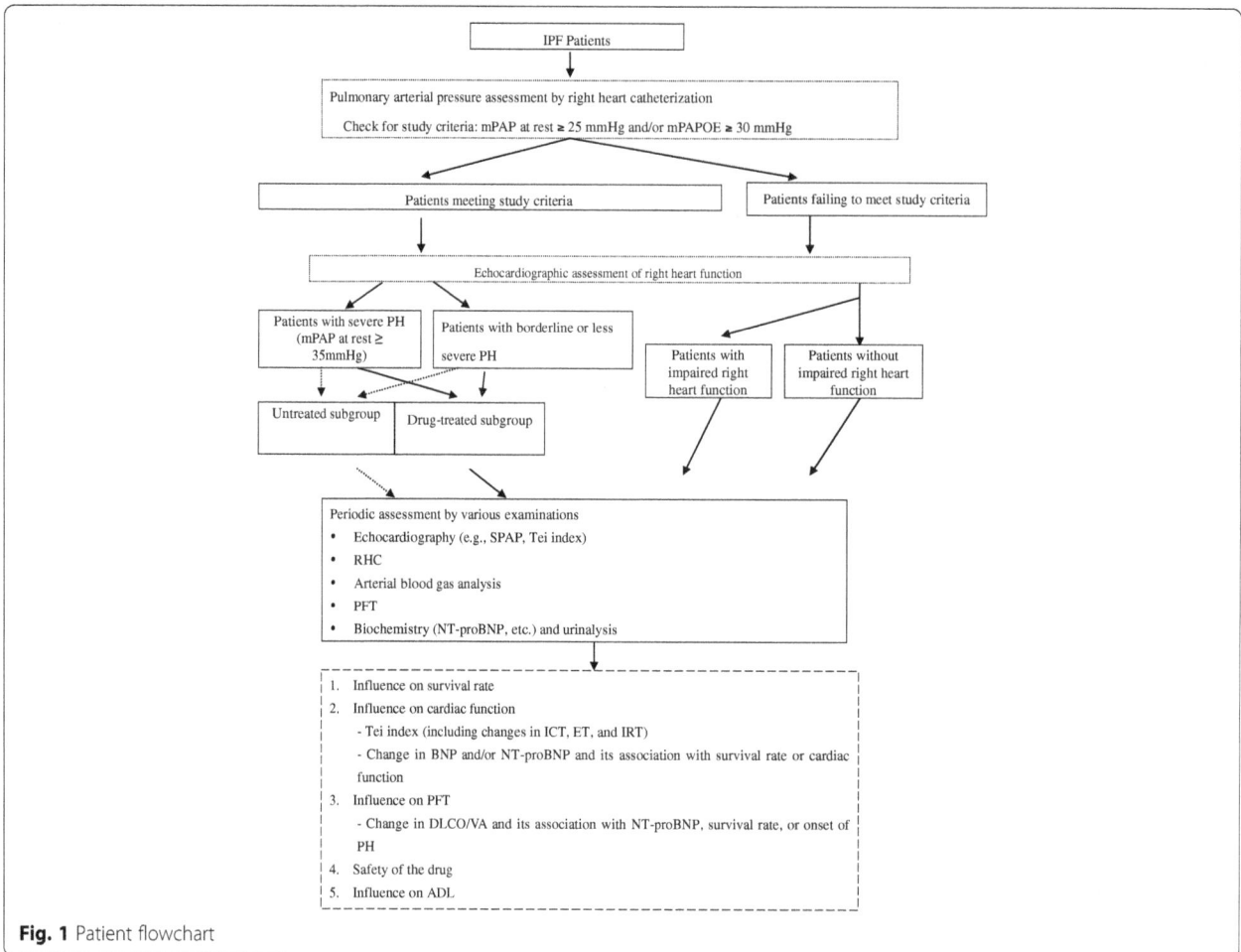

Fig. 1 Patient flowchart

Target sample size
See Additional file 2.

Outcome measures
ECG examinations were carried out during the run-in period* and every 6 months thereafter**. Complete two-dimensional, pulsed-wave, color-flow echocardiography was performed using the Toshiba ultrasound system Xario (TOSHIBA MEDICAL SYSTEMS CORPORATION, Tochigi, Japan) as previously described [14–25]. (See also Additional file 3).

Doppler measurements were carried out during the run-in period* and every 6 months**. (See also Additional file 3 and Additional file 4: Fig. S1).

RHC was carried out during the run-in period* and every 6 months thereafter**. Hemodynamic parameters (systolic PAP [SPAP]; diastolic PAP [DPAP]; mean PAP [mPAP]; systolic PAWP [SPAWP]; diastolic pulmonary capillary wedge pressure [DPAWP]; mean PAWP [mPAWP]; systolic right ventricular pressure [SRVP]; diastolic RVP [DRVP]; mean RVP [mRVP]; systolic right atrial pressure [SRAP]; diastolic RAP [DRAP]; mean RAP [mRAP]; and cardiac output [CO]) and pulmonary vascular resistance (PVR) were measured, with the patient in the supine position, via the internal jugular vein and using a Swan-Ganz continuous cardiac output (CCO) thermodilution flow-directed pulmonary artery catheter (Edwards Lifesciences LLC, USA). Cardiac output was measured by the thermodilution method using a Vigilance hemodynamic monitor (Edwards Lifesciences LLC, USA).

Systolic PAP on effort (SPAPOE), diastolic PAP on effort (DPAPOE) and mean PAP on effort (mPAPOE) were measured while patients were clasping and opening both hands repeatedly by putting a full strain on the body. Furthermore, mixed venous blood gas analysis was performed.

Survival analysis
Hospital-free survival and overall survival were determined by the duration of survival from week 0 (start of assessment), i.e., as the date treatment started for the drug-treated group and 2 weeks after RHC for the untreated group. Even for those unable to undergo the periodic assessments due to change of their attending physician, etc., this survival analysis was continued by contacting the patient's current physician to have his/her survival status confirmed. Patients were censored from hospital-free

survival if they could no longer continue ambulatory treatment and were admitted to another hospital or if they could no longer present to our hospital for progression of respiratory failure.

Adverse events

All patients were assessed for adverse events during the run-in period* and every 4 weeks thereafter**, as well as based on their medical records on unscheduled visits to our outpatient clinic. Even for those unable to undergo the periodic assessments due to change of their attending physician, adverse events were assessed by contacting their current physician to have these events confirmed.

Other parameters

Pulmonary function test (PFT) was carried out during the run-in period* and every 6 months thereafter**. (See also Additional file 3).

ADL assessments including exercise tolerance test [26–28] were performed during the run-in period* and every 6 months thereafter**. (See also Additional file 3 and Additional file 5: Figure S2). Those in whom LTOT was in place to ensure adequate oxygen inhalation during 6MWT (deemed equivalent to IPF patients receiving routine therapy in clinical practice to allow them to be monitored for changes in their condition, prognosis and functional capacity for ADL) were assessed for treadmill exercise test (TMET) with LTOT in place.

Arterial blood gas (ABG), arterial plasma lactate, brain natriuretic peptide (BNP) and N-terminal (NT)-proBNP were determined during the run-in period and every 6 months thereafter. [29] (See also Additional file 3).

Hematology, biochemistry and urinalysis were performed during the run-in period* and every 4 weeks thereafter**.

*Run-in period: Within 2 weeks after written informed consent was obtained from each patient.

**Every 6 months: Consecutive 6 months with a ± 1-week window counting from week 0 (start of assessment) defined as the date drug treatment started for the drug-treated group and 2 weeks after RHC for the untreated group. However, the periodic assessments not conducted in patients as planned based on the attending physician's judgement were deemed acceptable, unless they met any of the criteria for discontinuation of the study (e.g., pneumonia, etc.) (Fig. 1 and Additional file 6: Figure S3).

Study drug

Bosentan was administered, as a rule, according to the approved dosage and administration. Bosentan is to be usually initiated in adults at a dose of 62.5 mg twice daily after breakfast and dinner for 4 weeks and increased to a dose of 125 mg twice daily after breakfast and dinner from week 5 of treatment onwards with the dosage adjusted according to the patient's symptoms and tolerability, but not exceeding 250 mg per day. In this study conducted in routine clinical settings, however, it was acceptable to continue treatment at the initial dosage if deemed by the investigator to be appropriate based on the patient's condition (see also Additional file 7).

Concomitant drugs and therapies

Drugs allowed for use in the study included drugs intended for the treatment of the underlying disease (IPF) and drugs, other than drugs specific for PAH, for the treatment of PH as required for aggravation of PH. Drugs prohibited for use included cyclosporine, tacrolimus, glibenclamide and other drugs specific for PAH (e.g., PDE-5 inhibitors, endothelin receptor antagonists and prostaglandins) as well as any other investigational drug.

Study period

The study was conducted for 24 months between September 2010 and September 2022 with patient enrollment lasting until January 2020 (see Additional file 8).

Statistical analysis

Data are expressed as the mean ± standard deviation (SD). Changes from baseline in individual outcome measures were compared between drug-treated and untreated patients, and analyzed for statistical significance. Analysis on paired data was performed using Mann-Whitney U test. Changes in trend over time were analyzed using the Residual Maximum Likelihood (REML) or least squares method. All statistical analyses were performed using JMP version 11.2.1 (SAS Institute Inc., Cary, NC). A two-sided P value of <0.5 was considered to indicate a statistically significant change.

Results

Patients

This report presents the results of an interim analysis of the IPF patients in this study. A total of 32 IPF patients were enrolled in this study between February 2011 and June 2016, who comprised all the outpatients who had met the study entry criteria. At the time of their initial presentation to our hospital, all patients were confirmed to have chronic fibrotic idiopathic interstitial pneumonia (IIP) based on high-resolution CT findings of completely organized honeycomb lung with basal predominance in bilateral subpleural regions for which no effective therapy exists. Patients chiefly complained of symptoms of progressive respiratory failure. While all patients confirmed to have no progressive pulmonary fibrosis on CT were given detailed explanations as to the potential adverse effects associated with the use of antifibrotics, such as pirfenidone or nitentanib, which has only recently been launched in Japan and indicated for very few patients, as well as the costs due under current health insurance, none were confirmed to have received any treatment specific for IPF (e.g., pirfenidone or nintentanib) within 3 months prior to their enrollment or wished to receive any antifibrotic drug after the first 3 months or later, and none dropped out because of any treatment given, other than symptomatic treatment, for PH as the underlying disease, such as calcium channel blockers.

Of these 32 patients, the following 3 patients were excluded from the study: 1 who was found to have cancer during the study, which had probably existed at the time of enrollment (untreated, borderline or less severe PH group), 1 who developed symptoms of disc hernia during the run-in period (non-PH group), and 1 who died from aspiration pneumonia during the run-in period before the start of bosentan therapy (drug-treated, borderline or less severe PH group). The remaining 29 patients who had completed the study or were still on the study treatment were included in the present analyses. Of these 29 patients, 3 (including 1 female) had no borderline PH or PH (non-borderline PH/ PH) and the remaining 26 patients with boarderline or less severe PH, or severe PH were randomized to receive or not to receive bosentan therapy. Of these, 13 were in the drug-treated group and the other 13 were in the untreated group, including 1 in each group confirmed to have mPAP at rest $\geq$35 mmHg (severe PH), and 12 in the drug-treated group (age range, 56–76 years old) and 12 in the untreated group (age range, 51–80 years old) confirmed to have mPAP at rest <35 mmHg (borderline or less severe PH).

Patient demographics and characteristics were similar between the untreated, borderline or less severe PH group and the drug-treated, borderline or less severe PH group (Table 1).

Adverse events (Table 2)
Exacerbation of subjective symptoms of dyspnea (Table 2, Figure 2a)
Of the 12 untreated patients with borderline or less severe PH, 7 were confirmed to have experienced exacerbation of subjective symptoms of dyspnea based on the data obtained at the cut-off date, with the time to exacerbation of dyspnea being 152.00 ± 89.94 days (mean ± SD). Of 12 the drug-treated patients with borderline or less severe PH, 3 were confirmed to have experienced exacerbation of dyspnea based on the data obtained at the cut-off date, with the time to exacerbation being 259.00 ± 49.87 days (mean ± SD). Proportional hazard analysis showed that the risk ratio of the drug-treated group to the untreated group was 0.32, but with no significant difference.

Increase of O₂ dose (Table 2, Figure 2b)
Of the 12 untreated patients with borderline or less severe PH, 5 were confirmed to have required an increase of the O_2 dose based on the data obtained on the cut-off date. Of the 12 drug-treated patients with borderline or less severe PH, 3 were confirmed to have required an increase of the O_2 dose based on the data obtained on the cutoff date. The risk ratio analysis showed that the hazard ratio of the drug-treated group to the untreated group was 0.58, with the time to O_2 dose increase at the time of analysis being 357.71 ± 50.83 days in the untreated group versus 438.20 ± 34.61 days in the drug-treated group, which was not significantly different despite the fact that the results favored the drug-treated group. Only 1 patient with borderline or less severe PH in the drug-treated group achieved a decrease of the O_2 dose on day 243 because of improved respiratory function.

Hospital-free survival (Table 2, Figure 2c)
Of the 12 untreated patients with borderline or less severe PH, 8 were confirmed to have been hospitalized based on the data obtained on the cut-off date.

In contrast, of the 12 drug-treated patients with borderline or less severe PH, 2 were confirmed to have been hospitalized based on the data obtained on the cutoff date.

At the time of survival time analysis, hospital-free survival was 358.87 ± 68.65 days (mean ± SE) (median, 331 days) in the untreated group, which was significantly different from that in the drug-treated group (603.44 ± 50.074 days) as assessed by proportional hazard analysis (hazard ratio of the drug-treated group to the untreated group, 0.19, $P = 0.017$; log-rank test, $P = 0.019$; and Wilcoxon test, $P = 0.014$).

Overall survival (Table 2, Figure 2d)
Of the 12 untreated patients with borderline or less severe PH, 7 were confirmed dead (event) based on the data obtained on the cut-off date. Of the 12 drug-treated patients with borderline or less severe PH, 1 was confirmed dead with the time to event being 671 days.

At the time of survival analysis, the time to event was 433.78 ± 66.98 days (mean ± SE) in the untreated group, which was shown to be significantly different from that in the drug-treated group as assessed by proportional hazard analysis (hazard ratio of the drug-treated group to the untreated group, 0.10, $P = 0.0082$; log-rank test, $P = 0.011$; and Wilcoxon test, $P = 0.011$).

Clinical course
Eight of the 12 untreated patients received LTOT. Of the 12 patients, 1 completed the 2-year treatment period, 2 were still on the study (with one having completed regular examinations up to month 12 and the other up to month 18), and 1 was not available for the periodic assessments from month 18 onwards due to change of the attending

Table 1 Clinical characteristics of subjects with borderline or less severe PH (mPAP <35 mmHg)

	Untreated borderline or less severe PH	Drug-treated borderline or less severe PH	P^*
No. (male/female)	12(8/4)	12(9/3)	0.66
Age (y.o.)	70.50 ± 7.97	66.92 ± 6.45	0.11
Height (cm)	160.04 ± 10.11	160.87 ± 10.07	0.84
Weight (kg)	62.067 ± 12.17	54.95 ± 12.72	0.25
No. of patients with LTOT	8	7	0.67
ADL including exercise tolerance test			
WHO functional class	2.67 ± 0.78	2.83 ± 0.83	0.78
mMRC score	2.42 ± 1.084	2.33 ± 1.44	0.98
SGRQ score			
Symptoms	56.10 ± 22.87	45.78 ± 28.96	0.52
Activity	61.60 ± 22.35	55.18 ± 33.21	0.98
Impact	37.53 ± 23.11	34.38 ± 22.18	0.91
Total	49.42 ± 21.27	43.93 ± 26.41	0.77
SF36			
Physical functioning (PF)	45.83 ± 21.41	60.42 ± 26.41	0.11
Role physical (RP)	38.58 ± 21.96	51.058 ± 39.16	0.56
Bodily pain (BP)	72.17 ± 26.30	80.00 ± 25.23	0.45
General health (GH)	40.67 ± 18.34	46.75 ± 20.067	0.49
Vitality (VT)	49.34 ± 20.55	58.36 ± 29.23	0.40
Social functioning (SF)	56.25 ± 26.38	68.75 ± 33.50	0.35
Role emotional (RE)	62.51 ± 30.048	67.36 ± 37.69	0.52
Mental health (MH)	63.75 ± 19.67	65. 00 ± 27.88	0.62
Right heart cardiography			
mPAP (mmHg)	20.83 ± 5.75	21.17 ± 7.73	0.93
mPAPOE (mmHg)	42.67 ± 12.78	42.58 ± 8.87	0.45
mPAWP (mmHg)	6.83 ± 3.79	6.28 ± 3.57	0.76
mRVP (mmHg)	14.42 ± 3.58	14.083 ± 6.57	0.31
mRAP (mmHg)	2.50 ± 1.68	3.00 ± 2.13	0.45
CO (L/min)	4.80 ± 1.12	5.10 ± 1.27	0.82
CI (L/min/m^2)	2.90 ± 0.56	3.21 ± 0.63	0.38
PVR (wood)	3.12 ± 1.65	3.022 ± 2.0031	0.95
PVRI	5.073 ± 2.67	4.58 ± 2.61	1.00
Mixed venous			
PHv	7.39 ± 0.029	7.40 ± 0.026	0.45
PvCO$_2$ (mmHg)	49.34 ± 6.036	48.15 ± 4.22	0.82
PvO$_2$ (mmHg)	36.69 ± 3.89	37.55 ± 3.93	0.60
SVO$_2$ (%)	68.77 ± 5.47	70.53 ± 5.71	0.66
PFT			
%VC (%)	68.34 ± 16.92	69.55 ± 22.62	0.98
FVC (L)	2.0033 ± 0.57	2.087 ± 0.80	0.86
%DLCO (%)	30.72 ± 16.0019	27.37 ± 23.76	0.25
TTE			
ET (msec)	299.71 ± 55.95	263.83 ± 36.16	0.18
PAAcT (msec)	98.67 ± 32.65	94.75 ± 11.65	0.58
AcT/ET	0.33 ± 0.087	0.37 ± 0.060	0.23

Table 1 Clinical characteristics of subjects with borderline or less severe PH (mPAP <35 mmHg) *(Continued)*

	Untreated borderline or less severe PH	Drug-treated borderline or less severe PH	P^*
PEP (msec)	92.71 ± 12.65	87.42 ± 18.62	0.12
ICT (msec)	17.083 ± 19.96	21.75 ± 21.73	0.70
IRT (msec)	55.71 ± 45.0023	52.42 ± 36.49	0.95
ICT + IRT (msec)	87.79 ± 64.54	72.82 ± 46.34	0.69
TEI index	0.32 ± 0.27	0.30 ± 0.25	0.98
TAPSE(cm)	2.32 ± 0.47	2.27 ± 0.55	0.75
Diastolic RA area (cm^2)	8.20 ± 3.21	10.64 ± 4.91	0.29
Diastolic RA major axis (cm)	4.35 ± 2.0037	4.20 ± 2.018	0.66
Systolic RA area (cm^2)	4.74 ± 2.10	5.46 ± 2.60	0.60
Systolic RA major axis (cm)	2.95 ± 0.99	2.65 ± 0.55	0.25
Diastolic RV area (cm^2)	16.090 ± 6.57	15.39 ± 7.96	0.33
Diastolic RV major axis (cm)	6.38 ± 1.28	6.22 ± 1.098	0.49
Systolic RV area (cm^2)	9.27 ± 3.47	9.38 ± 4.38	0.64
Systolic RV major axis (cm)	4.98 ± 1.42	4.95 ± 0.89	0.60
RVEF (%)	58.91 ± 12.45	51.98 ± 13.29	0.13
Aortic Blood data at rest			
pH	7.41 ± 0.027	7.42 ± 0.022	0.25
PO$_2$ (mmHg)	76.84 ± 10.091	82.46 ± 7.93	0.11
Aortic oxygen saturation (%)	95.02 ± 1.55	95.85 ± 1.20	0.12
BNP (pg/ml)	29.42 ± 20.26	20.76 ± 13.10	0.34
NT-proBNP (pg/ml)	93.33 ± 60.15	69.67 ± 48.21	0.45
LA (mg/dl)	11.82 ± 4.082	10.00 ± 3.53	0.33
TMET			
METS	3.55 ± 1.89	3.96 ± 2.54	0.81
Post-TMET Aortic Blood data			
Post-TMET pH	7.34 ± 0.061	7.36 ± 0.069	0.45
Post-TMET PCO$_2$ (mmHg)	46.94 ± 12.22	43.017 ± 6.75	0.66
Post-TMET PO$_2$ (mmHg)	54.075 ± 15.93	67.23 ± 14.71	0.18
Post-TMET oxygen-Sat (%)	80.35 ± 18.077	90.85 ± 4.42	0.14
Post-TMET BNP (pg/ml)	40.20 ± 34.88	35.62 ± 46.66	0.27
Post-TMETNT-proBNP (pg/ml)	102.83 ± 67.48	108.67 ± 124.95	0.64
LA post TMET − LA at rest (mg/dl)	24.68 ± 20.012	22.82 ± 18.88	0.98
6MWD	246.18 ± 104.27	296.63 ± 128.0090	0.31
Post-6 MW Aortic Blood data			
Post-6MWT pH	7.39 ± 0.021	7.40 ± 0.039	0.15
Post-6 MW-PCO$_2$ (mmHg)	41.042 ± 8.32	42.64 ± 5.42	0.53
Post-6 MW-PO$_2$ (mmHg)	77.20 ± 30.98	72.067 ± 15.79	0.91
Post-TMET Oxygen-Sat (%)	92.58 ± 4.13	90.00 ± 8.35	0.69
Post-6 MW-BNP (pg/ml)	34.52 ± 25.66	25.080 ± 23.95	0.33
Post-6 MW-NT-proBNP (pg/ml)	98.50 ± 75.13	80.67 ± 72.41	0.47
LA post-6 MW − LA at rest (mg/dl)	8.60 ± 8.31	5.42 ± 8.34	0.14

Data presented as mean ± SD
$^*P$ value for Mann-Whitney U test to assess the difference between the untreated and drug-treated patients with borderline or less severe PH

Table 2 Adverse events observed in untreated and drug-treated patients with borderline or less severe PH

	Untreated borderline or less severe PH	Drug-treated borderline or less severe PH
Exacerbation of dyspnea	7	3
Time to exacerbation of dyspnea (mean ± SD) (days)	152.00 ± 89.94	259.00 ± 49.37
Increase of the O_2 dose	5	2
Time to O_2 dose increase (mean ± SE) (days)	199.00 ± 132.90,	335.00 ± 182.43
Decrease of the O_2 dose	0	1
Hospitalization (hospital-free survival)	8 (241.50 ± 192.24)	2 (239.002 ± 169.00)
Death (survival)	7 (309.29 ± 195.13)	1 (671)
Other adverse events	3[a]	6[b]

[a] Gastrointestinal hemorrhage ($n = 1$), pneumonia ($n = 1$), and ileus ($n = 1$)
[b] Pneumothorax ($n = 3$), CHF ($n = 2$), and liver dysfunction ($n = 1$)

physician after change of address. Of the remaining 8 patients, 7 were censored from hospital-free survival analysis due to progression of respiratory failure, including 5 and 1 who were not available for the periodic assessments other than mMRC, 6MWD and TMET from months 6 and 18 onwards, respectively, and were later confirmed dead. One patient was confirmed alive at the time of analysis but was not available for the periodic assessments other than mMRC, 6MWD and TMET from month 12 onwards. The remaining 1 patient developed ileus and was confirmed to have died due to a disease other than lung disease at another hospital and was completely excluded from the periodic assessments from month 6 onwards.

As for the periodic assessments with mMRC, TMET and 6MWT, of the 11 patients assessed by mMRC at month 6, 9 each were further assessed at month 12 and 8 were further assessed at month 18, and 7 completed the assessments at month 24, including 1 patient who was assessed at months 18 and 24 by contacting the patient's current physician after change of address. Of the 11 patients assessed by TMET and 6MWT at month 6, 8 were further assessed at month 12, and 7 completed the assessments at months 18 and 24.

Seven of the 12 drug-treated patients included in the analysis received LTOT. Four patients completed the study after finishing the assessments at month 48 and 1 of the remaining 8 patients withdrew from the study before month 6 due to hepatic dysfunction. Another patient withdrew from the study due to lung cancer detected on day 518. The last two patients were censored from hospital-free survival analysis due to exacerbation of respiratory failure on days 641 and 303, respectively, with the former confirmed dead on day 671. The remaining 4 patients were still on the study treatment (with 1 having completed regular examinations at baseline alone, 1 up to month 6, 2 up to month 12, and 1 up to month 18).

Lung function and RHC
Drug-treated patients with borderline or less severe PH
Compared with baseline (Table 1b), significant changes were noted in lung function %DLCO at months 6 and 12 (month 6, +7.011, $P = 0.010$; month 12, +12.18, $P = 0.0025$) (See Additional file 9: Figure %DLCO).

Compared with baseline (Table 2b), there was a decreasing trend in mPAP at months 6 and 12 although no significant difference was noted (month 6, −2.60, $P = 0.098$, $R = 0.84$; month 12, −1.71, $P = 0.38$, $R = 0.83$). A similar trend was observed for PVR (month 6, −0.69, $P = 0.11$, $R = 0.88$; month 12, −0.41, $P = 0.41$, $R = 0.87$). Compared with baseline, there was a significant improvement in mixed venous saturation of oxygen at month 6 (+4.78, $P = 0.037$, $R = 0.45$), but no significant change was noted from baseline to month 12.

Moreover, significant differences were observed in the drug-treated patients with borderline or less severe PH with regard to changes in mPAP, PVR and PVRI from baseline to month 6 (untreated vs. drug-treated: mPAP, +4.71 vs. -2.60 mmHg, $P = 0.0035$; PVR, +1.60 vs. -0.69 woods, $P = 0.0020$) (Fig. 3).

It will be a long time, however, before comparisons of data can be made between the groups for month 12 onwards, with many untreated patients with borderline or less severe PH having been censored from hospital-free survival analysis with an even smaller number of patients available for the periodic assessments.

Results for other assessment parameters (See Additional file 10, Additional file 11: Figure ADL, Additional file 12: Figure TTE, and Additional file 13: Figure Arterial blood analysis).

Overall, while drug-treated patients with borderline or less severe PH tended to fare better than untreated patients with borderline or less severe PH, it was difficult to draw any conclusion due to the small number of patients currently available for analysis, especially in untreated patients with borderline or less severe PH.

Thus, while the study appears to provide potentially valuable findings at this stage, their relevance and/or validity require to be closely examined when the final data of this trial become available.

Discussion
Many patients with IPF experience a rapid elevation of PAP as well as progression of IPF [7] and elevated PAP is shown to be associated with poor prognosis [7]. Therapies currently available for slowing the progression of fibrosis, such as pirfenidone, cannot be expected to improve IPF [30]. Besides, for any honeycomb lung that has become completely organized, no realistic treatment options are available, other than symptomatic relief with LTOT, to neutralize the progression of respiratory failure.

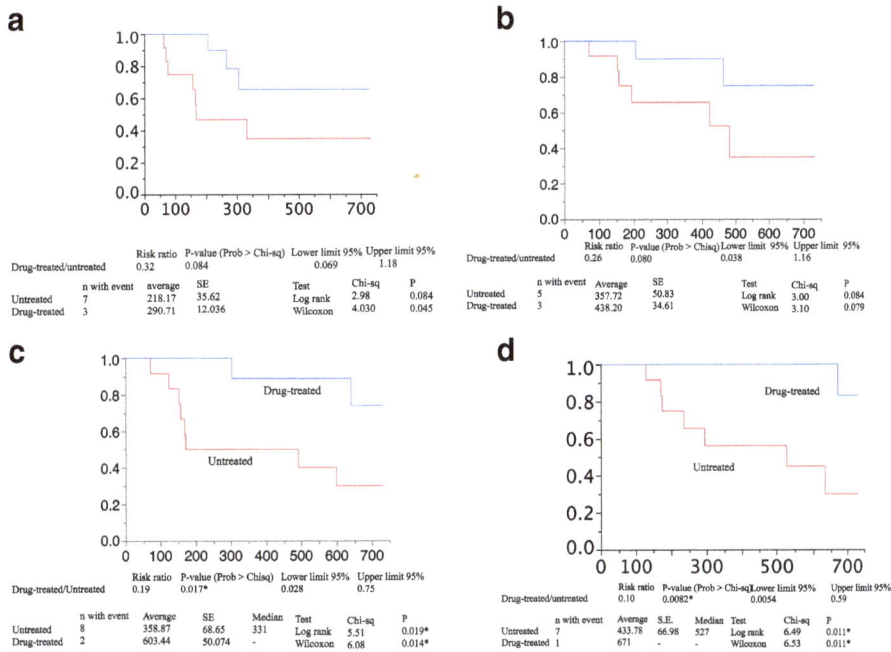

a

Drug-treated/untreated	Risk ratio	P-value (Prob > Chi-sq)	Lower limit 95%	Upper limit 95%
	0.32	0.084	0.069	1.18

	n with event	average	SE	Test	Chi-sq	P
Untreated	7	218.17	35.62	Log rank	2.98	0.084
Drug-treated	3	290.71	12.036	Wilcoxon	4.030	0.045

b

Drug-treated/untreated	Risk ratio	P-value (Prob > Chisq)	Lower limit 95%	Upper limit 95%
	0.26	0.080	0.038	1.16

	n with event	Average	SE	Test	Chi-sq	P
Untreated	5	357.72	50.83	Log rank	3.00	0.084
Drug-treated	3	438.20	34.61	Wilcoxon	3.10	0.079

c Drug-treated / Untreated

Drug-treated/Untreated	Risk ratio	P-value (Prob > Chisq)	Lower limit 95%	Upper limit 95%
	0.19	0.017*	0.028	0.75

	n with event	Average	SE	Median	Test	Chi-sq	P
Untreated	8	358.87	68.65	331	Log rank	5.51	0.019*
Drug-treated	2	603.44	50.074	-	Wilcoxon	6.08	0.014*

d Drug-treated / Untreated

Drug-treated/untreated	Risk ratio	P-value (Prob > Chi-sq)	Lower limit 95%	Upper limit 95%
	0.10	0.0082*	0.0054	0.59

	n with event	Average	S.E.	Median	Test	Chi-sq	P
Untreated	7	433.78	66.98	527	Log rank	6.49	0.011*
Drug-treated	1	671	-	-	Wilcoxon	6.53	0.011*

Fig. 2 Analysis of survival by adverse event. **a** Analysis of the time to exacerbation of subjective dyspnea. Among the untreated patients with borderline or less severe PH, the time to exacerbation of dyspnea was 152.00 ± 89.94 days (mean ± SD) in 7 of 12 patients confirmed to have experienced exacerbation of subjective symptoms of dyspnea by the data obtained on the cut-off date. Among the drug-treated patients with borderline or less severe PH, the time to exacerbation of dyspnea was 259.00 ± 49.87 days (mean ± SD) in 3 of 12 patients confirmed to have experienced exacerbation of dyspnea by the data obtained on the cut-off date. Proportional hazard analysis showed that the risk ratio of the drug-treated to untreated groups was 0.58, but with no significant difference noted. The time to exacerbation of dyspnea at the time of analysis was 218.17 ± 35.62 days (mean ± SE) in the untreated group and 290.71 ± 12.036 days in the drug-treated group, but with no significant difference noted. **b** Analysis of the time to an increase in the dose of O_2 (event). Increase of the O_2 dose: In the untreated patients with borderline or less severe PH, the time to the dose increase was 199.00 ± 132.90 days (mean ± SD) in 5 of 12 patients confirmed to have required an increase of the dose of O_2 by the data obtained on the cutoff date. In the drug-treated patients with borderline or less severe PH, the time to the dose increase was 335.00 ± 182.43 days (mean ± SD) in 3 of 12 patients confirmed to have required an increase of the O_2 dose based on the data obtained on the cut-off date. The risk ratio analysis showed that the hazard ratio of the drug-treated to untreated groups was 0.58. The time to O_2 dose increase at the time of analysis was 357.71 ± 50.83 days in the untreated group and 438.20 ± 34.61 days in the drug-treated group with no significant difference between the groups, despite the results favoring the drug-treated group. In addition, only 1 drug-treated patient with borderline or less severe PH achieved a decrease of the O_2 dose on day 243 due to an improvement of respiratory function. **c** Hospital-free survival. Of the 12 untreated patients with borderline or less severe PH, 8 were confirmed to have been hospitalized (event) by the data obtained on the cut-off date with the time to hospitalization being 241.50 ± 192.24 days (mean ± SD). Of the 12 drug-treated patients with borderline or less severe PH, 2 was confirmed to have been hospitalized by the data obtained on the cut-off date with the time to hospitalization being 239.002 ± 169.00 days. At the time of survival time analysis, hospital-free survival in the untreated group was 358.87 ± 68.65 days (mean ± SE) (median, 331 days), which was shown to be significantly different from that in the drug-treated group (603.44 ± 50.074) by proportional hazard analysis (hazard ratio [HR] of the drug-treated to untreated groups, 0.10; P = 0.017). **d** Overall survival. Of the 12 untreated patients with borderline or less severe PH, 7 were confirmed dead (event) by the data obtained on the cut-off date with the time to event being 309.29 ± 195.13 days (mean ± SD); of the drug-treated patients with borderline or less severe PH, 1 was confirmed dead by the data on the cut-off date with the time to event being 671 days. At the time of survival analysis, the time to event in the untreated group was 433.78 ± 66.98 days (mean ± SE), which was significantly different from that in the drug-treated group by proportional hazard analysis (HR of the drug-treated to untreated groups, 0.10; P = 0.0082)

In addition, it remains largely unclear how IPF and associated PH may interact to influence each other. Again, in agreement with the ATS/ERS/JRS/ALAT Clinical Practice Guideline 2015 that remains inconclusive with regard to the effect of drugs for PAH on IPH except in a subset of cases, recommending dual ERAs in patients with IPF recommended as "worthwhile considerations" and bosentan as "a conditional recommendation against use" [31], our study provided no definite clue as to how IPF and associated PH may interact. Furthermore, while our study did not allow PH and lung fibrosis to be examined for any relationship due to its small sample size, it did show no significant correlation between FVC and mPAP, suggesting that how PH and lung fibrosis interact may not readily lend itself to clarification.

Against this background, bosentan was shown to be efficacious in a subset of IIP patients in the BUILD-1 study, and this is in contrast to the results of a number of randomized controlled trials [10, 32, 33], including the BUILD-3 and ARTEMIS trials, conducted in a wide range of biopsy-proven IPF patients (where the pathology of IPF studied, including the pathologic activity,

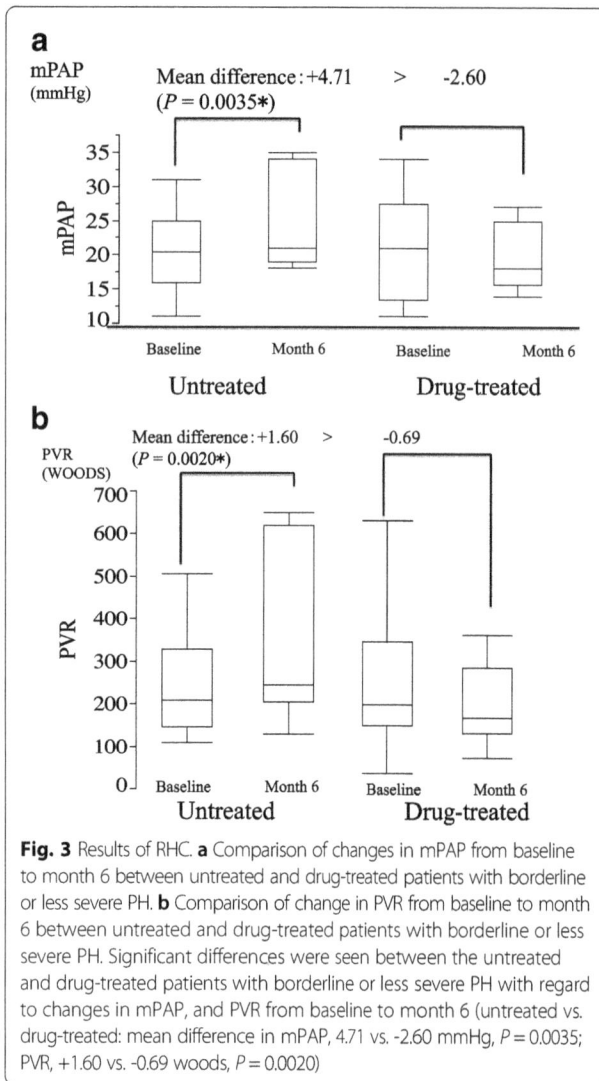

Fig. 3 Results of RHC. **a** Comparison of changes in mPAP from baseline to month 6 between untreated and drug-treated patients with borderline or less severe PH. **b** Comparison of change in PVR from baseline to month 6 between untreated and drug-treated patients with borderline or less severe PH. Significant differences were seen between the untreated and drug-treated patients with borderline or less severe PH with regard to changes in mPAP, and PVR from baseline to month 6 (untreated vs. drug-treated: mean difference in mPAP, 4.71 vs. -2.60 mmHg, $P = 0.0035$; PVR, +1.60 vs. -0.69 woods, $P = 0.0020$)

varied widely, i.e., those with fibrotic IIP, f-NSIP, elevated PAP and decreased CI), which argued against the use of bosentan in patients with PH and f-IIP. Of note, these studies failed to evaluate bosentan in patients perfectly matched for background IPF, suggesting that early intervention with bosentan in those with mildly elevated PAP may not have been sufficiently explored, while the patient background factors may have additively or synergistically contributed to the unfavorable outcomes reported in these studies.

With these considerations in mind, we enrolled patients with completely organized honeycomb lung in this study to ensure that all study subjects were as nearly matched for IPF background as possible and that they had pathologically inactive IPF (i.e., they had no active inflammatory lesion, such as GGO) that would require no change of treatment during the study. Since the subjects of this study were required to regularly visit our hospital, patients who presented to our hospital for the

first time with symptoms of progressive respiratory failure were enrolled (those without symptoms of progressive respiratory failure were not eligible for treatment at regular intervals at our hospital and were followed up at some other nearby hospital).

The present study included IPF patients with completely organized pulmonary fibrosis alone in an attempt to rule out the potential influence of IPF-associated interstitial inflammation and inter-individual differences in IPF status. As a result, the majority of patients enrolled in the study were found to have borderline to less severe PH. While it remains unclear why these patients comprised the majority, in retrospect, ambulatory patient enrollment may have led to those IPF patients who required no emergency or acute intensive care, i.e., those with only honeycomb lesions accompanied by gradually progressive dyspnea, being included in the study, who could therefore represent a selected segment of the entire IPF population. Thus, the present bosentan study was conducted in IPF patients with progressive dyspnea despite minimal IPF pulmonary lesion activity, thus ruling out the additive or synergistic influence of IPF lesions on progression of dyspnea to unequivocally demonstrate the impact of therapeutic intervention for PH in progressive dyspnea and to investigate treatment-associated pathophysiological changes in cardiac function using ECG, as well as the long-term efficacy and safety of early therapeutic intervention in PH with bosentan, with borderline PH defined as mean PAP on effort (mPAPOE) $\geq$ 30 mmHg (including mPAP at rest <25 mmHg).

At its early phase involving a small number of patients, this study demonstrated a greater-than-expected significant difference in prognosis between bosentan-treated and untreated patients with progressive respiratory failure who were confirmed to have completely organized honeycomb lung. Based on this finding, we performed an ad hoc interim analysis, which demonstrated that bosentan therapy led to a clearly better prognosis in patients with honeycomb lung suffering from symptoms of progressive respiratory failure than that in untreated patients, which was very poor. At the same time, study results reconfirmed that patients with progressive respiratory failure with completely organized honeycomb lung have a really poor prognosis. Although the possible imbalance in patient characteristics between the two groups may have affected the study results, this study adhered to randomization with the envelope method, thus making such possibility rather unlikely.

The main limitation of this study is the small number of patients included in the analysis, but this interim report was prepared following detection of a significant difference in prognosis in patients with borderline or less severe PH treated with bosentan when only half the number of patients targeted had completed the study. Again, with this study still at an exploratory stage, we have no sufficient information to determine the sample size, but an earlier bosentan repeated-dose study (AC-052-111 trial) of patients with PAH (WHO functional class III or above) conducted in Japan provided the rationale for the sample size required (i.e., 11 patients required to conduct a two-sided t-test for AUC with two-sided significance level of 5% and 90% power). Given the current state of clinical trials in this field, the sample size of this study appears to be never too small. It is highly likely that the favorable prognosis seen in the bosentan-treated patients with borderline or less severe PH might have been affected by inclusion of those with IPF experiencing a rapid elevation of PAP (not always seen among the untreated patients with borderline or less severe PH undergoing the periodic assessments). It is also possible, however, that rapid PAP elevation may have led to many patients being excluded from periodic assessments, while slowly progressive PAP elevation may have allowed patients to undergo the periodic assessments, although it is difficult to prove one way or the other.

Despite this limitation, however, our study has raised the following possibilities. First, targeting patients with completely organized honeycomb lung and symptoms of progressive respiratory failure might help select patients with rapid PAP elevation. Second, the use of bosentan may be associated with improved prognosis in selected patients similar to those included in this study. Moreover, although previous reports have failed to demonstrate a significant difference in prognosis in the entire IPF patient population with any of the drugs tested, as therapeutic options capable of suppressing the pathology of IPF become available in the future, the use of bosentan in combination with any such option might contribute further to improvements in prognosis.

In addition, while the study data remain yet to mature at present, the available data demonstrate improvements in exercise tolerance over time in bosentan-treated patients compared with untreated patients thus favoring bosentan therapy, although many untreated patients were censored from hospital-free survival analysis and excluded from the periodic assessments. If these effects on exercise tolerance can be replicated through accumulation of data from continuation of this study, bosentan may have a role to play in protecting against declines in exercise tolerance by working at various levels. Moreover, changes in respiratory conditions among the drug-treated patients suggest that bosentan therapy may have corrected abnormal breath patterns that tended toward hyperventilation. These results suggest a potential role for bosentan in delaying the progression of respiratory failure and that a decrease in respiratory rate from relief of dyspnea may be linked to a trend toward increased

PO_2, decreased PCO_2 and increased PH after exercise tolerance and stress testing, which corresponded to improvements seen in breathing efficiency after stress testing, despite no significant change in 6MWD in which the patients were assessed at the pace each patient felt comfortable. Otherwise, while the study data also suggest improvements in RV function on TTE in patients with borderline or less severe PH treated with bosentan, this finding requires to be examined at the completion of the study (see Additional file 10).

Again, while the drug-treated group did not require LTOT or increasing the O_2 inhalation dose, the untreated group reached the endpoint of hospital survival in a very short time with progressive dyspnea.

Another limitation of the study is that, among the exercises leading to increased PAP during RHC, it included clasping and opening both hands repeatedly with a full strain exerted on the body, which allowed PAP to be monitored but made it rather difficult to continue the exercise during CO measurement thus making PVR, the most critical of all parameters, less amenable to measurement. While the reasons for the observed increases in PAP during exercise in the study can only be surmised, they may include changes in PAP or increases in pulmonary blood flow associated with PVR during exercise [34–36] and intrathoracic pressure associated with straining on the part of the patients being evaluated.

A still further limitation of the study is that all patients with lower values of PAP (mPAP <25 or mPAPOE <30) were included in the untreated group, while all patients should have been randomized. Health insurance in Japan made it hardly feasible, however, to design this study as a randomized trial in which patients without PH would also be randomized to bosentan or any other drug specific for PAH. Again, given that patients with IPF might show variable outcomes, e.g., rapid declines, frequent exacerbations, or slow declines, thus representing a heterogeneous population, patients may have had to be enrolled only after their lung function has been shown to be stable for many years. However, it was simply unfeasible to enroll patients only after their lung function had been shown to be stable for some time. Instead, we have further refined the definition of eligible patients as those confirmed to have completely organized honeycomb lung and to have no active inflammatory lesion, such as GGO.

In addition, the inclusion criteria initially defined the patient age as ranging between 20 and 40 years old to exclude familial pulmonary fibrosis. Given that this could also exclude IPF, however, the patient age may have been better defined as 40 years old or older and may have led to different outcomes. Indeed, a retrospective analysis of all patients enrolled confirmed that they ranged in age between 51 and 80 years old, which has led us to redefine the patient age as 40 years old or older.

While all patients confirmed to have no progressive pulmonary fibrosis on CT were given detailed explanations as to the potential adverse effects associated with the use of antifibrotics, such as pirfenidone or nitentanib, which has only recently been launched in Japan and indicated for very few patients, as well as the costs due under current health insurance, none of these patients had previously received any medical treatment for IPF within 3 months prior to their visit and none wished to receive any antifibrotic after the first 3 months or later. Thus, further study is warranted to investigate whether various treatment options, including combination therapy with bosentan and an antifibrotic, may lead to further improvements in prognosis in these patients.

Conclusions

This was an interim report of our ongoing long-term study conducted to evaluate the effects of bosentan, as a PAH-specific drug, on IPF-associated PH based on detailed data analysis. Despite its limitations, the study appears to suggest that the bosentan-treated group fared remarkably better than the untreated group, while it was thought likely that those without borderline PH or PH receiving no treatment were associated with poor prognosis, and those with borderline PH or PH receiving bosentan therapy were associated with better prognosis. Again, study findings suggest that there exists a subset of IPF patients who might benefit from bosentan therapy with regard to improvements in IPF and prognosis. The authors plan to prepare a final report after accrual of further patients required to complete the study.

Abbreviations

6MWT: 6-min walk test; ABG: Arterial blood gas; ADL: Activities of daily living; BNP: Brain natriuretic peptide; CCO: Continuous cardiac output; CI: Cardiac index; CO: Cardiac output; CT: Computed tomography; DPAOE: Diastolic pulmonary arterial pressure on effort; ECG: Echocardiography; f-IIP: Fibrotic idiopathic interstitial pneumonia; f-NSIP: Fibrotic nonspecific interstitial pneumonia; HPV: Hypoxic pulmonary vasoconstriction; IPF: Idiopathic pulmonary fibrosis; LTOT: Long-term oxygen therapy; mPAP: Mean pulmonary arterial pressure; mPAPOE: Mean pulmonary arterial pressure on effort; PAH: Pulmonary arterial hypertension; PaO$_2$: Partial pressure of oxygen in arterial blood; PAP: Pulmonary arterial pressure; PAWP: Pulmonary capillary wedge pressure; PDE-5: Phosphodiesterase type 5; PH: Pulmonary hypertension; PVR: Pulmonary vascular resistance; RAP: Right arterial pressure; RVP: Right ventricular pressure; SPAPOE: Systolic pulmonary arterial pressure on effort

Acknowledgements

We thank Professor Marius M Hoeper, MD, Department of Respiratory Medicine, Hannover Medical School and German Centre of Lung Research (DZL), Hannover, Germany for his helpful advice.

Funding

This research did not receive any specific grant from funding agencies in the public, commercial, or not-for-profit sectors.

Authors' contributions

YT: participated in the conception and design of the study, and the analysis and interpretation of data. MH: participated in the conception and design of the study, and the interpretation of data. AG: participated in the conception and design of the study, the interpretation of data, drafting of the article, and critical revisions of important intellectual content. All authors read and approved the final manuscript.

Competing interests

The authors declare that they have no competing interests.

Author details

[1]Department of Respiratory Medicine, Nippon Medical School, Chiba Hokusoh Hospital, 1715 Kamagari, Inzai, Chiba 270-1694, Japan. [2]Department of Pulmonary Medicine and Oncology, Graduate School of Medicine, Nippon Medical School, 1-1-5 Sendagi, Bunkyo-ku, Tokyo 113-8603, Japan.

References

1. Seeger W, Adir Y, Barberà JA, Champion H, Coghlan JG, Cottin V, De Marco T, Galiè N, Ghio S, Gibbs S, Martinez FJ, Semigran MJ, Simonneau G, Wells AU, Vachiéry JL. Pulmonary hypertension in chronic lung diseases. J Am Coll Cardiol. 2013;62:D109–16.
2. Hamada K, Nagai S, Tanaka S, Handa T, Shigematsu M, Nagao T, Mishima M, Kitaichi M, Izumi T. Significance of pulmonary arterial pressure and diffusion capacity of the lung as prognosticator in patients with idiopathic pulmonary fibrosis. Chest. 2007;131:650–6.
3. Kimura M, Taniguchi H, Kondoh Y, Kimura T, Kataoka K, Nishiyama O, Sakamoto K, Hasegawa Y. Pulmonary hypertension as a prognostic indicator at the initial evaluation in idiopathic pulmonary fibrosis. Respiration. 2013; 85:456–63.
4. Behr J, Ryu JH. Pulmonary hypertension in interstitial lung disease. Eur Respir J. 2008;31:1357–67.
5. Minai OA, Santacruz JF, Alster JM, Budev MM, McCarthy K. Impact of pulmonary hemodynamics on 6-min walk test in idiopathic pulmonary fibrosis. Respir Med. 2012;106:1613–21.
6. Nathan SD, Shlobin OA, Ahmad S, Koch J, Barnett SD, Ad N, Burton N, Leslie K. Serial development of pulmonary hypertension in patients with idiopathic pulmonary fibrosis. Respiration. 2008;76:288–94.
7. Shorr AF, Wainright JL, Cors CS, Lettieri CJ, Nathan SD. Pulmonary hypertension in patients with pulmonary fibrosis awaiting lung transplant. Eur Respir J. 2007;30:715–21.
8. Carlsen J, Hasseriis Andersen K, Boesgaard S, Iversen M, Steinbrüchel D, Bøgelund AC. Pulmonary arterial lesions in explanted lungs after transplantation correlate with severity of pulmonary hypertension in chronic obstructive pulmonary disease. J Heart Lung Transplant. 2013;32:347–54.
9. Günther A, Enke B, Markart P, Hammerl P, Morr H, Behr J, Stähler G, Seeger W, Grimminger F, Leconte I, Roux S, Ghofrani HA. Safety and tolerability of bosentan in idiopathic pulmonary fibrosis: an open label study. Eur Respir J. 2007;29:713–9.
10. King TE Jr, Behr J, Brown KK, du Bois RM, Lancaster L, de Andrade JA, Stähler G, Leconte I, Roux S, Raghu G. BUILD-1: a randomized placebo-controlled trial of bosentan in idiopathic pulmonary fibrosis. Am J Respir Crit Care Med. 2008;177:75–81.
11. King TE Jr, Brown KK, Raghu G, du Bois RM, Lynch DA, Martinez F, Valeyre D, Leconte I, Morganti A, Roux S, Beehr J. BUILD-3: a randomized, controlled trial of bosentan in idiopathic pulmonary fibrosis. Am J Respir Crit Care Med. 2011;184:92–9.
12. Valerio G, Bracciale P, Grazia D'AA. Effect of bosentan upon pulmonary hypertension in chronic obstructive pulmonary disease. Ther Adv Respir Dis. 2009;3:15–21.
13. Han MK, Muellerova H, Curran-Everett D, Dransfield MT, Washko GR, Regan EA, Bowler RP, Beaty TH, Hokanson JE, Lynch DA, Jones PW, Anzueto A, Martinez FJ, Crapo JD, Silverman EK, Make BJ. GOLD 2011 disease severity classification in COPD gene: a prospective cohort study. Lancet Respir Med. 2013;1(1):43–50.

14. Tei C, Dujardin KS, Hodge DO, Bailey KR, McGoon MD, Tajik AJ, Seward SB. Doppler echocardiographic index for assessment of global right ventricular function. J Am Soc Echocardiogr. 1996;9:838–47.

15. Yamaguchi K, Miyahara Y, Yakabe K, Kiya T, Nakatomi M, Shikuwa M, Kohno S. Right ventricular impairment in patients with chronic respiratory failure on home oxygen therapy–non-invasive assessment using a new Doppler index. J Int Med Res. 1998;26:239–47.

16. Nishimura E, Ikeda S, Naito T, Yamaguchi K, Yakabe K, Iwasaki T, Yoshinaga T, Shikuwa M, Miyahara Y, Kohno S. Evaluation of right-ventricular function by Doppler echocardiography in patients with chronic respiratory failure. J Int Med Res. 1999;27:65–73.

17. Vonk MC, Sander MH, van den Hoogen FH, van Riel PL, Verheugt FW, van Dijk AP. Right ventricle Tei-index: a tool to increase the accuracy of non-invasive detection of pulmonary arterial hypertension in connective tissue diseases. Eur J Echocardiogr. 2007;8:317–21.

18. Graettinger WF, Greene ER, Voyles WF. Doppler predictions of pulmonary artery pressure, flow, and resistance in adults. Am Heart J. 1987;113:1426–37.

19. Rudski LG, Lai WW, Afilalo J, Hua L, Handschumacher MD, Chandrasekaran K, Solomon SD, Louie EK, Schiller NB. Guidelines for the echocardiographic assessment of the right heart in adults: a report from the American Society of Echocardiography endorsed by the European Association of Echocardiography, a registered branch of the European Society of Cardiology, and the Canadian Society of Echocardiography. J Am Soc Echocardiogr. 2010;23:685–713. quiz 786-8

20. Badesch DB, Champion HC, Sanchez MA, Hoeper MM, Loyd JE, Manes A, McGoon M, Naeije R, Olschewski H, Oudiz RJ, Torbicki A. Diagnosis and assessment of pulmonary arterial hypertension. J Am Coll Cardiol. 2009;54(1 Suppl):S55–66.

21. Grifoni S, Olivotto I, Cecchini P, Pieralli F, Camaiti A, Santoro G, Conti A, Agnelli G, Berni G. Short-term clinical outcome of patients with acute pulmonary embolism, normal blood pressure, and echocardiographic right ventricular dysfunction. Circulation. 2000;101:2817–22.

22. Tanaka Y, Hino M, Mizuno K, Gemma A. Evaluation of right ventricular function in patients with COPD. Respir Care. 2013;58(5):816–23.

23. Tanaka Y, Hino M, Mizuno K, Gemma A. Assessment of the relationship between right ventricular function and the severity of obstructive sleep-disordered breathing. Clin Respir J. 2014;8(2):145–51.

24. Narasimhan M, Koenig SJ, Mayo PH. Advanced echocardiography for the critical care physician: part 2. Chest. 2014;145(1):135–42.

25. Serra W, Chetta A, Santilli D, Mozzani F, Dall'Aglio PP, Olivieri D, Cattabiani MA, Ardissino D, Gherli T. Echocardiography may help detect pulmonary vasculopathy in the early stages of pulmonary artery hypertension associated with systemic sclerosis. Cardiovasc Ultrasound. 2010;8:25.

26. Celli BR, Cote CG, Marin JM, Casanova C, Montes de Oca M, Mendez RA, Pinto Plata V, Cabral HJ. The body-mass index, airflow obstruction, dyspnea, and exercise capacity index in chronic obstructive pulmonary disease. N Engl J Med. 2004;350(10):1005–12.

27. Rutten-van Mölken M, Roos B, Van Noord JA. An empirical comparison of the St George's respiratory questionnaire (SGRQ) and the chronic respiratory disease questionnaire (CRQ) in a clinical trial setting. Thorax. 1999;54(11):995–1003.

28. Akashiba T, Horie T. Exercise stress test. Research group on respiratory failure (MHW specified disease) ed., respiratory failure – guideline for diagnosis and treatment. Tokyo: Medical Review Co., Ltd.; 1996. p. 16–23. Method to apply to cases of Hugh-Jones class IV

29. Tanaka Y, Hino M, Morikawa T, Takeuchi K, Mizuno K, Kudoh S. Arterial blood lactate is a useful guide to when rehabilitation should be instigated in COPD. Respirology. 2008;13(4):564–8.

30. Azuma A, Nukiwa T, Tsuboi E, Suga M, Abe S, Nakata K, Taguchi Y, Nagai S, Itoh H, Ohi M, Sato A, Kudoh S. Double-blind, placebo-controlled trial of pirfenidone in patients with idiopathic pulmonary fibrosis. Am J Respir Crit Care Med. 2005;171(9):1040–7.

31. Raghu G, Rochwerg B, Zhang Y, Garcia CA, Azuma A, Behr J, Brozek JL, Collard HR, Cunningham W, Homma S, Johkoh T, Martinez FJ, Myers J, Protzko SL, Richeldi L, Rind D, Selman M, Theodore A, Wells AU, Hoogsteden H, Schünemann HJ, American Thoracic Society; European Respiratory society; Japanese Respiratory Society; Latin American Thoracic Association. An official ATS/ERS/JRS/ALAT clinical practice guideline: treatment of idiopathic pulmonary fibrosis. An update of the 2011 clinical practice guideline. Am J Respir Crit Care Med. 2015;192(2):e3–19.

32. Raghu G, Behr J, Brown KK, Egan JJ, Kawut SM, Flaherty KR, Martinez FJ, Nathan SD, Wells AU, Collard HR, Costabel U, Richeldi L, de Andrade J, Khalil N, Morrison LD, Lederer DJ, Shao L, Li X, Pedersen PS, Montgomery AB, Chien JW, O'Riordan TG, ARTEMIS-IPF Investigators. Treatment of idiopathic pulmonary fibrosis with ambrisentan: a parallel, randomized trial. Ann Intern Med. 2013;158(9):641–9.

33. Corte TJ, Keir GJ, Dimopoulos K, Howard L, Corris PA, Parfitt L, Foley C, Yanez-Lopez M, Babalis D, Marino P, Maher TM, Renzoni EA, Spencer L, Elliot CA, Birring SS, O'Reilly K, Gatzoulis MA, Wells AU, Wort SJ, BPHIT Study Group. Bosentan in pulmonary hypertension associated with fibrotic idiopathic interstitial pneumonia. Am J Respir Crit Care Med. 2014;190(2):208–17. doi:10.1164/rccm.201403-0446OC.

34. Argiento P, Chesler N, Mulè M, D'Alto M, Bossone E, Unger P, Naeije R. Exercise stress echocardiography for the study of the pulmonary circulation. Eur Respir J. 2010;35(6):1273–8.

35. Stamm A, Saxer S, Lichtblau M, Hasler ED, Jordan S, Huber LC, Bloch KE, Distler O, Ulrich S. Exercise pulmonary haemodynamics predict outcome in patients with systemic sclerosis. Eur Respir J. 2016;48(6):1658–67.

36. Saggar R, Lewis GD, Systrom DM, Champion HC, Naeije R. Pulmonary vascular responses to exercise: a haemodynamic observation. Eur Respir J. 2012;39(2):231–4.

8

Prevalence of pre-transplant anti-HLA antibodies and their impact on outcomes in lung transplant recipients

Ji Eun Park[1,3], Chi Young Kim[1], Moo Suk Park[1], Joo Han Song[1], Young Sam Kim[1], Jin Gu Lee[2], Hyo Chae Paik[2] and Song Yee Kim[1*]

Abstract

Background: Previous studies have suggested that antibodies against human leukocyte antigen (HLA) are associated with worse outcomes in lung transplantation. However, little is known about the factors associated with outcomes following lung transplantation in Asia. Accordingly, we investigated the prevalence of anti-HLA antibodies in recipients before transplantation and assessed their impact on outcomes in Korea.

Methods: A single-center retrospective study was conducted. The study included 76 patients who received a lung transplant at a tertiary hospital in South Korea between January 2010 and March 2015.

Results: Nine patients (11.8%) had class I and/or class II panel-reactive antibodies greater than 50%. Twelve patients (15.8%) had anti-HLA antibodies with a low mean fluorescence intensity (MFI, 1000–3000), 7 (9.2%) with a moderate MFI (3000–5000), and 12 (15.8%) with a high MFI (> 5000). Ten patients (13.2%) had suspected donor-specific antibodies (DSA), and 60% (6/10) of these patients had antibodies with a high MFI. In an analysis of outcomes, high-grade (≥2) primary graft dysfunction (PGD) was more frequent in patients with anti-HLA antibodies with moderate-to-high MFI values than in patients with low MFI values (39.4% vs. 14.0%, $p = 0.011$). Of 20 patients who survived longer than 2 years and evaluated for pBOS after transplant, potential bronchiolitis obliterans syndrome (pBOS) or BOS was more frequent in patients with anti-HLA antibodies with moderate-to-high MFI than in patients with low MFI, although this difference was not statistically significant (50.0% vs. 14.3%, $p = 0.131$).

Conclusions: The prevalence of anti-HLA antibodies with high MFI was not high in Korea. However, the MFI was relatively high in patients with DSA. Anti-HLA antibodies with moderate-to-high MFI values were related to high-grade PGD. Therefore, recipients with high MFI before lung transplantation should be considered for desensitization and close monitoring.

Keywords: Anti-HLA antibodies, Donor-specific antibodies, Lung transplantation, Outcomes

Background

Lung transplantation is the ultimate therapeutic option for patients with end-stage lung disease. Despite improvements in transplantation techniques and immunosuppression therapy, the current 5-year survival rate is only 57% [1]. The presence of antibodies against human leukocyte antigens (HLA) prior to transplantation is

reported to be associated with worse post-transplant outcomes [2–6]. However, evidence for this association in lung transplantation is not as strong as that for other types of solid organ transplantation.

Elevated panel-reactive antibody (PRA) levels before lung transplant are linked to adverse graft outcomes and post-transplant survival. Several studies have found that lung transplant recipients with elevated pre-transplant PRA tend to exhibit more ventilator days after transplant, development of bronchiolitis obliterans syndrome, and a low graft survival rate [7–14]. However, there is no consensus about the cutoff PRA level or the appropriate mean

---
* Correspondence: dobie@yuhs.ac
[1]Division of Pulmonology, Department of Internal Medicine, Severance Hospital, Institute of Chest Diseases, Yonsei University College of Medicine, 50-1, Yonsei-ro, Seodaemun-gu, Seoul, Republic of Korea
Full list of author information is available at the end of the article

fluorescence intensity (MFI) threshold for identifying anti-HLA antibodies or assessing their impact on outcomes in lung transplant recipients. A recent study has reported an association between pre-transplant anti-HLA antibodies with high MFI values (i.e., > 3000) and a high rate of antibody-mediated rejection [15].

Limited data exist regarding the distribution and impact of anti-HLA antibodies before lung transplantation in Asia, despite the increasing number of lung transplantations in the region, indicating the importance of these analyses. The objectives of this study were (1) to investigate the prevalence of pre-transplant anti-HLA antibodies for a wide spectrum of thresholds in patients prior to lung transplant and (2) to assess their impact on outcomes in lung transplant recipients in Korea.

Methods

Study design and population

In this retrospective study, the medical records of consecutive lung transplant recipients at one tertiary care hospital in South Korea between January 2010 and March 2015 were reviewed. Pediatric cases (< 16 years of age) and heart-lung transplantation cases were excluded. In total, 76 lung transplant recipients, who were followed through September 2015, were included.

Immunologic evaluation

Before transplantation, all patients underwent panel reactive antibody (PRA) class I and class II identification (Immucor, Stamford, CT, USA). The anti-HLA antibodies specificity is classified into 1000, 3000, and 10,000 based on the MFI value. MFI < 1000 is very weak, $1000 \leq MFI < 3000$ is weak, $3000 \leq MFI < 10,000$ is moderate, and above 10,000 is strong. The cut off value of MFI considered to be anti HLA Ab positive is 1000. The highest mean fluorescence intensity (MFI) was recorded as the MFI. Anti-HLA antibodies against donor HLA was defined as donor-specific antibodies (DSA). DSA was quantified based on MFI, the cutoff value of MFI considered as DSA positive is 500.

Clinical settings

The transplantation was performed regardless of the status of DSA because of the problem of donor shortage. And we considered desensitization protocol including plasma exchange and immunoglobulin after lung transplantation in patients with pre-transplant DSA and MFI ≥ 3000.

All patients received induction therapy with high-dose steroids (methylprednisolone, 500 mg), followed by standard triple immunosuppressive therapy consisting of tacrolimus, mycophenolate, and prednisolone after lung transplant. Pre-transplant immunological results did not affect the choice of immunosuppressant regimen.

Clinical outcomes

Clinical outcomes included primary graft dysfunction (PGD) and bronchiolitis obliterans syndrome (BOS). PGD after lung transplantation represents an injury to the transplanted lung that develops in the first 72 h after transplantation. The severity of PGD is graded based on the ratio of arterial oxygen pressure to the inspired oxygen concentration (PaO_2/FiO_2) and the presence of infiltration on chest radiographs according to the International Society for Heart and Lung Transplantation (ISHLT) criteria [16]. BOS was identified as a progressive decline in forced expiratory volume in 1 s (FEV_1) after excluding other etiologies. BOS was diagnosed according to the criteria of ISHLT. A potential BOS (pBOS) stage defined by a 10% to 19% decrease in FEV_1 and/or by $a \geq 25\%$ decrease in FEF_{25-75} from baseline [17, 18]. The incidence of BOS could not be determined because the study period was relatively short; accordingly, pBOS was used as an outcome, instead of BOS. pBOS was analyzed in patients who survived longer than 2 years after lung transplantation.

Statistical analysis

All analyses were performed using SPSS (version 20.0) (SPSS, Inc., Chicago, IL, USA). Continuous variables are reported as means and standard deviations, and categorical variables are reported as counts and percentages. Recipient characteristics in groups distinguished by anti-HLA antibodies were compared using Fisher's exact tests and Mann–Whitney U tests for categorical and continuous variables, respectively. A two-tailed p-value of < 0.05 was considered statistically significant.

Ethics

Informed consent was waived because this was a retrospective study. The research protocol was approved by the Institutional Review Board (IRB) of Severance Hospital (IRB No. 4–2013-0770).

Results

In total, 76 lung transplant recipients were included in the analysis. Patients were followed from the time of lung transplantation until death or the end of the study period.

Baseline characteristics

Table 1 summarizes the baseline characteristics of recipients. The median patient age was 52.0 years (range, 17–75 years) and 42 recipients (55.3%) were male. Primary diagnosis consisted of 37 cases of idiopathic pulmonary fibrosis (48.7%), 4 cases of chronic obstructive lung disease (COPD) (5.3%), 1 of pulmonary artery hypertension (1.3%), 4 of destroyed lung by tuberculosis (5.3%), 5 of interstitial lung disease with connective tissue disease (6.6%), 9 of lymphangioleiomyomatosis

Table 1 Recipients characteristics of patients with class I/II panel reactive antibody < 50% and ≥50%

	All recipients (n = 76)	PRA < 50% (n = 67)	PRA ≥ 50% (n = 9)	p-value
Age, median (range), yrs	52.0 (17–75)	53.0 (18–75)	44.0 (17–52)	0.013
Male, n (%)	42 (55.3)	39 (58.2)	3 (33.3)	0.284
BMI, median (IQR), kg/m^2	19.1 (17.4–21.6)	19.0 (17.4–21.6)	19.8 (16.1–21.6)	0.981
ABO, n (%)				0.413
A	26 (34.2)	24 (35.8)	2 (22.2)	
B	26 (34.2)	23 (34.3)	3 (33.3)	
AB	6 (7.9)	4 (6.0)	2 (22.2)	
O	18 (23.7)	16 (23.9)	2 (22.2)	
Primary diagnosis, n (%)				0.277
COPD/emphysema	4 (5.3)	3 (4.5)	1 (11.1)	
IPF	37 (48.7)	35 (52.2)	2 (22.2)	
IPAH	1 (1.3)	1 (1.5)	0 (0)	
IIP other than IPF*	3 (3.9)	2 (3.0)	1 (11.1)	
Bronchiectasis/ destroyed lung by TB	4 (5.3)	4 (6.0)	0 (0)	
BOS after HSCT	11 (14.5)	9 (14.9)	2 (22.2)	
Interstitial lung disease related with CTD	5 (6.6)	4 (6.0)	1 (11.1)	
LAM	9 (11.8)	7 (10.4)	2 (22.2)	
Others**	2 (2.6)	2 (3.0)	0 (0)	
Smoking, n (%)				0.141
Smoker	30 (39.5)	29 (43.3)	1 (11.1)	
≥ 20 pack-years	22 (28.9)	21 (31.3)	1 (11.1)	
< 20 pack-years	8 (10.6)	8 (12.0)	0 (0)	
Never smoker	46 (60.5)	38 (56.7)	8 (88.9)	
Bilateral lung transplantation, n (%)	62 (81.6)	53 (79.1)	9 (100)	0.197

*NSIP and AIP were included
**Others: diffuse panbronchiolitis, langerhans cell histiocytosis
BMI, body mass index; COPD, chronic obstructive pulmonary disease; IPF, idiopathic pulmonary fibrosis; IPAH, Idiopathic pulmonary arterial hypertension; IIP, Idiopathic interstitial pneumonia; TB, tuberculosis; BOS, Bronchiolitis obliterans syndrome; CTD, connective tissue disease; LAM, Lymphangioleiomyomatosis; NSIP, non-specific interstitial pneumonia; AIP, acute interstitial pneumonia; HSCT, hematopoietic stem cell transplantation

(11.8%), 3 of idiopathic interstitial pneumonia other than idiopathic pulmonary fibrosis (IPF) (3.9%), 11 of bronchiolitis obliterans after stem cell transplantation (14.5%), and 2 cases of others diseases, such as diffuse panbronchiolitis and Langerhans cell histiocytosis (2.6%). The most common transplantation type was a bilateral lung transplantation (62 patients, 81.6%).

When divided into two groups based on a class I/II PRA value of < 50% and ≥50%, the only factor that differed significantly between groups was age; patients in the PRA ≥50% group were younger than those in the PRA < 50% group (53 vs. 44 years, $p = 0.013$). Patient subgroups dichotomized according to PRA levels were similar with respect to recipient characteristics, except age (Table 1).

Prevalence of anti-HLA antibodies
Among 76 patients, high levels of class I or class II PRA (≥50%) were detected in 9 patients (11.8%). In terms of

the distribution of MFI, 12 patients (15.8%) had anti-HLA antibodies with a low MFI (1000–3000), 7 (9.2%) had a moderate MFI (3000–5000), and 12 (15.8%) had a high MFI (> 5000). The proportion of patients with a high PRA and the distribution of MFI were relatively similar between Class I and Class II (Table 2).

At the time of lung transplantation, all recipients were screened for DSA based on the presence of antibodies to HLA of the respective donor, as determined by PRA. Ten patients (13.2%) had DSA. Most of the 10 DSA-positive recipients (7/10, 70%) had high PRA and 60% (6/10) had high MFI (> 5000) anti-HLA antibodies. In contrast, only 3% of patients without DSA had high PRA, and 9.1% of patients without DSA (6/66) had high MFI. However, there were no differences in non-immunological factors, such as age, sex, BMI, underlying disease, and surgery type of lung transplantation, between patients with and without DSA (Table 3).

Table 2 Prevalence of pre-transplant panel reactive antibody and donor-specific antibodies

	Recipients (n = 76)
Total	
cPRA	
Not detected	41 (54.0)
PRA < 50%	26 (34.2)
PRA ≥ 50%	9 (11.8)
Anti-HLA Ab (MFI)	
< 1000	45 (59.2)
1000 ≤ MFI < 3000	12 (15.8)
3000 ≤ MFI < 5000	7 (9.2)
≥ 5000	12 (15.8)
Class I	
cPRA	
Not detected	50 (65.8)
Class I PRA < 50%	20 (26.3)
Class I PRA ≥ 50%	6 (7.9)
Anti-HLA Ab (MFI)	
< 1000	54 (71.1)
1000 ≤ MFI < 3000	11 (14.5)
3000 ≤ MFI < 5000	2 (2.6)
≥ 5000	10 (13.2)
Class II	
cPRA	
Not detected	54 (71.0)
Class I PRA < 50%	18 (23.7)
Class I PRA ≥ 50%	4 (5.3)
Anti-HLA Ab (MFI)	
< 1000	59 (77.6)
1000 ≤ MFI < 3000	9 (11.8)
3000 ≤ MFI < 5000	6 (7.9)
≥ 5000	3 (3.9)

cPRA, calculated panel reactive antibody; PRA, panel reactive antibody; HLA, human leukocyte antigen; MFI, mean fluorescence intensity

Outcomes

According to the grade of PGD, patients were divided into 2 groups, i.e., non-high-grade PGD (grade 0–1) and high-grade PGD (grade ≥ 2). High-grade PGD developed in 33 patients (43.3%). High-grade PGD developed in more patients with anti-HLA antibodies of moderate or high MFI values (≥3000) than in patients with low MFI values (39.4% vs. 14.0%, $p = 0.011$). High PRA titers or the presence of DSA was not associated with the development of high-grade PGD (Table 4).

Table 5 shows the association between pre-transplanted anti-HLA antibodies and pBOS or BOS. Twenty patients who survived longer than 2 years after

transplantation and underwent pulmonary function test for BOS evaluation were evaluated, and pBOS or BOS developed in 6 of these patients (30%) among 20 patients. Four (20%) patients had pBOS and 2 (10%) patients had BOS. pBOS or BOS was more frequent in patients with anti-HLA antibodies of moderate or high MFI (≥3000) than in patients with low MFI (< 3000), although this difference was not statistically significant (50.0% vs. 14.3%, $p = 0.131$). Additionally, the associations between high PRA and pBOS or BOS and the associations between the presence of DSA and pBOS or BOS were not significant, respectively. Non-immune initiated factors such as cytomegalovirus (CMV) infection, *Pseudomonas* airway colonization, and airway ischemia, which may affect rejection after transplantation [19–21] were also evaluated, however, there was no difference between two groups.

Discussion

In this study, we performed a detailed immunological assessment of a cohort of patients who underwent lung transplantation and revealed the relationship between the degree of pre-transplant sensitization and post-transplant clinical outcomes.

We investigated sensitization before lung transplantation, as defined either by (i) high PRA and/or high MFI antibodies against class I and/or class II HLA or (ii) the presence of HLA class I and/or class II DSA. The proportion of patients with high PRA (> 50%) (class I, 7.9%; class II, 5.3%; total 11.8%) and high MFI (≥5000) (class I, 13.2%; class II, 3.9%; total 15.8%) were not high in Korea. DSA was observed in 13.2% of patients and was correlated with a high PRA or high MFI.

The presence of HLA antibodies differs among studies. In a retrospective study by Hadjiliadis et al., 101 of 656 lung transplantation recipients (15.4%) showed a PRA greater than 0 before transplantation, 37 (5.6%) patients had a PRA greater than 10%, and 20 (3.0%) patients had a PRA greater than 25% using cell-based complement dependent cytotoxicity (CDC) techniques [7]. As another solid organ, Gebel et al. reported that 25%–50% of patients on the waiting list for kidney transplantation have a PRA level of higher than 20% based on both CDC and flow cytometry [22]. In an analysis of heart transplantation, Tambur et al. reported that 5.5% of recipients had high PRA levels (PRA > 10%) before transplant by CDC. However, 72 patients (32.9%) had pre-transplant anti-HLA antibodies detectable by a flow cytometric approach to PRA testing (class I, 34 patients; class II, 7 patients; class I and II, 31 patients) [2]. Historically, anti-HLA antibodies were detected using the complement-dependent cytotoxicity (CDC) assays. This technique is complemented by solid phase assays using Luminex apparatus. Luminex assay is more sensitive

Table 3 Recipients characteristics with or without Donor Specific Antibody

	Donor Specific Antibody		p-value
	Yes (n = 10)	No (n = 66)	
Anti-HLA Ab (%)			< 0.001
PRA ≥ 50%	7 (70.0)	2 (3.0)	
Anti-HLA Ab (MFI)			< 0.001
< 1000	0 (0)	45 (68.2)	
1000 ≤ MFI < 3000	3 (30.0)	9 (13.6)	
3000 ≤ MFI < 5000	1 (10.0)	6 (9.1)	
≥ 5000	6 (60.0)	6 (9.1)	
Age, median (range), yrs	48.5 (17–57)	52.0 (17–75)	0.180
Male, n (%)	5 (50.0)	37 (56.1)	0.745
BMI, median (IQR), kg/m^2	18.4 (14.3–20.0)	19.3 (17.5–22.2)	0.161
ABO, n (%)			0.708
A	2 (20.0)	24 (36.4)	
B	4 (40.0)	22 (33.3)	
AB	1 (10.0)	5 (7.6)	
O	3 (30.0)	15 (22.7)	
Primary diagnosis, n (%)			0.321
COPD/emphysema	2 (20.0)	2 (3.0)	
IPF	3 (30.0)	34 (51.5)	
IPAH	0 (0)	1 (1.5)	
IIP other than IPF*	0 (0)	3 (4.5)	
Bronchiectasis/destroyed lung by TB	0 (0)	4 (6.1)	
BOS after HSCT	2 (20.0)	9 (13.6)	
Interstitial lung disease related with CTD	1 (10.0)	4 (6.1)	
LAM	2 (20.0)	7 (10.6)	
Others**	0 (0)	2 (3.0)	
Smoking, n (%)			0.733
Smoker	3 (30.0)	26 (39.4)	
≥ 20 pack-years	3 (30.0)	19 (28.8)	
< 20 pack-years	0 (0)	7 (10.6)	
Never smoker	7 (70.0)	40 (60.6)	
Bilateral lung transplantation, n (%)	9 (90.0)	53 (80.3)	0.678

*NSIP and AIP were included
**Others: diffuse panbronchiolitis, langerhans cell histiocytosis
BMI, body mass index; COPD, chronic obstructive pulmonary disease; IPF, idiopathic pulmonary fibrosis; IPAH, Idiopathic pulmonary arterial hypertension; IIP, Idiopathic interstitial pneumonia; TB, tuberculosis; BOS, Bronchiolitis obliterans syndrome; CTD, connective tissue disease; LAM, Lymphangioleiomyomatosis; NSIP, non-specific interstitial pneumonia; AIP, acute interstitial pneumonia; HSCT, hematopoietic stem cell transplantation

than the conventional CDC method [23–25]. A recent report by Goldberg et al. on the basis of results using Luminex assays showed that 30% of subjects had circulating class I HLA antibodies alone, 4% Class II, and 14.4% class I and class II at MFI > 1000 [26]. According to Chung et al., of 129 patients who were waiting for a kidney transplant in Korea, 56 patients (43.4%) had PRA ≥ 20% by solid phase Luminex PRA, 45 patients (34.9%) had anti-HLA antibodies based on a Luminex single antigen assay, and 25 patients (44.6%) had HLA-DSA [27]. Although the prevalence of anti-HLA antibodies differed depending on the test method, similar results were obtained when the same test method was used, including this study. In our analysis, the proportion of high PRA or anti-HLA Ab titer is not high compared to previous studies.

The lower median age in the group with PRA ≥ 50% may be explained by the young age of the two patients with BOS after hematopoietic stem cell transplantation (HSCT), i.e., 17 and 18 years old. There are no similar

Table 4 Association of pre-transplant panel reactive antibody with primary graft dysfunction status

	PGD 0–1 (n = 43)	PGD 2–3 (n = 33)	p-value
Total			
cPRA			> 0.999
Not detected or PRA < 50%, n (%)	38 (88.4)	29 (87.9)	
PRA ≥ 50%, n (%)	5 (11.6)	4 (12.1)	
Anti-HLA Ab (MFI)			0.011
Not detected or MFI < 3000, n (%)	37 (86.0)	20 (60.6)	
MFI ≥ 3000, n (%)	6 (14.0)	13 (39.4)	
Class I			0.394
cPRA			
Not detected or PRA < 50%, n (%)	41 (95.3)	29 (87.9)	
PRA ≥ 50%, n (%)	2 (4.7)	4 (12.1)	
Anti-HLA Ab (MFI)			0.077
Not detected or MFI < 3000, n (%)	39 (90.7)	25 (75.8)	
MFI ≥ 3000, n (%)	4 (9.3)	8 (24.2)	
Class II			
cPRA			
Not detected or PRA < 50%, n (%)	40 (93.0)	32 (97.0)	0.628
PRA ≥ 50%, n (%)	3 (7.0)	1 (3.0)	
Anti-HLA Ab (MFI)			0.071
Not detected or MFI < 3000, n (%)	41 (95.3)	27 (81.8)	
MFI ≥ 3000, n (%)	2 (4.7)	6 (18.2)	
Donor Specific Antibody			0.739
Yes, n (%)	5 (11.6)	5 (15.2)	
No, n (%)	38 (88.4)	28 (84.8)	

cPRA, calculated panel reactive antibody; PRA, panel reactive antibody; HLA, human leukocyte antigen; MFI, mean fluorescence intensity; PGD, primary graft dysfunction; CMV, cytomegalovirus; R, recipient; D, donor

reports; additionally, our results could be explained by an impact of previous HSCT on PRA.

The distribution of DSA positivity differs among studies. Brugiere et al. reported that 14%, 20%, and 32% of patients had class I, II, and I and II DSA, respectively, in France and the proportion of patients with DSA was somewhat higher than that in our study [28]. In contrast, Song et al. reported that 32 (14.5%) recipients were positive for DSAs against donor HLAs by PRA among 219 living donor liver transplant recipients in Korea [29]. In a study in which Rose et al. reported cardiac transplantation, 53 (9.4%) of 565 patients had DSA detectable by Luminex assays before transplant [30]. These discrepancies among studies may be related to differences in race or methodological differences. In our study, the DSA-positive group showed significantly higher levels of class I and II PRA than those of the DSA-negative group, consistent with previous results. Eventually, patients with high PRA (%) and high MFI values for anti-HLA antibodies should be considered as having a high probability of DSA, regardless of donor.

Many studies have shown that high PRA before transplantation increases the risk of mortality with acute and chronic transplant rejection after solid organ transplantation [7, 31, 32]. In particular, the presence of anti-HLA antibodies promotes BOS, the predominant cause of mortality in patients exhibiting long-term survival after lung transplantation [33–35]. Lau et al. reported that sensitized patients experience a significantly higher incidence of bronchiolitis obliterans syndrome than that of non-sensitized patients (56% vs. 23%, p = 0.044). Additionally, 2-year survival decreased (58% vs. 73%, p = 0.31) and pathology suggesting antibody-mediated injury in lung transplant recipients was related to an elevated pre-transplant PRA [10]. Furthermore, Shah et al. reported an increased mortality when total PRA levels exceeded 25% [8].

Our analysis of the effect of anti-HLA antibodies on post-transplant outcomes showed that high-grade PGD was related to a high MFI. In a literature review, a direct correlation between high anti-HLA antibodies and PGD incidence has not been reported; however, the cause of

Table 5 Association of pre-transplant panel reactive antibody with potential BOS

	BOS 0 (n = 14)	≥pBOS (n = 6)	p-value
Total			
cPRA			> 0.999
Not detected or PRA < 50%, n (%)	12 (85.7)	5 (83.3)	
PRA ≥ 50%, n (%)	2 (14.3)	1 (16.7)	
Anti-HLA Ab (MFI)			0.131
Not detected or MFI < 3000, n (%)	12 (85.7)	3 (50)	
MFI ≥ 3000, n (%)	2 (14.3)	3 (50)	
Class I			
cPRA			> 0.999
Not detected or PRA < 50%, n (%)	12 (85.7)	5 (83.3)	
PRA ≥ 50%, n (%)	2 (14.3)	1 (16.7)	
Class I anti-HLA Ab (MFI)			0.549
Not detected or MFI < 3000, n (%)	12 (85.7)	4 (66.7)	
MFI ≥ 3000, n (%)	2 (14.3)	2 (33.3)	
Class II			
cPRA			–
Not detected or PRA < 50%, n (%)	14 (100)	6 (100)	
PRA ≥ 50%, n (%)	–	–	
Class II anti-HLA Ab (MFI)			0.079
Not detected or MFI < 3000, n (%)	14 (100)	4 (66.7)	
MFI ≥ 3000, n (%)	0 (0)	2 (33.3)	
Donor Specific Antibody			> 0.999
Yes, n (%)	2 (14.3)	1 (16.7)	
No, n (%)	12 (85.7)	5 (83.3)	
CMV status			
Donor + / Recipient -, n (%)	0 (0)	0 (0)	–
Donor + / Recipient +, n (%)	14 (100)	6 (100)	–
Donor BAL culture +, n (%)	9 (64.3)	2 (33.3)	0.336
Pseudomonas aeruginosa colonization, n (%)	1 (7.1)	1 (16.7)	0.521
Ischemic time, min (mean ± SD)	213.2 ± 62.8	197.0 ± 55.6	0.386

cPRA, calculated panel reactive antibody; PRA, panel reactive antibody; HLA, human leukocyte antigen; MFI, mean fluorescence intensity; BOS, bronchiolitis obliterans syndrome; pBOS, potential bronchiolitis obliterans syndrome; CMV, cytomegalovirus; BAL, bronchoalveolar lavage

PGD is considered multifactorial and could include the inflammatory response associated with anti-HLA. Hadjiliadis et al. reported that an elevated pre-transplant PRA in lung transplant recipients is associated with poor survival, especially during the early post-transplant period; this was attributed to a direct effect of anti-HLA antibodies on the allograft [7]. Bharat et al. reported that PGD is associated with an inflammatory cascade that augments the anti-HLA response that predisposes patients to BOS. Based on many previous studies as well as the results of this study, an immunological response may be one of the mechanisms among the multifactorial causes of PGD [26].

Similar results have been reported for other solid organ transplant types. Perera et al. found that pre-existing DSA may result in early morbidity in liver transplant recipients. In a renal transplant study, Caro-Oleas et al. reported that patients with existing or de novo anti-HLA-DSA had the highest likelihood of rejection episodes. In this study, patients with DSA-positive results were more likely to have a high MFI and therefore had a high risk of acute rejection. Therefore, in patients with a high MFI, the occurrence of PGD immediately after lung transplantation should be closely monitored.

The majority of recipients with elevated PRA had risk factors for humoral sensitization. In particular, humoral immune responses after transplant are associated with BOS development according to several studies, emphasizing the need for the monitoring of anti-HLA antibodies prior to lung transplantation. Andres et al. suggested that the development of anti-HLA antibodies after lung transplant plays an important role in the development of BOS [36]. However, based on our results, we cannot definitively confirm the relationship between high PRA or DSA and pBOS or BOS. The short follow-up duration or the inclusion of pBOS could explain the differences between our results and those of previous studies.

This study had some limitations. First, this was a retrospective cohort study, with a limited number of patients at a single center. Second, the follow-up duration was relatively short; accordingly, long-term outcomes are unclear. Third, single antigen assays were not performed in all patients; therefore, some DSA could be missed. Finally, we did not determine the proximal mechanism underlying the observed link between high PRA and outcome.

Despite these limitations, this study was the first to evaluate the distribution of pre-lung transplantation anti-HLA antibodies in Asia, where a relatively small volume of lung transplants has been performed. Since there is very little data reported on the status of pBOS or BOS after lung transplantation in Asia, it may be meaningful in spite of these limitations.

Considering the results of this study, patients with a high MFI before lung transplantation should be considered for desensitization, close observation and careful post-op management because high-grade PGD, which is highly related to short-term mortality, was more common in patients with high MFI than in those with low MFI in Asia.

Conclusions
The proportion of patients with high PRA and high MFI were not high in lung transplant recipients in Korea, and high MFI was related to high-grade PGD, but not to pBOS or BOS. Caution is needed in the management of sensitized patients and further prospective and long-term studies are required.

Abbreviations
BMI: body mass index; BOS: bronchiolitis obliterans syndrome; CDC: complement dependent cytotoxicity; CMV: cytomegalovirus; COPD: chronic obstructive lung disease; DSA: donor-specific antibodies; FEF_{25-75}: forced expiratory flow at 25–75%; FEV_1: forced expiratory volume in 1 s; HLA: human leukocyte antigen; HSCT: hematopoietic stem cell transplantation; IPF: idiopathic pulmonary fibrosis; IRB: Institutional Review Board; ISHLT: International Society for Heart and Lung Transplantation; MFI: mean fluorescence intensity; PGD: primary graft dysfunction; PRA: panel-reactive antibodies; TB: tuberculosis

Acknowledgements
None

Funding
None

Authors' contributions
SYK and JEP conceived and designed the study. All authors contributed to participant recruitment, and data collection. MSP, JHS, CYK and YSK described the usual care procedure and management. HCP and JGL are responsible for the intervention. SYK and JEP wrote the first draft of the manuscript. All authors critically evaluated the data, reviewed the manuscript, and approved the final manuscript.

Competing interests
The authors declare that they have no competing interests.

Author details
[1]Division of Pulmonology, Department of Internal Medicine, Severance Hospital, Institute of Chest Diseases, Yonsei University College of Medicine, 50-1, Yonsei-ro, Seodaemun-gu, Seoul, Republic of Korea. [2]Department of Thoracic and Cardiovascular Surgery, Severance Hospital, Yonsei University College of Medicine, Seoul, Republic of Korea. [3]Department of Pulmonary and Critical Care Medicine, Ajou University School of Medicine, Suwon, Republic of Korea.

References
1. Chambers DC, Yusen RD, Cherikh WS, Goldfarb SB, Kucheryavaya AY, Khusch K, Levvey BJ, Lund LH, Meiser B, Rossano JW, et al. The registry of the International Society for Heart and Lung Transplantation: thirty-fourth adult lung and heart-lung transplantation Report-2017; focus theme: allograft ischemic time. J Heart Lung Transplant. 2017;36(10):1047–59.
2. Tambur AR, Bray RA, Takemoto SK, Mancini M, Costanzo MR, Kobashigawa JA, D'Amico CL, Kanter KR, Berg A, Vega JD, et al. Flow cytometric detection of HLA-specific antibodies as a predictor of heart allograft rejection. Transplantation. 2000;70(7):1055–9.
3. Barama A, Oza U, Panek R, Belitsky P, MacDonald AS, Lawen J, McAlister V, Kiberd B. Effect of recipient sensitization (peak PRA) on graft outcome in haploidentical living related kidney transplants. Clin Transpl. 2000;14(3):212–7.
4. Bray RA, Nolen JD, Larsen C, Pearson T, Newell KA, Kokko K, Guasch A, Tso P, Mendel JB, Gebel HM. Transplanting the highly sensitized patient: the Emory algorithm. Am J Transplant Off J Am Soc Transplant Am Soc Transplant Surg. 2006;6(10):2307–15.
5. Appel JZ 3rd, Hartwig MG, Cantu E 3rd, Palmer SM, Reinsmoen NL, Davis RD. Role of flow cytometry to define unacceptable HLA antigens in lung transplant recipients with HLA-specific antibodies. Transplantation. 2006; 81(7):1049–57.
6. Leffell MS, Cherikh WS, Land G, Zachary AA. Improved definition of human leukocyte antigen frequencies among minorities and applicability to estimates of transplant compatibility. Transplantation. 2007;83(7):964–72.
7. Hadjiliadis D, Chaparro C, Reinsmoen NL, Gutierrez C, Singer LG, Steele MP, Waddell TK, Davis RD, Hutcheon MA, Palmer SM, et al. Pre-transplant panel reactive antibody in lung transplant recipients is associated with significantly worse post-transplant survival in a multicenter study. J Heart Lung Transplant. 2005;24(7 Suppl):S249–54.
8. Shah AS, Nwakanma L, Simpkins C, Williams J, Chang DC, Conte JV. Pretransplant panel reactive antibodies in human lung transplantation: an analysis of over 10,000 patients. Ann Thorac Surg. 2008;85(6):1919–24.
9. Gammie JS, Pham SM, Colson YL, Kawai A, Keenan RJ, Weyant RJ, Griffith BP. Influence of panel-reactive antibody on survival and rejection after lung transplantation. J Heart Lung Transplant. 1997;16(4):408–15.
10. Lau CL, Palmer SM, Posther KE, Howell DN, Reinsmoen NL, Massey HT, Tapson VF, Jaggers JJ, D'Amico TA, Davis RD Jr. Influence of panel-reactive antibodies on posttransplant outcomes in lung transplant recipients. Ann Thorac Surg. 2000;69(5):1520–4.
11. Smith MA, Sundaresan S, Mohanakumar T, Trulock EP, Lynch JP, Phelan DL, Cooper JD, Patterson GA. Effect of development of antibodies to HLA and cytomegalovirus mismatch on lung transplantation survival and development of bronchiolitis obliterans syndrome. J Thorac Cardiovasc Surg. 1998;116(5):812–20.

12. Wisser W, Wekerle T, Zlabinger G, Senbaclavaci O, Zuckermann A, Klepetko W, Wolner E. Influence of human leukocyte antigen matching on long-term outcome after lung transplantation. J Heart Lung Transplant. 1996;15(12):1209–16.

13. Love RB, Meyer KC, Devito-Haynes LD, Ulschmid S, Leverson GE, Van Der Bij W, De Boer WJ, Hepkema BG, Cornwell RD, Woolley DS, et al. Effect of HLA-DR mismatch on lung transplant outcome. J Heart Lung Transplant. 2001; 20(2):177.

14. Quantz MA, Bennett LE, Meyer DM, Novick RJ. Does human leukocyte antigen matching influence the outcome of lung transplantation? An analysis of 3,549 lung transplantations. J Heart Lung Transplant. 2000;19(5):473–9.

15. Kim M, Townsend KR, Wood IG, Boukedes S, Guleria I, Gabardi S, El-Chemaly S, Camp PC, Chandraker AK, Milford EL, et al. Impact of pretransplant anti-HLA antibodies on outcomes in lung transplant candidates. Am J Respir Crit Care Med. 2014;189(10):1234–9.

16. Christie JD, Edwards LB, Kucheryavaya AY, Benden C, Dipchand AI, Dobbels F, Kirk R, Rahmel AO, Stehlik J, Hertz MI. The registry of the International Society for Heart and Lung Transplantation: 29th adult lung and heart-lung transplant report-2012. J Heart Lung Transplant. 2012;31(10):1073–86.

17. Verleden GM, Raghu G, Meyer KC, Glanville AR, Corris P. A new classification system for chronic lung allograft dysfunction. J Heart Lung Transplant. 2014; 33(2):127–33.

18. Estenne M, Maurer JR, Boehler A, Egan JJ, Frost A, Hertz M, Mallory GB, Snell GI, Yousem S. Bronchiolitis obliterans syndrome 2001: an update of the diagnostic criteria. J Heart Lung Transplant. 2002;21(3):297–310.

19. Botha P, Archer L, Anderson RL, Lordan J, Dark JH, Corris PA, Gould K, Fisher AJ. Pseudomonas aeruginosa colonization of the allograft after lung transplantation and the risk of bronchiolitis obliterans syndrome. Transplantation. 2008;85(5):771–4.

20. Heng D, Sharples LD, McNeil K, Stewart S, Wreghitt T, Wallwork J. Bronchiolitis obliterans syndrome: incidence, natural history, prognosis, and risk factors. J Heart Lung Transplant. 1998;17(12):1255–63.

21. Snell GI, Westall GP. The contribution of airway ischemia and vascular remodelling to the pathophysiology of bronchiolitis obliterans syndrome and chronic lung allograft dysfunction. Current opinion in organ transplantation. 2010;15(5):558–62.

22. Gebel HM, Bray RA. Sensitization and sensitivity: defining the unsensitized patient. Transplantation. 2000;69(7):1370–4.

23. Patel JK, Kobashigawa JA. Thoracic organ transplantation: laboratory methods. Methods in molecular biology (Clifton, NJ). 2013;1034:127–43.

24. Couzi L, Araujo C, Guidicelli G, Bachelet T, Moreau K, Morel D, Robert G, Wallerand H, Moreau JF, Taupin JL, et al. Interpretation of positive flow cytometric crossmatch in the era of the single-antigen bead assay. Transplantation. 2011;91(5):527–35.

25. Smith JD, Ibrahim MW, Newell H, Danskine AJ, Soresi S, Burke MM, Rose ML, Carby M. Pre-transplant donor HLA-specific antibodies: characteristics causing detrimental effects on survival after lung transplantation. J Heart Lung Transplant. 2014;33(10):1074–82.

26. Zazueta OE, Preston SE, Moniodis A, Fried S, Kim M, Townsend K, Wood I, Boukedes S, Guleria I, Camp P, et al. The presence of Pretransplant HLA antibodies does not impact the development of chronic lung allograft dysfunction or CLAD-related death. Transplantation. 2017;101(9):2207–12.

27. Chung BH, Choi BS, Oh EJ, Park CW, Kim JI, Moon IS, Kim YS, Yang CW. Clinical impact of the baseline donor-specific anti-human leukocyte antigen antibody measured by Luminex single antigen assay in living donor kidney transplant recipients after desensitization therapy. Transplant international : official journal of the European Society for Organ Transplantation. 2014;27(1):49–59.

28. Brugiere O, Thabut G, Suberbielle C, Reynaud-Gaubert M, Thomas P, Pison C, Saint Raymond C, Mornex JF, Bertocchi M, Dromer C, et al. Relative impact of human leukocyte antigen mismatching and graft ischemic time after lung transplantation. J Heart Lung Transplant. 2008;27(6):628–34.

29. Song SH, Kim MS, Lee JJ, Ju MK, Lee JG, Lee J, Choi JS, Choi GH, Kim SI, Joo DJ. Effect of donor-specific antibodies and panel reactive antibodies in living donor liver transplant recipients. Annals of surgical treatment and research. 2015;88(2):100–5.

30. Rose ML, Smith JD. Clinical relevance of complement-fixing antibodies in cardiac transplantation. Hum Immunol. 2009;70(8):605–9.

31. Schulman LL, Weinberg AD, McGregor C, Galantowicz ME, Suciu-Foca NM, Itescu S. Mismatches at the HLA-DR and HLA-B loci are risk factors for acute rejection after lung transplantation. Am J Respir Crit Care Med. 1998;157(6 Pt 1):1833–7.

32. Peltz M, Edwards LB, Jessen ME, Torres F, Meyer DM. HLA mismatches influence lung transplant recipient survival, bronchiolitis obliterans and rejection: implications for donor lung allocation. J Heart Lung Transplant. 2011;30(4):426–34.

33. Sundaresan S, Mohanakumar T, Smith MA, Trulock EP, Lynch J, Phelan D, Cooper JD, Patterson GA. HLA-A locus mismatches and development of antibodies to HLA after lung transplantation correlate with the development of bronchiolitis obliterans syndrome. Transplantation. 1998; 65(5):648–53.

34. van den Berg JW, Hepkema BG, Geertsma A, Koeter GH, Postma DS, de Boer WJ, Lems SP, van der Bij W. Long-term outcome of lung transplantation is predicted by the number of HLA-DR mismatches. Transplantation. 2001; 71(3):368–73.

35. Chalermskulrat W, Neuringer IP, Schmitz JL, Catellier DJ, Gurka MJ, Randell SH, Aris RM. Human leukocyte antigen mismatches predispose to the severity of bronchiolitis obliterans syndrome after lung transplantation. Chest. 2003;123(6):1825–31.

36. Jaramillo A, Smith MA, Phelan D, Sundaresan S, Trulock EP, Lynch JP, Cooper JD, Patterson GA, Mohanakumar T. Development of ELISA-detected anti-HLA antibodies precedes the development of bronchiolitis obliterans syndrome and correlates with progressive decline in pulmonary function after lung transplantation. Transplantation. 1999;67(8):1155–61.

9

A case of allergic bronchopulmonary aspergillosis successfully treated with mepolizumab

Takeshi Terashima*[iD], Taro Shinozaki, Eri Iwami, Takahiro Nakajima and Tatsu Matsuzaki

Abstract

Background: Allergic bronchopulmonary aspergillosis (ABPA) is an allergic pulmonary disease comprising a complex hypersensitivity reaction to *Aspergillus fumigatus*. Clinical features of ABPA are wheezing, mucoid impaction, and pulmonary infiltrates. Oral corticosteroids and anti-fungal agents are standard therapy for ABPA, but long-term use of systemic corticosteroids often causes serious side effects.

Case presentation: A 64-year-old woman was diagnosed with ABPA based on a history of bronchial asthma (from 40 years of age), elevated total IgE, the presence of serum precipitating antibodies and elevated specific IgE antibody to *A. fumigatus*, and pulmonary infiltration. Bronchoscopy showed eosinophilic mucoid impaction. Systemic corticosteroid therapy was initiated, and her symptoms disappeared. Peripheral eosinophilia and pulmonary infiltration recurred five months after cessation of corticosteroid treatment. Systemic corticosteroids were re-initiated and itraconazole was added as an anti-fungal agent. The patient was free of corticosteroids, aside from treatment with a short course of systemic corticosteroids for asthma exacerbation, and clinically stable with itraconazole and asthma treatments for 3 years. In 2017, she experienced significant deterioration. Laboratory examination revealed marked eosinophilia (3017/μL) and a chest computed tomography (CT) scan demonstrated pulmonary infiltration in the left upper lobe and mucoid impaction in both lower lobes. The patient was treated with high-dose inhaled corticosteroid/long-acting beta-agonist, a long-acting muscarinic antagonist, a leukotriene receptor antagonist, and theophylline; spirometry revealed a forced expiratory volume in 1 s (FEV_1) of 1.01 L. An uncontrolled asthma state was indicated by an Asthma Control Test (ACT) score of 18. Mepolizumab, 100 mg every 4 weeks, was initiated for the treatment of severe bronchial asthma with ABPA exacerbation. Bronchial asthma symptoms dramatically improved, and ACT score increased to 24, by 4 weeks after mepolizumab treatment. Peripheral eosinophil count decreased to 174/μL. Spirometry revealed improvement of lung function (FEV_1: 1.28 L). A chest CT scan demonstrated the disappearance of pulmonary infiltration and mucoid impaction.

Conclusions: To our knowledge, this is the first case of ABPA to be treated with mepolizumab. Dramatic improvements were observed in symptoms, lung function, peripheral eosinophil counts, and chest images. Mepolizumab could serve as an alternative treatment with the potential to provide a systemic corticosteroid-sparing effect.

Keywords: Mepolizumab, Allergic bronchopulmonary aspergillosis, Bronchial asthma, Eosinophilia

* Correspondence: terasima@tdc.ac.jp
Department of Respiratory Medicine, Tokyo Dental College Ichikawa General Hospital, 5-11-13, Sugano, Ichikawa, Chiba 272-0824, Japan

Background

Allergic bronchopulmonary aspergillosis (ABPA) is an allergic pulmonary disease with a complex hypersensitivity reaction to *Aspergillus fumigatus*. Clinical characteristics of ABPA include recurrent asthma exacerbations; chest images of affected patients reveal mucoid impaction, pulmonary eosinophilic infiltrates, and bronchiectasis. Allergic immune reactions can be observed, such as peripheral eosinophilia and elevated total IgE, as well as the presence of serum precipitating antibodies and elevated specific IgE antibody to *A. fumigatus* [1, 2]. Because ABPA is caused by a hypersensitivity reaction to bronchial colonization by *A. fumigatus*, standard therapy comprises a combination of systemic corticosteroids (to attenuate allergic inflammation) and anti-fungal agents (to reduce the fungal load). Serious side effects of corticosteroids are a notable risk in patients undergoing long-term treatment. In this report, we describe a case of severe bronchial asthma with ABPA that was successfully treated with mepolizumab, a recombinant anti-IL-5 antibody.

Case presentation

A 64-year-old woman was diagnosed with bronchial asthma at 40 years of age. Initially, her symptoms were mild and controlled with a moderate dose of inhaled corticosteroid (ICS) and a short-acting beta-agonist. She reported a medical history of eosinophilic rhinitis. At 60 years of age, she experienced frequent wheezing exertion; spirometry revealed forced expiratory volume in 1 s (FEV_1)/forced vital capacity (FVC) of 62.6%, FEV_1 of 0.92 L, and peak expiratory flow of 3.37 L/s. She was diagnosed with severe bronchial asthma and treated with an ICS/long-acting beta-agonist (LABA), a long-acting muscarinic antagonist (LAMA), a leukotriene receptor antagonist (LTRA), and theophylline. The patient exhibited purulent sputum, despite these medications, for 3 months and was referred to our hospital in 2013 because of persistent fever that had lasted 2 weeks. Laboratory examination showed a white blood cell count of 12,700/µL (27% eosinophils), C-reactive protein level of 11.79 mg/dL, serum IgE level of 3400 IU/mL, and positive *Aspergillus*-specific IgE (6.24 UA/mL). Serum proteinase-3 anti-neutrophil cytoplasmic antibody (ANCA) and myeloperoxidase-ANCA were negative (< 1.0 U/mL). Precipitating antibody to *Aspergillus* was positive by the technique of Ouchterlony. A chest radiograph showed opacity in the right lower field; a computed tomography (CT) scan showed infiltration in the right middle and lower lobes, as well as mucoid impaction in both lower lobes (Fig. 1). Bronchoscopy revealed a mucoid impaction in the right middle lobe bronchus (Fig. 2); the differential specimen count obtained by bronchial washing from the right middle lobe was

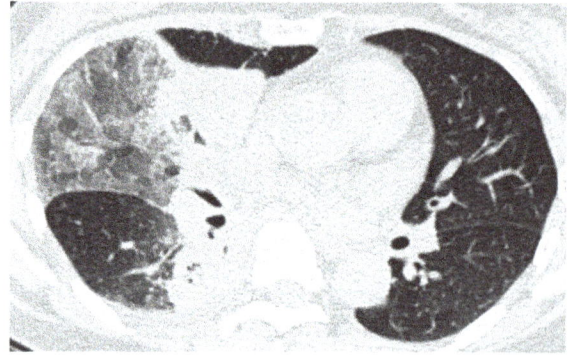

Fig. 1 Computed tomography image of the chest showing infiltration in the right middle and lower lobes

composed of 38% eosinophils. Notably, the bronchial washing culture yielded no bacteria or fungus. The patient was diagnosed with ABPA based on the history of bronchial asthma, elevated total IgE, the presence of serum precipitating antibody and elevated specific IgE antibody to *A. fumigatus*, and pulmonary infiltration. Systemic corticosteroid therapy (prednisone 30 mg/day) was initiated, and the patient's symptoms dissipated. The corticosteroids were gradually tapered, then discontinued after 3 months. The patient developed "moon face" as a consequence of corticosteroid treatment; peripheral eosinophilia and pulmonary infiltration appeared again, 5 months after the cessation of corticosteroid treatment. Systemic corticosteroids (prednisone 10 mg/day) were re-initiated, and itraconazole (200 mg/day) was added as

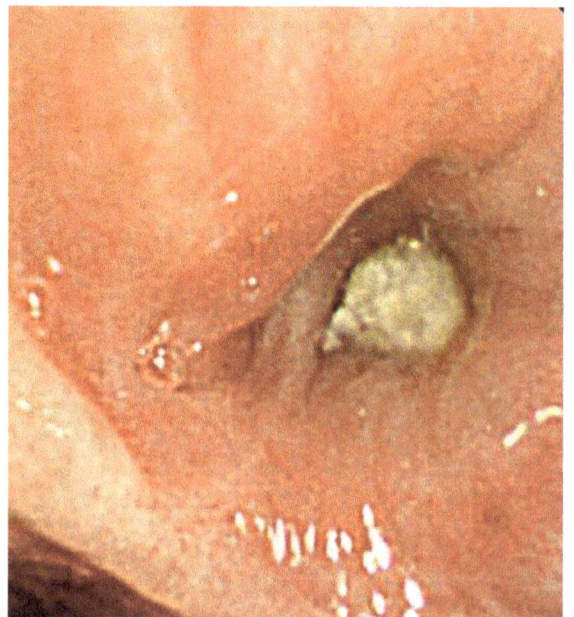

Fig. 2 Bronchoscopic findings showing mucus plugging within the right middle lobe bronchus

an anti-fungal agent. Systemic corticosteroid treatment was again tapered and discontinued after 4 weeks. The patient was free of corticosteroids, aside from treatment with a short course of systemic corticosteroids for asthma exacerbation, and clinically stable with itraconazole and asthma treatments for 3 years.

In 2017, the patient experienced significant deterioration. She complained of wheezing, productive cough, and dyspnea on effort. Laboratory examination revealed marked peripheral eosinophilia ($3017/\mu L$) and a chest CT scan demonstrated pulmonary infiltration in the left upper lobe, as well as mucoid impaction in both lower lobes (Fig. 3). The patient was treated with high-dose ICS/LABA, LAMA, LTRA, and theophylline; spirometry showed severe airway obstruction (FEV_1/FVC: 66.9%; FEV_1: 1.01 L). An uncontrolled asthma state was indicated by an Asthma Control Test (ACT) score of 18. Mepolizumab (100 mg every 4 weeks) was initiated for the treatment of severe bronchial asthma with ABPA exacerbation. Bronchial asthma symptoms were dramatically improved, and ACT score was increased to 24 at 4 weeks after mepolizumab treatment. Peripheral eosinophil count decreased from $3017/\mu L$ to $230/\mu L$ and $174/\mu L$, 1 and 4 weeks after mepolizumab, respectively. Spirometry showed improvement of lung function (FEV_1/FVC: 69.8%; FEV_1: 1.25 L after 1 week; FEV_1/FVC: 69.2%, FEV_1: 1.28 L after 4 weeks). The serum level of IgE did not change after mepolizumab. A chest CT scan demonstrated the disappearance of pulmonary infiltration and mucoid impaction (Fig. 3).

Discussion and conclusions

To our knowledge, this is the first case of ABPA to be treated with mepolizumab. Dramatic improvements were observed in symptoms, lung function, peripheral eosinophil counts, and chest images.

Our patient was diagnosed with ABPA because the observed clinical, radiologic, and laboratory findings met essential criteria for ABPA that were proposed in 2013, which include: 1) predisposing conditions: asthma or cystic fibrosis; 2) obligatory criteria: total baseline serum IgE > 1000 IU/mL, as well as positive immediate hypersensitivity skin test or elevated specific IgE to *A. fumigatus*; 3) supportive criteria: eosinophilia > 500 cells/μL, serum precipitating or IgG antibodies to *A. fumigatus*, and consistent radiologic opacities [1]. The radiologic features include transient (consolidation, nodules, and tram-track or gloved-finger appearance) or permanent (bronchiectasis or fibrosis) pulmonary opacities. Although persistent fever, which was seen in our case, is not a common symptom of ABPA, fever is included as one of the symptoms of ABPA [1, 3]. Differential diagnoses in our case included eosinophilic pneumonia and eosinophilic granulomatosis with polyangiitis. The predominant patterns of CT findings in acute eosinophilic pneumonia are consolidation

and/or ground-glass opacity, frequently accompanied by interlobular septal thickening [4]. Positive IgE against *A. fumigatus* and mucoid impaction (as documented by imaging and bronchoscopy) suggested ABPA, rather than acute eosinophilic pneumonia, in our case. The absence of extrathoracic manifestation and negative ANCA excluded the possibility of eosinophilic granulomatosis with polyangiitis.

ABPA is a severe type of allergic asthma that occurs in approximately 10% of patients with severe asthma. Although a combination of systemic corticosteroids and antifungal agents is a standard therapy, there is a risk of serious side effects with long-term use of systemic corticosteroids, such as "moon face," immunosuppression, diabetes, gastric ulcer, and osteoporosis. Omalizumab, a monoclonal antibody against IgE, has been used in ABPA treatment [5]. Reviews of ABPA cases, including 17 bronchial asthma cases that were treated with omalizumab, have shown beneficial effects such as reduced symptoms, decreased exacerbation rates, and corticosteroid-sparing effects [6]. The dose of omalizumab is determined by a patient's baseline total IgE level and body weight. The upper limit of the total IgE level is 1500 IU/mL; omalizumab can be administered up to a maximum dose of 600 mg every 2 weeks [7]. Notably, many patients with ABPA exceed the current dosing parameters of omalizumab because of their high total IgE levels, which is a limitation of omalizumab therapy [8].

Mepolizumab is a monoclonal antibody against interleukin-5, a cytokine that releases eosinophils from bone marrow and activates their functions [9]. Mepolizumab has been shown to reduce the frequency of asthma exacerbations in patients with severe eosinophilic asthma [10]. Moreover, mepolizumab exhibited a corticosteroid-sparing effect in eosinophilic asthma patients who require daily systemic corticosteroids [11]. A post hoc analysis showed that mepolizumab was effective for patients, regardless of prior history of omalizumab use; moreover, most patients in the prior omalizumab use subgroup reported that omalizumab was ineffective [12]. Total IgE level at the start of therapy does not affect the efficacy or adverse effects of mepolizumab, and mepolizumab is recommended as one of the therapeutic options in cases of severe eosinophilic asthma with total IgE > 1500 IU/mL [13].

The mechanisms underlying ABPA exacerbation are complex. The increased secretion of interleukin-4 and interleukin-5 from peripheral cells from patients with ABPA suggests that TH2 inflammation contributes to the pathogenesis of ABPA [14]. Notably, elevated levels of IgE and specific antibody against *A. fumigatus* suggested that clinical benefits may result from treatment with omalizumab; additionally, a marked eosinophilia in peripheral blood and bronchial washing suggested that beneficial effects may result from treatment with mepolizumab. The

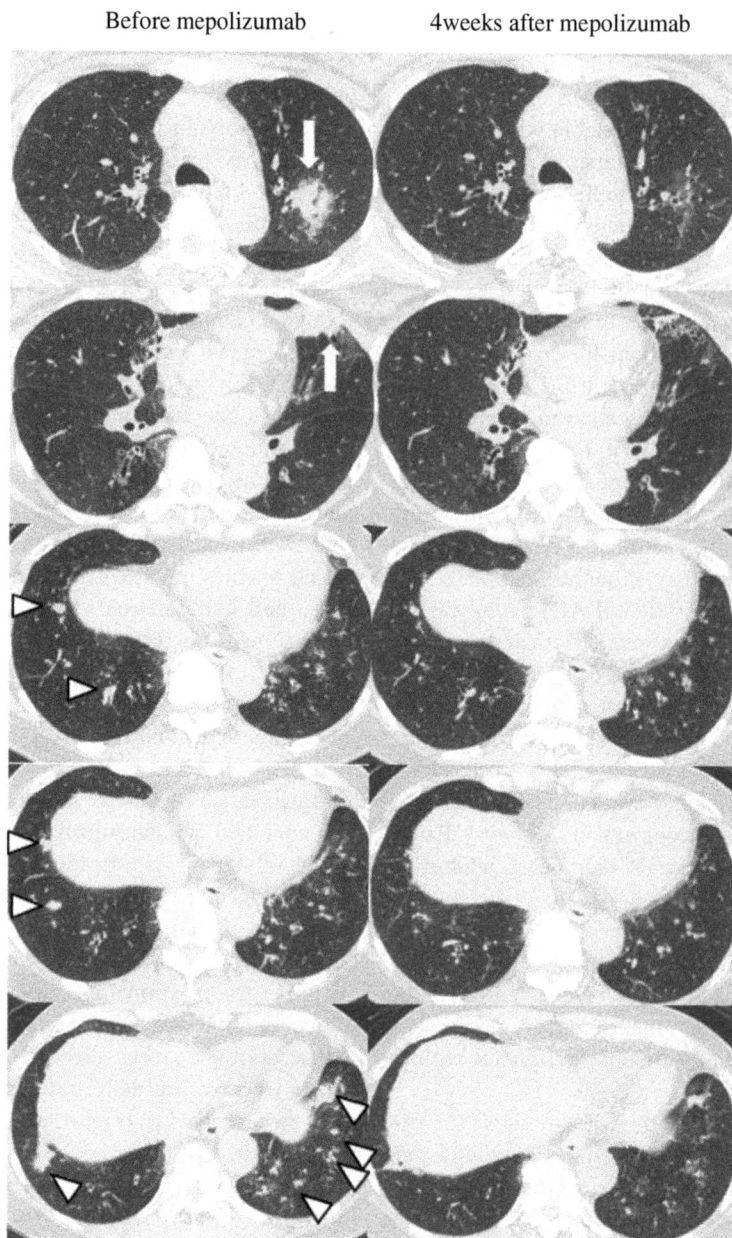

Fig. 3 High resolution computed tomography image of the chest showing pulmonary opacities (arrows) in the left upper lobe and mucus plugging (arrow heads) within both lower lobes, prior to mepolizumab treatment. These opacities and mucus plugging were attenuated at 4 weeks after mepolizumab treatment

synergistic effects of omalizumab and mepolizumab have been reported in a patient with severe and steroid-dependent ABPA [15]. Our case showed that a single dose of mepolizumab alone induced a 6-point increase in ACT score, 270-mL increase in FEV_1 and a 94% reduction in peripheral eosinophil counts; moreover, it attenuated pulmonary infiltration and mucoid impaction. An ACT score of ≤19 indicates uncontrolled asthma and a 3-point change in ACT score is clinically significant [16]. The improvement of lung function in our case appears to be dramatic, compared with the study of patients with severe eosinophilic asthma, in which the mean increase in FEV_1 was 100 mL after mepolizumab therapy [10].

It has been reported that an attempt to discontinue omalizumab resulted in exacerbation, which was resolved with reinstitution of omalizumab [6]. In our case, we have maintained mepolizumab as treatment for severe asthma with ABPA. Further observation is necessary to determine the optimal period of mepolizumab treatment.

In this report, we described a case of severe bronchial asthma with ABPA that was successfully treated with mepolizumab. Mepolizumab could serve as an alternative treatment with the potential for systemic corticosteroid-sparing effects. Double-blind, placebo-controlled trials are necessary to establish the efficacy and safety of this novel therapeutic intervention for ABPA.

Abbreviations

ABPA: Allergic bronchopulmonary aspergillosis; ACT: Asthma control test; ANCA: Anti-neutrophil cytoplasmic antibody; CT: Computed tomography; FEV_1: Forced expiratory volume in 1 s; FVC: Forced vital capacity; ICS: Inhaled corticosteroid; LABA: Long-acting beta-agonist; LAMA: Long-acting muscarinic antagonist; LTRA: Leukotriene receptor antagonist

Acknowledgements
Not applicable.

Funding
The authors declare that no funding was received for this study.

Authors' contributions
TT contributed to decision of treatment, collecting clinical data, data analysis, and writing the manuscript. TS, EI, TN, and TM contributed to the interpretation of clinical data and chest images. All authors have read and approved the final manuscript.

Competing interests
The authors declare that they have no competing interests.

References

1. Agarwal R, Chakrabarti A, Shah A, Gupta D, Meis JF, Guleria R, et al. Allergic bronchopulmonary aspergillosis: review of literature and proposal of new diagnostic and classification criteria. Clin Exp Allergy. 2013;43:850–73.
2. Knutsen AP. Allergic bronchopulmonary aspergillosis in asthma. Expert Rev Clin Immunol. 2017;13:11–4.
3. Shah A, Panjabi C. Allergic bronchopulmonary aspergillosis: a perplexing clinical entity. Allergy Asthma Immunol Res. 2016;8:282–97.
4. Yeon JJ, Kim K-I, Im JS, Chang HL, Ki NL, Ki NK, et al. Eosinophilic lung diseases: a clinical, radiologic, and pathologic overview. Radiographics. 2007;27:617–37.
5. Van Der Ent CK, Hoekstra H, Rijkers GT. Successful treatment of allergic bronchopulmonary aspergillosis with recombinant anti-IgE antibody. Thorax. 2007;62:276–7.
6. Li J-X, Fan L-C, Li M-H, Cao W-J, Xu J-F. Beneficial effects of omalizumab therapy in allergic bronchopulmonary aspergillosis: a synthesis review of published literature. Respir Med. 2017;122:33–42.
7. Jaffe JS, Massanari M. In response to dosing omalizumab in allergic asthma. J Allergy Clin Immunol. 2007;119:255–6.
8. Agarwal R, Gupta D, Aggarwal AN, Saxena AK, Chakrabarti A, Jindal SK. Clinical significance of hyperattenuating mucoid impaction in allergic bronchopulmonary aspergillosis: an analysis of 155 patients. Chest. 2007;132:1183–90.
9. Sanderson CJ. Interleukin-5, eosinophils, and disease. Blood. 1992;79:3101–9.
10. Ortega HG, Liu MC, Pavord ID, Brusselle GG, FitzGerald JM, Chetta A, et al. Mepolizumab treatment in patients with severe eosinophilic asthma. New Engl J Med. 2014;371:1198–207.
11. Bel EH, Wenzel SE, Thompson PJ, Prazma CM, Keene ON, Yancey SW, et al. Oral glucocorticoid-sparing effect of mepolizumab in eosinophilic asthma. New Engl J Med. 2014;371:1189–97.
12. Magnan A, Bourdin A, Prazma CM, Albers FC, Price RG, Yancey SW, et al. Treatment response with mepolizumab in severe eosinophilic asthma patients with previous omalizumab treatment. Allergy Eur J Allergy Clin Immunol. 2016;71:1335–44.
13. Menzella F, Galeone C, Bertolini F, Castagnetti C, Facciolongo N. Innovative treatments for severe refractory asthma: how to choose the right option for the right patient? J Asthma Allerg. 2017;10:237.
14. Rathore VB, Johnson B, Fink JN, Kelly KJ, Greenberger PA, Kurup VP. T cell proliferation and cytokine secretion to T cell epitopes of asp f 2 in ABPA patients. Clin Immunol. 2001;100:228–35.
15. Itman MC, Lenington J, Bronson S, Ayars AG. Combination omalizumab and mepolizumab therapy for refractory allergic bronchopulmonary aspergillosis. J Allergy Clin Immunol Pract. 2017;5:1137–9.
16. Schatz M, Kosinski M, Yarlas AS, Hanlon J, Watson ME, Jhingran P. The minimally important difference of the asthma control test. J Allergy Clin Immunol. 2009;124:719–23.

10

Acute effects of combined exercise and oscillatory positive expiratory pressure therapy on sputum properties and lung diffusing capacity in cystic fibrosis

Thomas Radtke[1,2*], Lukas Böni[3], Peter Bohnacker[3], Marion Maggi-Beba[2], Peter Fischer[3], Susi Kriemler[1], Christian Benden[4] and Holger Dressel[2]

Abstract

Background: Regular airway clearance by chest physiotherapy and/or exercise is critical to lung health in cystic fibrosis (CF). Combination of cycling exercise and chest physiotherapy using the Flutter® device on sputum properties has not yet been investigated.

Methods: This prospective, randomized crossover study compared a single bout of continuous cycling exercise at moderate intensity (experiment A, control condition) vs a combination of interval cycling exercise plus Flutter® (experiment B). Sputum properties (viscoelasticity, yield stress, solids content, spinnability, and ease of sputum expectoration), pulmonary diffusing capacity for nitric oxide ($DLNO$) and carbon monoxide ($DLCO$) were assessed at rest, directly and 45 min post-exercise (recovery) at 2 consecutive visits. Primary outcome was change in sputum viscoelasticity (G', storage modulus; G", loss modulus) over a broad frequency range ($0.1–100$ rad.s^{-1}).

Results: 15 adults with CF (FEV_1 range 24–94% predicted) completed all experiments. No consistent differences between experiments were observed for G' and G" and other sputum properties, except for ease of sputum expectoration during recovery favoring experiment A. $DLNO$, $DLCO$, alveolar volume (V_A) and pulmonary capillary blood volume (V_{cap}) increased during experiment A, while $DLCO$ and V_{cap} increased during experiment B (all $P < 0.05$). We found no differences in absolute changes in pulmonary diffusing capacity and its components between experiments, except a higher V_A immediately post-exercise favoring experiment A ($P = 0.032$).

Conclusions: The additional use of the Flutter® to moderate intensity interval cycling exercise has no measurable effect on the viscoelastic properties of sputum compared to moderate intensity continuous cycling alone. Elevations in diffusing capacity represent an acute exercise-induced effect not sustained post-exercise.

Keywords: Lung disease, Sputum viscoelasticity, Diffusing capacity for nitric oxide, Exercise, Airway clearance, Mucus

* Correspondence: thomas.radtke@uzh.ch
[1]Epidemiology, Biostatistics and Prevention Institute (EBPI), University of Zurich, Zurich, Switzerland
[2]Division of Occupational and Environmental Medicine, University of Zurich and University Hospital Zurich, Zurich, Switzerland
Full list of author information is available at the end of the article

Background

Cystic fibrosis (CF) is the most common genetic life-limiting disease in Caucasians caused by abnormalities in CF conductance transmembrane protein function. Depletion of airway surface liquid, dehydrated mucus, chronic inflammation and infection contribute to accumulation of secretions and subsequent progressive lung damage in CF [1]. Regular airway clearance is therefore of critical importance to lung health in CF. Exercise and chest physiotherapy are accepted airway clearance techniques (ACT's) in CF, belonging to the current top ten research priorities [2]. There are a number of different ACT's such as the active cycle of breathing technique, high-frequency chest wall oscillations, positive expiratory pressure (PEP) and oscillatory PEP. Oscillatory PEP with the Flutter® is equally effective compared to other ACT's [3] and has been shown to favorably alter respiratory flow [4], to increase sputum expectoration [5] and to reduce sputum viscoelasticity [6, 7] in CF.

Exercise alone or in combination with chest physiotherapy improves airway clearance and sputum expectoration [6, 8], but the exact mechanisms are not fully understood. Moreover, acute exercise is thought to facilitate mucociliary clearance by increased shear stress on airway epithelium and ciliary beat frequency as a result of an increased ventilation [9], improved water content of mucus [10] and increased trunk oscillations during weight bearing exercises such as walking or running [11]. Recently, moderate intensity exercise has been identified as 'optimal training intensity' for individuals with mild to moderate CF lung disease due to improvements in bronchodilation and pulmonary diffusing capacity and prevention of airflow restriction compared to vigorously intense exercise [12]. Enhanced mucus clearance might potentially (at least in part) result in an improvement in pulmonary gas diffusion.

The aim of this study was to compare a single bout of moderate intensity cycling exercise incorporating a breathing therapy device, the Flutter®, with a single bout of moderate intensity cycling exercise alone on sputum viscoelasticity (primary endpoint) and pulmonary diffusing capacity in adults with CF. We hypothesized that the combination of a high ventilation during cycling exercise in combination with increased oscillatory shear stress (Flutter®) yields greater improvements in sputum viscoelasticity compared to cycling exercise alone.

Methods

Study design

We conducted a prospective, randomized, controlled crossover trial (Clinicaltrials.gov, NCT02750722). Adults with CF were invited to our laboratory facility on three different occasions. At the first study visit, the patients provided a sputum sample, performed pulmonary function testing and cardiopulmonary exercise testing (CPET). At the second and third study visit, patients provided sputum samples, performed pulmonary function testing and, depending on randomization, performed either continuous cycling exercise at moderate intensity without Flutter® (Experiment A, control condition) or moderate intensity interval cycling exercise incorporating Flutter® therapy (Experiment B, experimental condition). The detailed exercise protocol including measurements and assessments during study visit 2 and 3 are shown in Fig. 1.

Study participants

Individuals with CF were recruited from the Adult CF Center at the University Hospital Zurich, Switzerland, between June 2016 and January 2017. Patients aged 18 years and older with a confirmed diagnosis of CF able to provide sputum samples were included. Exclusion criteria were as follows: i) listing for lung transplantation or status post lung transplantation, ii) chronic pulmonary infection with *Burkholderia* cepacia complex, iii) unstable clinical condition (i.e., major hemoptysis or pneumothorax within the last 3 months, acute pulmonary exacerbation [13], intravenous antibiotic treatment during the last 4 weeks, change in pulmonary medication during the study period); iv) cardiac arrhythmias with exercise and v) requirement of additional oxygen with exercise. Ethical approval was obtained from the Cantonal Ethics Committee of Zurich (2015–00153), Switzerland. All patients provided written informed consent.

Randomization

We used central randomization to randomly allocate patients to the different experimental conditions (Experiment A or B). A person not involved in the study generated a list of random numbers using the statistical software package STATA (Version 12, StataCorp. 2012, College Station, Texas, USA). The list consisted of 30 random numbers, where even numbers represented the experimental condition 'A' and odd numbers the condition 'B'. The order of the experiments at study visit 2 and 3 was either 'A-B' or 'B-A'. At the first study visit, after written informed consent was obtained, the principal investigator (TR) called the person creating the list of random numbers to obtain information on the order of the exercise experiments for visit 2 and 3, respectively. The patient was immediately informed about the testing order for the following study visits.

Assessments

All tests were scheduled at the same time of the day (+ – 1 h deviation) to avoid any potential impact of diurnal variation on pulmonary function measurements [14]. The time period between study visit 1 and 3 was 8 ± 2 days, respectively. Patients were told to abstain from fatty meals (for 3 h), caffeine-containing substances (for 4 h) and to avoid vigorous physical exercise during the last 24-h prior to the study visits, respectively. Moreover, patients were told to abstain

Experiment A
Moderate continuous exercise

75% HR$_{peak}$

50%
HR$_{peak}$

Rest | Warm
up

0   30   0   3   6   12   16   30   0   45 (min)

Experiment B
Moderate interval exercise
plus Flutter®

75%   75%   75%   75%
HR$_{peak}$ HR$_{peak}$ HR$_{peak}$ HR$_{peak}$

50%
HR$_{peak}$

Rest | Warm
up   Flutter®   Flutter®   Flutter®   Flutter®

0   30   0   3   6   10   12   16   18   22   24   28   30   0   45 (min)

- Diffusing   - HR   - HR   - Diffusing capacity   - Diffusing capacity
  capacity   - V'O$_2$ - V'O$_2$ - Sputum sample   - Sputum sample
- Spirometry   - V'CO$_2$ - V'CO$_2$ - Ease of sputum   - Ease of sputum
- Sputum sample   - V'E   - V'E   expectoration   expectoration
- Ease of sputum   - VT   - VT   - SpO$_2$ - SpO$_2$
  expectoration   - f$_R$ - f$_R$
- Health status
- SpO$_2$

Fig. 1 Experimental study design. f$_R$, respiratory frequency; HR, heart rate; SpO$_2$, oxygen saturation; V'CO$_2$, carbon dioxide production; V'E, minute ventilation; V'O$_2$, oxygen consumption; VT, tidal volume. The grey shaded area represents the periods when the participants breathed through the mouthpiece for metabolic cart measurements

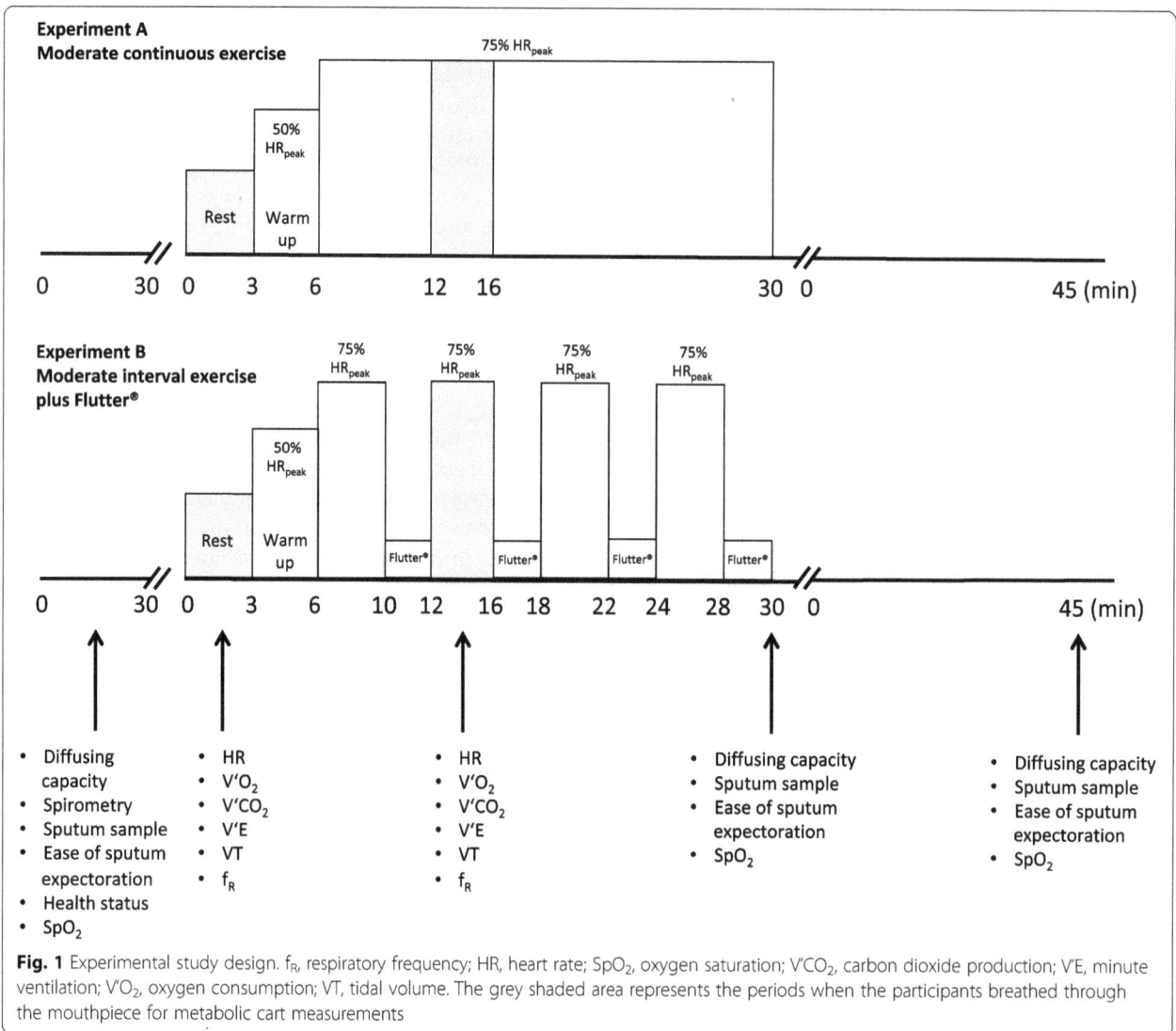

from their regular inhalation and airway clearance therapy on the day of the study visits. The following provides a short description of assessments methods.

Sputum samples

At the beginning of each study visit, one sputum sample was collected. At study visits 2 and 3, two additional samples were collected immediately post-exercise and again 45 min post-exercise, referred to as recovery (Fig. 1). Sputum was gently expectorated and collected into sterile and coded containers (cryotubes 5 mL, VWR). The containers were immediately stored at − 4 °C and transferred on ice into a deep freezer (− 80 °C) after each study visit.

Sputum rheology

Rheological measurements were performed on a MCR 702 rheometer (Anton Paar, Austria) in parallel plate mode, using sandblasted 25 mm diameter stainless steel plates

(PP25 S Anton Paar, Austria) and a gap size of 0.5 mm. First, a frequency sweep was performed (0.1–100 rad s^{-1}, γ = 1%) followed by an amplitude sweep (0.1–1000%, ω = 1 rad s^{-1}). The snap frozen sputum samples (− 80 °C) were transferred to the fridge (4 °C) at least 6 h before the measurement. The slowly thawed samples were then transferred from the cryotubes to the lower measuring plate using a 1 mL micropipette. The micropipette tips were cut in the front with a scalpel to have a larger die, thus minimizing shear on the sample. The upper plate was slowly lowered onto the sputum, and a solvent trap containing moist sponges was placed over the sample. Prior to measurements, the sputum was let to rest for five minutes. All measurements were performed temperature controlled at 20 °C. Inertia calculations are based on equations reported by Ewoldt et al. [15].

The spinnability of sputum describes its ability to form filaments, which provides valuable information about cohesion forces in the sputum [16]. At the end of each rheological measurement, the upper plate was separated from the lower plate at a constant velocity of 3.6 mm s^{-1} [17], which was filmed (iPhone 6, Apple) at 120 fps (Fig. 2a). The sputum formed a filament between the separating plates. The separation distance at which the sample broke ('spinnability') was extracted from the movie by counting the amount of frames from the onset of separation until filament breaking.

To estimate sputum solids content, 0.25 mL aliquots of sputum were filled in 1.5 mL HPLC vials (VWR, Switzerland) and weighed with a high precision scale (Mettler AE 163, Mettler Toledo, Switzerland). The samples were then dried for 24 h at 50 °C and a pressure of 100 mbar using a vacuum drying oven (SalvisLab, Switzerland) and subsequently weighed again. All rheological measurements were done by a person (PB) who was blinded with respect to the two different experimental conditions.

Ease of sputum expectoration was assessed on a 10 cm visual analogue scale (0 = very difficult and 10 = very easy). A blinded assessor, not involved in the study, measured the distance for all scales after completion of all study experiments.

Spirometry

Spirometry was always performed before diffusing capacity measurements with the patient in sitting position using a commercially available system (MasterScreen™ PFT Pro, Jaeger, PanGas AG Healthcare, Switzerland) according to American Thoracic Society/European Respiratory Society Standards [18]. All tests were performed pre-bronchodilation (i.e., withheld of short-acting bronchodilators and

anticholinergic drugs for at least 4 h, long-acting bronchodilators for at least 12 h, and once-daily, long-acting bronchodilators for at least 24 h). We calculated percent-predicted values for forced expiratory volume in 1 s (FEV$_1$) using reference equations from Quanjer et al. [19].

Pulmonary diffusing capacity

Details on the methods can be found elsewhere [20]. In brief, pulmonary diffusing capacity measurements were done in triplicate at rest and for the measurements done 45 min post-exercise (visit 2 and 3). If intra-session reproducibility criteria were not fulfilled additional measurements were performed [21]. Two maneuvers were performed immediately post-exercise (see Fig. 1 in the publication). In general, a 5 min pause was done between consecutive maneuvers to assure adequate elimination of test gas from the lungs [22]. For the analysis, we used the average value of the first two single-breaths tests for maneuvers performed at rest and 45 min post-exercise, when intra-session acceptability criteria were fulfilled [21]. If intra-session acceptability criteria were not fulfilled [21], the third single-breath test was considered and the average of the two highest test results was used. For the measurements immediately post-exercise (see Fig. 1 in the publication), the first test was used for statistical analysis. We calculated percent-predicted values for diffusing capacity for nitric oxide (DLNO) and carbon monoxide (DLCO), pulmonary capillary blood volume (V$_{cap}$) and the alveolar-capillary membrane diffusing capacity for carbon monoxide (DMCO) according to references equations published by Zavorsky et al. [21].

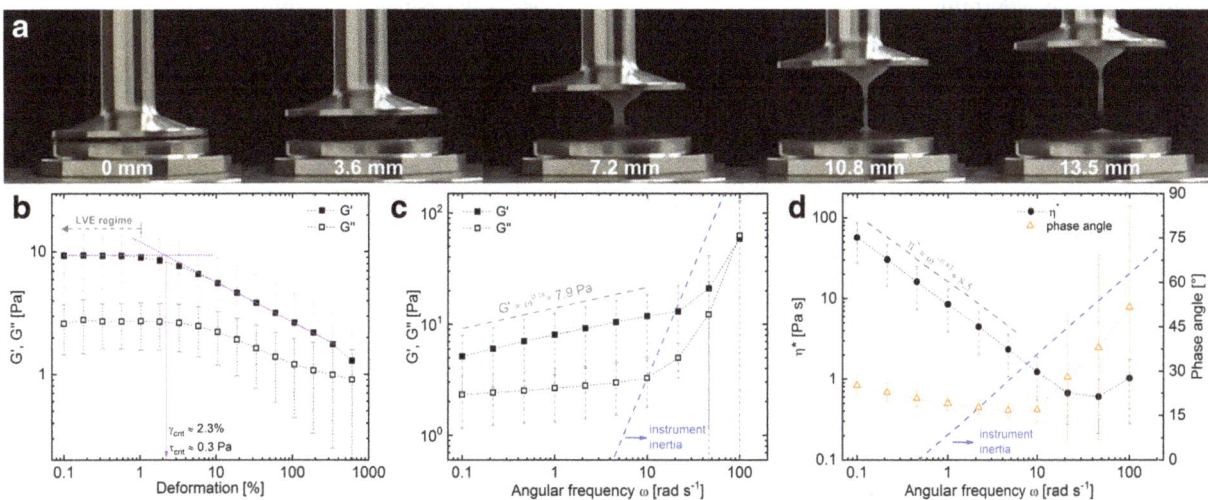

Fig. 2 Rheology and spinnability of cystic fibrosis sputum. (**a**) Spinnability of sputum was assessed at the end of rheological measurements by lifting up the upper plate at a constant velocity of 3.6 mm s^{-1}. (**b**) Amplitude sweep (at 1 rad s^{-1}) showing a linear viscoelastic (LVE) regime up to about 1% deformation. The dashed violet lines show the graphical determination of the dynamic yield point / stress. (**c, d**) Frequency sweeps depicting G′ (storage modulus), G″ (loss modulus) and η* (complex viscosity). The grey dashed lines represent the vertically shifted fitting curves (fitting between 0.1–10 rad s^{-1}). The blue dashed lines in (**b, c**) indicate the calculated instrument inertia limit

Cardiopulmonary exercise testing

Cardiopulmonary exercise testing (CPET) was performed on a cycle ergometer (custo ec 3000e, custo med GmbH, Ottobrunn, Germany) using the Godfrey Protocol [23]. The test started with a three-minute rest period followed by three-minutes of unloaded pedaling at 60–70 rpm. Afterwards, the workrate (W, watts) was increased every minute according to the patient's height: 10 W (< 120 cm), 15 W (120–150 cm) or 20 W (> 150 cm) [23]. The increment was individually adapted for patients with severely reduced lung function (i.e., $FEV_1 < 30\%$ predicted). After the patients had reached their maximal exercise performance, he/she rested for another three-minutes on the cycle ergometer (recovery phase).

The metabolic cart (Metalyzer®, Cortex Biophysik GmbH, Leipzig, Germany) was calibrated with gases of known standard concentrations before each test. Heart rate was measured with a Polar heart rate monitor (Polar RS400, Polar Electro, Oy, Kempele, Finland) and oxygen saturation (SpO_2) was continuously measured at the earlobe (Nonin® Xpod® Pure-SAT®,Nonin Medical, Inc, USA). Ratings of perceived exertion and dyspnea were evaluated at peak exercise by means of a 0–10 Borg scale [24]. One of the following criteria had to be fulfilled to ensure the test was maximal: 1) plateau in oxygen consumption ($V'O_2$) despite an increase in workrate; 2) peak heart rate over 85% of predicted [25], 3) respiratory exchange ratio (RER) > 1.05, 4) peak ventilation exceeded predicted maximum voluntary ventilation (calculated as $FEV_1 \times 35$) and 5) subjective impression of the supervisor. Maximal heart rates were used to calculate exercise intensities (50 and 75% of peak heart rate) for the cycling experiments at visit 2 and 3.

Patient-reported health status

Patient-reported health status was assessed with the Feeling Thermometer. The Feeling Thermometer is part of the EQ-5D, a common instrument used for healthy economic analyses and established by the EuroQol group [26]. The Feeling Thermometer is a modified visual analogue scale in form of a thermometer. The instrument has marked intervals from 0 (worst health state) to 100 (perfect health). We used the instrument to evaluate whether patients were in a stable health condition during the study.

Anthropometry

We measured each patient's height to the nearest 0.1 cm using a stadiometer (Seca). Body weight was measured to the nearest 0.5 kg at each study visit using a balanced scale (Seca, Model 791, Vogel & Halke).

Moderate cycling exercise with and without Flutter® therapy

At study visit 2 and 3, moderate intensity cycling exercise at 75% of the peak heart rate achieved during CPET was performed either continuously (experiment A) or in

4-min intervals (experiment B) interspersed with 2-min resting periods, during which breathing maneuvers were performed using the Flutter® (see Fig. 1). At rest and during cycling (minute 12–16′), patients respired through a mouthpiece connected to the metabolic cart to measure respiratory gases (Fig. 1). Heart rate was continuously monitored with a chest belt and heart rate monitor (Polar RS400, Polar Electro, Oy, Kempele, Finland) and SpO_2 with an earlobe pulse oximeter (Nonin® Xpod® PureSAT®,Nonin Medical, Inc, USA), respectively. The average value during 3 min at rest and during minutes 14–16 during exercise (steady-state conditions) were used for data analyses.

Flutter® breathing therapy

The Flutter® (VRP1, Eur. Patent. No: 0337990) is an airway clearance device providing oscillations during exhalation and vibrations of the airways aiming to facilitate mucus clearance in the airways. The Flutter® is a pipe like device with an oscillating stainless steel ball and a perforated cover. The device produces positive expiratory pressure and the angle at which the Flutter® is held determines the oscillation frequency of 6 to 20 Hz [27]. Exhalation through the Flutter® causes oscillation of the steel ball and produces rhythmic variations in positive expiratory pressure of 10 to 25 cm H_2O [28, 29]. Flutter® therapy increases peak expiratory flow and creates an expiratory airflow bias in CF [6], initiating mucociliary clearance mechanisms.

During experiment B, 6–10 breathing maneuvers were performed during each of the 2 min resting periods (Fig. 1) without forced expiratory technique. The breathing maneuvers started with a slightly deep inspiration, a 2–3 s end-inspiratory pause and a forced expiration lasting about 5 s while the patient was sitting on the cycle ergometer without pedaling. The Flutter® device was kept in neutral (horizontal) position to maximize the oscillation amplitude and to target a frequency range of 10–15 Hz [29], optimal for mucus clearance. All patients received proper instructions on the use of the device at the first study visit. Patients without experience with the Flutter® received a device at the end of visit 1 enabling practice at home before the second study visit.

Statistical analysis and sample size calculation

All statistical analyses were performed with the statistical software package SPSS version 23 (IBM Corp. Armont, NY, USA). Descriptive data are presented as median (interquartile range, IQR), mean ± SD or N (%). We used the non-parametric Friedman Test to test for differences in resting (pre-exercise) sputum properties, spirometry, pulmonary diffusing capacity and patient-reported health status between the three study visits. Differences in outcome variables between the three different time points (pre-exercise; immediately post-exercise and 45 min post-exercise, respectively) during each experimental condition were analyzed with the non-parametric Friedman test followed by a Wilcoxon-signed rank test, if changes over time in the Friedman test were significant ($P < 0.05$). We calculated absolute changes between the different time-points (i.e., post-exercise minus pre-exercise and 45 min post-exercise minus pre-exercise values) and compared the two experimental conditions using the non-parametric Mann-Whitney-U test. The level of statistical significance was set as $P < 0.05$.

No previous study has investigated changes in sputum viscoelasticity following a combination of cycling and Flutter® using the same instruments as in our study from which we could derive means and standard deviations (SD's) and on which we could base our power calculations. However, two previous studies using randomized crossover designs comparing i) an acute bout of cycling and treadmill exercise versus no exercise [11] or ii) Flutter® therapy with autogenic drainage [7] were able to demonstrate significant changes in sputum viscoelasticity in 14 individuals with CF in each study. We therefore aimed to include 16 patients in our study.

Results

Baseline patient characteristics are shown in Table 1 ($N = 16$).

During the study, one female patient requiring oral antibiotic therapy for treatment of a pulmonary exacerbation and was excluded from the analyses. All other patients completed all assessments without complications. There

Table 1 Patient baseline characteristics

Variables	
N	16
Sex (male/female)	7/9
Age (years)	23 (22, 25)
BMI (kg m^{-2})	20 (18, 21)
Cystic fibrosis-related diabetes (N (%))	8 (50)
Pancreatic insufficiency (N (%))	13 (81)
Chronic *Pseudomonas aeruginosa* infection (N (%))	7 (44)
FEV$_1$ (% predicted)	52 (43, 72)
DLNO (% predicted)	59 (51, 73)
DLCO (% predicted)	82 (69, 86)
V'O$_{2peak}$ (mL kg^{-1} min^{-1})	32.0 (30.3, 34.4)
Mechanical power (W kg^{-1})	2.9 (2.3, 3.1)
HR$_{peak}$ (beats min^{-1})	167 (163, 179)
RER	1.20 (1.15, 1.26)

Data are median (IQR) or N (%). *BMI* body mass index, *CF* cystic fibrosis, *DLCO* diffusing capacity of the lung for carbon monoxide, *DLNO* diffusing capacity of the lung for nitric oxide, *FEV$_1$* forced expiratory volume in one second, *HR$_{peak}$* peak heart rate, *RER* respiratory exchange ratio, *V'O$_{2peak}$* peak oxygen consumption

were no differences in pre-exercise sputum properties, pulmonary function data and patient-reported health status between the three study visits, respectively (Additional file 1: Table S1). Cardiorespiratory variables during exercise were comparable between both experiments (Additional file 2: Table S2), whereas patients had a higher respiratory frequency during experiment A compared to B ($P < 0.001$).

All patients were able to provide sputum samples at the requested time points during the study. 13/15 patients had previous experience using Flutter®, but only two were using the Flutter® on a regular basis.

CF sputum viscoelasticity and spinnability

The average of all sputum samples ($n = 45$) obtained at rest during each of the three visits showed spinnability (Fig. 2a) and viscoelastic behavior (Fig. 2b-d) characteristic for CF sputum [7, 30–32]. Details can be found in the online supplements (Additional file 3: Table S4). At high frequencies ($\omega > 10$ rad s^{-1}) G' and G'' as well as η^* (complex viscosity) and the phase angle increased due to instrument inertia, which causes artifacts in the sample signal. Consequently, the analysis of sputum viscoelasticity (G' and G'') was restricted to an angular frequency of 10 rad s^{-1}. Instrument inertia is further debated in the Discussion section and online supplements.

Changes in sputum rheological properties

Table 2 shows changes in sputum properties for each experimental condition. No time-course changes were found during either experiment A or B, except for sputum solids content during experimental condition A ($P = 0.038$). Individual raw data for G' at 1 and 10 rad s^{-1} are shown in Additional file 4: Figure S1 and Additional file 5: Figure S2 in the online supplements. In the experimental condition A, one study participant had very high values for G' at 1 and 10 rad s^{-1} immediately post-exercise. Of note, there was no technical problem during the rheological measurements, but the sputum sample was purulent and thick. A summary of all sputum rheological data excluding this particular participant is shown in Additional file 6: Table S3 in the online supplements.

No differences in sputum rheological properties (viscoelastic moduli G' and G'', yield stress, solids content) were found between experiments (Table 3), except differences in sputum spinnability comparing pre- versus 45´ post-exercise values between experiments. During recovery (absolute change, pre- vs. 45 min post-exercise), we noticed differences in patient reported ease of sputum expectoration, favoring experimental condition A ($P = 0.016$).

Changes in pulmonary diffusing capacity

Individual raw data for DLNO, DLCO, V$_A$ and V$_{cap}$ at different time points during experiments A and B are

Table 2 Changes in sputum properties, pulmonary diffusing capacity and oxygen saturation during experiments A and B ($N = 15$)

Variables	Experiment A				Experiment B			
	Pre-exercise	Post-exercise	45 min post-exercise	P-value	Pre-exercise	Post-exercise	45 min post-exercise	P-value
Sputum properties								
G' 1 rad s^{-1} (Pa)	6.7 (4.2, 9.7)	10.3 (6.0, 20.3)	14.1 (6.1, 19.0)	0.057	7.5 (4.1, 13.0)	8.8 (6.5, 13.8)	13.3 (7.1, 14.6)	0.085
G' 10 rad s^{-1} (Pa)	10.2 (6.4, 14.4)	15.9 (8.3, 28.1)	20.9 (9.7, 26.0)	0.062	11.5 (5.9, 20.1)	13.6 (8.8, 18.0)	20.0 (10.1, 23.0)	0.155
G'' 1 rad s^{-1} (Pa)	2.3 (1.7, 3.2)	3.1 (2.1, 5.9)	3.8 (2.0, 6.2)	0.085	2.6 (1.3, 3.6)	3.2 (2.3, 4.9)	4.5 (2.5, 4.9)	0.155
G'' 10 rad s^{-1} (Pa)	2.9 (2.2, 4.0)	3.7 (2.6, 6.6)	4.2 (2.6, 6.7)	0.085	3.6 (1.8, 4.3)	3.7 (2.8, 5.7)	5.3 (2.9, 6.1)	0.282
Dynamic yield stress (Pa)	0.20 (0.10, 0.30)	0.30 (0.20, 0.60)	0.30 (0.20, 0.40)	0.066	0.20 (0.10, 0.40)	0.20 (0.18, 0.33)	0.30 (0.2, 0.53)	0.074
Sputum solids content (%)	5.3 (3.9, 7.4)	6.2 (4.2, 9.7)	6.5 (4.4, 8.1)	0.038	4.5 (3.6, 5.8)	6.2 (4.1, 7.5)	6.9 (3.8, 8.4)	0.672
Spinnability (mm)	6.7 (6.4, 8.2)	7.7 (6.5, 21.0)	6.7 (6.3, 8.2)	0.155	9.2 (6.4, 12.4)	6.2 (5.8, 8.3)	8.9 (7.2, 31.0)	0.089
Ease of sputum expectoration (cm)	8.1 (5.2, 8.3)	7.7 (3.4, 9.3)	8.2 (4.7, 8.9)	0.180	7.1 (5.2, 8.7)	6.5 (4.4, 9.1)	5.3 (4.3, 9.2)	0.482
Pulmonary diffusing capacity								
DLNO (mL min^{-1} mmHg^{-1})	78.1 (68.4, 141.6)	86.9 (67.4, 140.6)	79.2 (65.6, 134.0)	0.015*	84.7 (64.8, 143.1)	83.8 (69.9, 135.2)	82.6 (69.4, 147.8)	0.482
DLNO/V$_A$ (mL min^{-1} mmHg^{-1} L^{-1})	21.1 (19.8; 22.4)	21.2 (20.0; 22.2)	20.7 (18.2; 21.8)	0.015#	21.1 (19.7; 22.7)	20.5 (19.2; 22.4)	20.7 (18.3; 22.3)	0.007#
DLCO (mL min^{-1} mmHg^{-1})	22.4 (20.3, 31.9)	24.6 (20.3, 36.2)	21.5 (19.5, 31.1)	0.002*	23.7 (19.6, 34.3)	24.2 (19.4, 34.0)	22.9 (19.3, 32.5)	0.011*
DLCO/V$_A$ (mL min^{-1} mmHg^{-1} L^{-1})	5.8 (5.2, 6.1)	6.1 (5.4, 6.5)	5.6 (5.3, 6.2)	0.047*	5.7 (5.4, 6.01)	6.0 (5.3, 6.2)	5.5 (5.0, 5.9)	<0.001*#
DLNO/DLCO ratio	3.8 (3.4, 4.1)	3.6 (3.4, 3.8)	3.6 (3.4, 4.1)	0.025	3.8 (3.4, 4.2)	3.5 (3.3, 3.9)	3.7 (3.3, 4.1)	0.005
DMCO (mL min^{-1} mmHg^{-1})	52 (42, 112)	56 (43, 88)	53 (43, 92)	0.612	58 (42, 106)	54 (45, 89)	56 (42, 118)	0.717
V$_A$ (L)	3.8 (3.4, 6.0)	4.2 (3.5, 6.1)	3.9 (3.4, 5.6)	0.001	3.9 (3.3, 5.9)	3.9 (3.5, 5.5)	4.0 (3.6, 6.0)	0.420
V$_{cap}$ (mL)	76 (69, 82)	91 (77, 91)	76 (67, 91)	<0.001*	75 (72, 94)	82 (76, 92)	75 (67, 83)	0.015*
Oxygen saturation								
SpO$_2$ (%)	97.0 (95.8, 97.0)	96.0 (94.8, 97.0)	96.0 (95.5, 97.0)	0.598	96.5 (96.0, 97.6)	96.0 (96.0, 97.3)	97.0 (96.8, 98.0)	0.125

Data are displayed as median (interquartile range, IQR). DLCO, diffusing capacity of the lung for carbon monoxide; DLNO, diffusing capacity of the lung for nitric oxide; DMCO, alveolar-capillary membrane diffusing capacity for carbon monoxide; G', storage modulus; G", loss modulus; SpO$_2$, oxygen saturation; V$_A$, alveolar volume; V$_{cap}$, pulmonary capillary blood volume. Pulmonary gas diffusion variables were measured in SI units (mmol min^{-1} kPa^{-1}) and converted to traditional units (mL min^{-1} mmHg^{-1}) by multiplying with 2.987. Differences in outcome variables between the three different time points during each experimental condition (experiment A and B) were analyzed using the non-parametric Friedman test followed by a Wilcoxon-signed rank test. The Wilcoxon signed-rank test was only performed, if changes over time were significant ($P < 0.05$)

*indicates significant differences between pre- and post-exercise values based on Wilcoxon signed-rank test ($P < 0.05$)

# indicates significant differences between pre- and 45' post-exercise values based on Wilcoxon signed-rank test ($P < 0.05$)

Table 3 Comparison of absolute changes in sputum properties, pulmonary diffusing capacity and oxygen saturation between experiments A and B (N = 15)

Variables	Experiment A		Experiment B		P-values	
	Absolute change pre- versus post-exercise	Absolute change pre- versus 45 min post-exercise	Absolute change pre- versus post-exercise	Absolute change pre- versus 45 min post exercise	Pre- versus post- exercise between A & B	Pre- versus 45 min post- exercise between A & B
Sputum properties						
G' 1 rad s⁻¹ (Pa)	1.98 (0.1, 9.9)	−0.27 (−3.3, 6.8)	0.87 (−2.8, 4.8)	3.21 (0.1, 7.2)	0.237	0.290
G' 10 rad s⁻¹ (Pa)	2.54 (1.1, 14.2)	11.35 (−1.0, 16.5)	1.22 (−3.9, 8.2)	2.90 (−0.4, 15.1)	0.290	0.725
G'' 1 rad s⁻¹ (Pa)	0.82 (−1.2, 3.1)	2.40 (−0.1, 4.1)	0.46 (−0.2, 1.63)	1.64 (−0.2, 3.3)	0.595	0.567
G'' 10 rad s⁻¹ (Pa)	0.85 (−0.3, 2.7)	2.52 (−0.1, 4.0)	0.61 (−0.6, 1.6)	1.82 (−0.2, 3.6)	0.468	0.576
Dynamic yield stress (Pa)	0.07 (0.0, 0.3)	0.20 (0.0, 0.3)	0.01 (−0.1, 0.1)	0.10 (0.0, 0.2)	0.217	0.713
Sputum solids content (%)	0.25 (−0.1, 3.5)	0.86 (0.4, 1.9)	1.11 (−1.2, 3.4)	0.94 (−1.6, 3.6)	0.967	0.653
Spinnability (mm)	1.00 (−0.2, 11.0)	−1.40 (−14.3, 0.4)	−1.25 (−3.9, 0.7)	1.20 (−1.1, 5.7)	0.077	0.009
Ease of sputum expectoration (cm)	0.50 (−0.2, 1.7)	0.80 (−0.1, 1.2)	−0.20 (−1.6, 1.3)	−1.1 (−1.8, 0.1)	0.276	0.016
Pulmonary diffusing capacity						
$DLNO$ (mL min⁻¹ mmHg⁻¹)	4.23 (−0.9, 8.8)	−0.90 (−2.8, 1.4)	1.40 (−5.7, 5.1)	−2.86 (−7.2, 5.0)	0.152	1.000
$DLNO/V_A$ (mL min⁻¹ mmHg⁻¹ L⁻¹)	−0.17 (−0.6, 0.2)	−1.04 (−1.5, −0.6)	−0.18 (−0.9, 0.3)	−1.16 (−1.8, −0.1)	0.934	0.967
$DLCO$ (mL min⁻¹ mmHg⁻¹)	2.16 (0.8, 4.5)	−0.12 (−0.8, 0.6)	1.87 (0.1, 2.3)	−0.76 (−2.1, 0.9)	0.110	0.351
$DLCO/V_A$ (mL min⁻¹ mmHg⁻¹ L⁻¹)	0.28 (0.1, 0.5)	−0.09 (−0.2, 0.1)	0.21 (0.0, 0.4)	−0.22 (−0.3, −0.1)	0.468	0.271
$DLNO/DLCO$ ratio	−0.16 (−0.3, −0.1)	−0.01 (−0.2, 0.1)	−0.17 (−0.4, 0.1)	−0.13 (−0.2, −0.0)	0.771	0.533
$DMCO$ (mL min⁻¹ mmHg⁻¹)	1.0 (−3.0, 3.0)	1.0 (−5.0, 2.0)	0.0 (−9.0, 3.0)	2.0 (−7.0, 5.0)	0.632	0.519
V_A (L)	0.26 (0.0, 0.4)	0.04 (−0.0, 0.2)	0.06 (−0.1, 0.3)	0.03 (−0.2, 0.2)	0.032	0.693
V_{cap} (mL)	12.0 (9.0, 17.0)	0.0 (−3.0, 3.0)	12.0 (1.0, 15.0)	−5.0 (−11.0, 4.0)	0.135	0.114
Oxygen saturation						
SpO_2 (%)	0.0 (−1.5, 1.0)	0.0 (−0.8, 0.5)	0.0 (−1.0, 0.0)	0.3 (−0.1, 1.0)	0.983	0.378

Data are displayed as median (interquartile range, IQR). DLCO, diffusing capacity of the lung for carbon monoxide; DLNO, diffusing capacity of the lung for nitric oxide; DMCO, alveolar-capillary membrane diffusing capacity for carbon monoxide; G', storage modulus; G", loss modulus; SpO₂, oxygen saturation; V_A, alveolar volume; V_{cap}, pulmonary capillary blood volume. Pulmonary gas diffusion variables were measured in SI units (mmol min⁻¹ kPa⁻¹) and converted to traditional units (mL min⁻¹ mmHg⁻¹) by multiplying with 2.987. Differences in outcome variables at different time points (pre-exercise versus post-exercise and pre-exercise versus 45′ post-exercise) between the two experimental conditions were analyzed using the non-parametric Mann-Whitney-U test shown in Additional file 7: Figure S3 and Additional file 8: Figure S4 in the online supplements. Time course changes in pulmonary diffusing capacity were observed during both experiments, while changes in $DLNO$ and V_A were only observed in experimental condition A (Table 2). No differences in pulmonary diffusing capacity were found between the two experimental conditions (Table 3), except a higher V_A comparing post-exercise and pre-exercise changes favoring experiment A ($P = 0.032$).

Discussion

This randomized controlled crossover study investigated acute effects of moderate intensity continuous cycling exercise versus interval cycling exercise incorporating the Flutter® device on sputum viscoelasticity (primary endpoint) and pulmonary diffusing capacity in adults with CF. This study provides three important findings. First, the addition of Flutter® to moderately intense stationary cycling has no measurable effect on sputum viscoelastic properties compared to stationary cycling alone. Second, our results highlight experimental challenges to simulate 'coughing' (i.e., 100 rad s^{-1} measurements or generally high frequency measurements) in a shear rheological setup due to instrument inertia effects. Third, the increase in pulmonary diffusing capacity over time reflects an acute exercise-induced effect, not sustained post-exercise.

Sputum rheological properties and exercise

In the present study, we found no differences in sputum viscoelasticity between the two experimental conditions, thus rejecting our initial hypothesis. Two previous studies reported altered sputum viscoelasticity after an acute bout of treadmill exercise or Flutter® and treadmill exercise compared to resting breathing in adults with CF [6, 11]. Treadmill but not cycling exercise reduced sputum viscoelasticity and trunk oscillations during treadmill running/walking have been postulated as a possible underlying mechanism [11]. One could argue that the chosen exercise mode in our study was not sufficient to improve viscoelastic properties of sputum in our patients and/or that the magnitude of effect from Flutter® was not large enough to produce greater changes in sputum viscoelastic properties compared to cycling alone. During exercise, our patients achieved approximately 47–49% of their maximal minute ventilation (90–97% of their maximal tidal volumes and 50–55% of their maximal respiratory frequencies, see Additional file 2: Table S2) suggestive of a high ventilatory demand. Higher exercise intensities (e.g., 90% of maximal heart rate) may induce significant airway narrowing [12] unlikely to be maintained by many patients when exercising for longer periods, in particular, in patients with advanced lung disease. With respect to Flutter®, our patients performed 6–10 breathing maneuvers during each of four cycles. Higher volumes of

Flutter® therapy (6 cycles à 15 breaths) combined with huffing and coughing (forced expiration technique, FET) improved sputum viscoelasticity compared to resting breathing in adults with CF [6]. It is important to note that we deliberately did not follow existing CF physiotherapy recommendations [27] suggesting to individually determine the angle of the Flutter® along with the performance of forced expiratory maneuvers. In this study, we were mainly interested in mechanistic effects of airway oscillations on sputum viscoelasticity [7] on top of high ventilation during exercise. We did not implement forced expiratory maneuvers due to potential interference with our cycling protocol and pulmonary gas exchange measurements. The authors hypothesize that a more intense Flutter® therapy, together with individual adaptation of the Flutter® angle, but not the lack of forced expiratory maneuvers, could explain the absence of additional effect in our study. Given the fact that positive expiratory pressure and oscillations are thought to mechanically impact on biophysical properties of mucus (i.e., reduction of viscoelasticity), huffing and coughing following Flutter® maneuvers assist in mobilization and transport of secretions from peripheral to central airways, but should not substantially change viscoelastic properties of sputum in addition. This hypothesis is supported by an in vitro experiment demonstrating that Flutter® oscillations alone augment sputum elasticity after 15 and 30 min, respectively [7].

It is important to mention that in comparison to our experimental study design, the study by Dwyer et al. [6] compared Flutter® therapy with resting breathing (no intervention), which likely increases the chance to observe effects between experimental conditions. Nevertheless, given the high variability of sputum properties [33] and differing intra- and interindividual responses to airway clearance therapy, a "no intervention" visit would have probably provided further insights into within-patient treatment responses.

Interestingly, and in line with findings by Dwyer et al. [11], ease of sputum expectoration was higher during recovery from continuous cycling versus cycling exercise with Flutter®. This suggests that patients perceive the benefit of airway clearance therapy not immediately but during recovery from exercise. However, the clinical meaningfulness of these findings cannot be interpreted due to the lack of a minimal important difference for the visual analogue scale.

Rheological measurements and inertia

We observed occurrence of inertia at high frequencies, causing experimental artifacts (see Additional file 9 for further discussion). King and Macklem suggested first that sputum rheology at high frequency simulates cough studying dog tracheal mucus [34]. The concept was then further elaborated suggesting that low frequency (1 rad s^{-1}) deformations are relevant when simulating ciliary transport [35] whereas high frequency (100 rad s^{-1})

deformations are more characteristic for cough clearance [36]. The 1 rad s^{-1} / 100 rad s^{-1} concept was initially elaborated using active microrheology but was later applied in shear rheology testing [6, 11, 37, 38]. We found a strong increase in moduli (G', G") and phase angles at frequencies >10 rad s^{-1} (Fig. 2c and d, Additional file 10: Figure S5a) and observed that sample torques deviated from the electrical torques (Additional file 10: Figure S5b), both strong indicators for inertia. The deviation of sample torque from electrical torque due to inertia is schematically represented in torque vector drawings in Additional file 10: Figure S5c. Also, we calculated the theoretical inertia limit of the rheometer, which agreed well with the observed onset of inertia. Further proof is obtained comparing our results to other findings that show a continuous trend of the dynamic moduli up to 50 Hz (≈ 314 rad s^{-1}) using passive microrheology [32], which is not affected by inertia at frequencies below 1 MHz [39]. Data generated in previous studies using shear rheology at 100 rad s^{-1} also showed signs of inertia [6, 11, 37, 38], revealed by a substantially increased loss modulus G" or complex modulus (G*) and high tan δ values compared to those measured at 1 rad s^{-1}. Future rheology measurements with sputum should be carefully checked for inertia, as in the worst-case scenario, false positive or false negative outcomes occur. We propose restricting frequencies to 10 rad s^{-1} to simulate the high frequency behavior of sputum in shear rheology.

Pulmonary diffusing capacity and exercise
In the present study, $DLNO$ and $DLCO$ increased during continuous cycling exercise, whereas interval cycling exercise interspersed with use of the Flutter® increased only $DLCO$ but not $DLNO$, most likely due to the absence of increase in V_A. It is well known that $DLNO$, $DLCO$, and V_{cap} increase linearly during exercise with respect to cardiac output [40]. In our study, continuous cycling increased post-exercise $DLNO$ by about 5%, but the effect was not sustained during recovery. We extend previous findings reporting a remarkable increase in $DLNO$ ($39 \pm 8\%$ from rest using rebreathing measurements) during moderate intensity cycling exercise in CF adults, with the authors questioning the duration of beneficial effects [12]. Our data demonstrate that increase in $DLNO$ is (only) an acute, exercise-induced effect, most likely the result of increased V_A and subsequently greater surface area for diffusion rather than improved mucociliary clearance mechanisms such as improved sputum hydration and/or viscoelastic properties.

This study has limitations. First, we did not measure expiratory flow during exercise [6, 11] to evaluate whether our experiments were sufficient to create an expiratory airflow bias, a mechanism potentially improving mucocili-

ary clearance. Furthermore, the sputum was sheared at 50 Pa in simple shear experiments prior to spinnability measurements. The shear homogenized the samples, theoretically disrupting sputum microstructure, which could have caused the comparably low spinnability values. Finally, our study patient cohort was small, limiting the generalizability of our findings to the overall CF population.

Conclusions
We conclude that the addition of Flutter® to moderate intensity interval cycling exercise has no measurable effect on the viscoelastic properties of sputum compared to moderate intensity continuous cycling alone. The higher pulmonary diffusing capacity represents an acute exercise-induced effect not sustained post-exercise.

Abbreviations
ACT: airway clearance techniques; BMI: body mass index; CF: cystic fibrosis; CPET: cardiopulmonary exercise testing; $DLCO$: pulmonary diffusing capacity for carbon monoxide; $DLNO$: pulmonary diffusing capacity for nitric oxide; $DLNO/DLCO$ ratio: ratio of pulmonary diffusing capacity for nitric oxide to pulmonary diffusing capacity for carbon monoxide; DMCO: alveolar-capillary membrane diffusing capacity for carbon monoxide; FEV_1: forced expiratory volume in 1 s; f_R: respiratory frequency; G*: complex modulus; G': storage modulus; G": loss modulus; LVE: linear viscoelasticity; PEP: positive expiratory pressure; RER: respiratory exchange ratio; SpO_2: oxygen saturation; tan δ: loss tangent; V'E: minute ventilation; $V'O_{2peak}$: peak oxygen consumption; V_A: alveolar volume; V_{cap}: pulmonary capillary blood volume; VT: tidal volume; η*: complex viscosity

Acknowledgments
We kindly thank André Königs from the University Hospital Zurich for his assistance in patient recruitment; Dario Kohlbrenner from the University Hospital Zurich for measuring the visual analogue scales; Simeon Zürcher for his support with the randomization and Dr. Julia Braun for statistical support (both University of Zurich). Moreover, we thank Evangelia Daviskas from the Department of Respiratory Medicine, Royal Prince Hospital Alfred Hospital, Sydney, Australia, for her advice with respect to the preparation of the sputum measurements and sample handling prior to the start of this study. The authors express their appreciation to Jörg Läuger from Anton Paar for his assistance with the interpretation of the inertia effects.

Funding
The Swiss Cystic Fibrosis Society (CFCH) funded the study. The sponsor had no role in the design of the study, data collection, analysis and interpretation, or the content of the manuscript.

Authors' contributions
TR takes responsibility for the overall content as guarantor. TR, SK, and HD contributed to the study design. TR and MMB conducted all experiments. LB, PB and PF were responsible for the sputum analysis. LB and PB measured and analyzed all sputum samples and were blinded to the patient's characteristics and experimental conditions. TR performed the data analysis. All authors contributed to the data interpretation and writing of the manuscript. TR wrote the first manuscript draft, all authors revised and approved the final manuscript version.

Competing interests
The authors declare that they have no competing interests.

Author details
[1]Epidemiology, Biostatistics and Prevention Institute (EBPI), University of Zurich, Zurich, Switzerland. [2]Division of Occupational and Environmental Medicine, University of Zurich and University Hospital Zurich, Zurich, Switzerland. [3]Department of Health Science and Technology, ETH Zurich, Zurich, Switzerland. [4]Division of Pulmonology, University Hospital of Zurich, Zurich, Switzerland.

References
1. Boucher RC. New concepts of the pathogenesis of cystic fibrosis lung disease. Eur Respir J. 2004;23:146–58.
2. Rowbotham NJ, Smith S, Leighton PA, Rayner OC, Gathercole K, Elliott ZC, Nash EF, Daniels T, Duff AJA, Collins S, Chandran S, Peaple U, Hurley MN, Brownlee K, Smyth AR. The top 10 research priorities in cystic fibrosis developed by a partnership between people with CF and healthcare providers. Thorax. 2018;73:388–90.
3. Morrison L, Innes S. Oscillating devices for airway clearance in people with cystic fibrosis. Cochrane Database Syst Rev. 2017;5:CD006842.
4. McCarren B, Alison JA. Physiological effects of vibration in subjects with cystic fibrosis. Eur Respir J. 2006;27:1204–9.
5. Konstan MW, Stern RC, Doershuk CF. Efficacy of the flutter device for airway mucus clearance in patients with cystic fibrosis. J Pediatr. 1994;124:689–93.
6. Dwyer TJ, Zainuldin R, Daviskas E, Bye PT, Alison JA. Effects of treadmill exercise versus flutter(R) on respiratory flow and sputum properties in adults with cystic fibrosis: a randomised, controlled, cross-over trial. BMC Pulm Med. 2017;17:14.
7. App EM, Kieselmann R, Reinhardt D, Lindemann H, Dasgupta B, King M, Brand P. Sputum rheology changes in cystic fibrosis lung disease following two different types of physiotherapy: flutter vs autogenic drainage. Chest. 1998;114:171–7.
8. Reix P, Aubert F, Werck-Gallois MC, Toutain A, Mazzocchi C, Moreux N, Bellon G, Rabilloud M, Kassai B. Exercise with incorporated expiratory manoeuvres was as effective as breathing techniques for airway clearance in children with cystic fibrosis: a randomised crossover trial. J Phys. 2012;58:241–7.
9. Basser PJ, McMahon TA, Griffith P. The mechanism of mucus clearance in cough. J Biomech Eng. 1989;111:288–97.
10. Hebestreit A, Kersting U, Basler B, Jeschke R, Hebestreit H. Exercise inhibits epithelial sodium channels in patients with cystic fibrosis. Am J Respir Crit Care Med. 2001;164:443–6.
11. Dwyer TJ, Alison JA, McKeough ZJ, Daviskas E, Bye PT. Effects of exercise on respiratory flow and sputum properties in patients with cystic fibrosis. Chest. 2011;139:870–7.
12. Wheatley CM, Baker SE, Morgan MA, Martinez MG, Liu B, Rowe SM, Morgan WJ, Wong EC, Karpen SR, Snyder EM. Moderate intensity exercise mediates comparable increases in exhaled chloride as albuterol in individuals with cystic fibrosis. Respir Med. 2015;109:1001–11.
13. Fuchs HJ, Borowitz DS, Christiansen DH, Morris EM, Nash ML, Ramsey BW, Rosenstein BJ, Smith AL, Wohl ME. Effect of aerosolized recombinant human DNase on exacerbations of respiratory symptoms and on pulmonary function in patients with cystic fibrosis. The Pulmozyme Study Group N Engl J Med. 1994;331:637–42.
14. Cinkotai FF, Thomson ML. Diurnal variation in pulmonary diffusing capacity for carbon monoxide. J Appl Physiol. 1966;21:539–42.
15. Ewoldt RH, Johnston MT, Caretta LM. Experimental challenges of shear rheology: how to avoid bad data. Biol Med Phys Biomed. 2015:207–41.
16. Burnett J, Glover FA, Blair GW. Field measurements of the "spinability" of bovine cervical mucus. Biorheology. 1967;4:41–5.
17. Critchfield AS, Yao G, Jaishankar A, Friedlander RS, Lieleg O, Doyle PS, McKinley G, House M, Ribbeck K. Cervical mucus properties stratify risk for preterm birth. PLoS One. 2013;8:e69528.
18. Miller MR, Hankinson J, Brusasco V, Burgos F, Casaburi R, Coates A, Crapo R, Enright P, van der Grinten CP, Gustafsson P, Jensen R, Johnson DC, MacIntyre N, McKay R, Navajas D, Pedersen OF, Pellegrino R, Viegi G, Wanger J. Standardisation of spirometry. Eur Respir J 2005;26:319–338.
19. Quanjer PH, Stanojevic S, Cole TJ, Baur X, Hall GL, Culver BH, Enright PL, Hankinson JL, Ip MS, Zheng J, Stocks J. Multi-ethnic reference values for spirometry for the 3-95-yr age range: the global lung function 2012 equations. Eur Respir J. 2012;40:1324–43.
20. Radtke T, Benden C, Maggi-Beba M, Kriemler S, van der Lee I, Dressel H. Intra-session and inter-session variability of nitric oxide pulmonary diffusing capacity in adults with cystic fibrosis. Respir Physiol Neurobiol. 2017;246:33–8.
21. Zavorsky GS, Hsia CC, Hughes JM, Borland CD, Guenard H, van der Lee I, Steenbruggen I, Naeije R, Cao J, Dinh-Xuan AT. Standardisation and application of the single-breath determination of nitric oxide uptake in the lung. Eur Respir J. 2017;49
22. Macintyre N, Crapo RO, Viegi G, Johnson DC, van der Grinten CP, Brusasco V, Burgos F, Casaburi R, Coates A, Enright P, Gustafsson P, Hankinson J, Jensen R, McKay R, Miller MR, Navajas D, Pedersen OF, Pellegrino R, Wanger J. Standardisation of the single-breath determination of carbon monoxide uptake in the lung. Eur Respir J 2005;26:720–735.
23. Godfrey S, Mearns M. Pulmonary function and response to exercise in cystic fibrosis. Arch Dis Child. 1971;46:144–51.
24. Borg GA. Psychophysical bases of perceived exertion. Med Sci Sports Exerc. 1982;14:377-81.
25. Balady GJ, Arena R, Sietsema K, Myers J, Coke L, Fletcher GF, Forman D, Franklin B, Guazzi M, Gulati M, Keteyian SJ, Lavie CJ, Macko R, Mancini D, Milani RV. Clinician's guide to cardiopulmonary exercise testing in adults: a scientific statement from the American Heart Association. Circulation. 2010;122:191–225.
26. EuroQol G. EuroQol–a new facility for the measurement of health-related quality of life. Health Policy. 1990;16:199–208.
27. International Physiotherapy Group for Cystic Fibrosis. Physiotherapy for people with cystic fibrosis: from infant to adult. 4th edition. 2009. Available online: https://www.cfww.org/docs/ipg-cf/bluebook/bluebooklet2009websiteversion.pdf accessed at April 27th 2018.
28. Homnick DN, Anderson K, Marks JH. Comparison of the flutter device to standard chest physiotherapy in hospitalized patients with cystic fibrosis - a pilot study. Chest. 1998;114:993–7.
29. Volsko TA, DiFiore J, Chatburn RL. Performance comparison of two oscillating positive expiratory pressure devices: acapella versus flutter. Respir Care. 2003;48:124–30.
30. Serisier DJ, Carroll MP, Shute JK, Young SA. Macrorheology of cystic fibrosis, chronic obstructive pulmonary disease & normal sputum. Respir Res. 2009;10:63.
31. Tomaiuolo G, Rusciano G, Caserta S, Carciati A, Carnovale V, Abete P, Sasso A, Guido S. A new method to improve the clinical evaluation of cystic fibrosis patients by mucus viscoelastic properties. PLoS One. 2014;9:e82297.
32. Hill DB, Vasquez PA, Mellnik J, McKinley SA, Vose A, Mu F, Henderson AG, Donaldson SH, Alexis NE, Boucher RC, Forest MG. A biophysical basis for mucus solids concentration as a candidate biomarker for airways disease. PLoS One. 2014;9
33. Radtke T, Böni L, Bohnacker P, Fischer P, Benden C, Dressel H. The many ways sputum flows - dealing with high within-subject variability in cystic fibrosis sputum rheology. Respir Physiol Neurobiol. 2018;254:36–9.
34. King M, Macklem PT. Rheological properties of microliter quantities of normal mucus. J Appl Physiol Respir Environ Exerc Physiol. 1977;42:797–802.
35. King M. Relationship between mucus viscoelasticity and ciliary transport in Guaran gel-frog palate model system. Biorheology. 1980;17:249–54.
36. King M. The role of mucus viscoelasticity in cough clearance. Biorheology. 1987;24:589–97.
37. Daviskas E, Anderson SD, Gomes K, Briffa P, Cochrane B, Chan HK, Young IH, Rubin BK. Inhaled mannitol for the treatment of mucociliary dysfunction in

Acute effects of combined exercise and oscillatory positive expiratory pressure therapy on sputum properties...

91

patients with bronchiectasis: effect on lung function, health status and sputum. Respirology. 2005;10:46–56.

38. Daviskas E, Anderson SD, Jaques A, Charlton B. Inhaled mannitol improves the hydration and surface properties of sputum in patients with cystic fibrosis. Chest. 2010;137:861–8.

39. Schnurr B, Gittes F, MacKintosh FC, Schmidt CF. Determining microscopic viscoelasticity in flexible and semiflexible polymer networks from thermal fluctuations. Macromolecules. 1997;30:7781–92.

40. Hsia CC. Recruitment of lung diffusing capacity: update of concept and application. Chest. 2002;122:1774–83.

11

Comparison of peak inspiratory flow rate via the Breezhaler®, Ellipta® and HandiHaler® dry powder inhalers in patients with moderate to very severe COPD

Pablo Altman[1]*, Luis Wehbe[2], Juergen Dederichs[3], Tadhg Guerin[4], Brian Ament[5], Miguel Cardenas Moronta[3], Andrea Valeria Pino[6] and Pankaj Goyal[3]

Abstract

Background: The chronic and progressive nature of chronic obstructive pulmonary disease (COPD) requires self-administration of inhaled medication. Dry powder inhalers (DPIs) are increasingly being used for inhalation therapy in COPD. Important considerations when selecting DPIs include inhalation effort required and flow rates achieved by patients. Here, we present the comparison of the peak inspiratory flow rate (PIF) values achieved by COPD patients, with moderate to very severe airflow limitation, through the Breezhaler®, the Ellipta® and the HandiHaler® inhalers. The effects of disease severity, age and gender on PIF rate were also evaluated.

Methods: This randomized, open-label, multicenter, cross-over, Phase IV study recruited patients with moderate to very severe airflow limitation (Global Initiative for Obstructive Lung Disease 2014 strategy), aged ≥40 years and having a smoking history of ≥10 pack years. No active drug or placebo was administered during the study. The inhalation profiles were recorded using inhalers fitted with a pressure tap and transducer at the wall of the mouthpiece. For each patient, the inhalation with the highest PIF value, out of three replicate inhalations per device, was selected for analysis. A paired t-test was performed to compare mean PIFs between each combination of devices.

Results: In total, 97 COPD patients were enrolled and completed the study. The highest mean PIF value (L/min ± SE) was observed with the Breezhaler® (108 ± 23), followed by the Ellipta® (78 ± 15) and the HandiHaler® (49 ± 9) inhalers and the lowest mean pressure drop values were recorded with the Breezhaler® inhaler, followed by the Ellipta® inhaler and the HandiHaler® inhaler, in the overall patient population. A similar trend was consistently observed in patients across all subgroups of COPD severity, within all age groups and for both genders.

Conclusions: Patients with COPD were able to inhale with the least inspiratory effort and generate the highest mean PIF value through the Breezhaler® inhaler when compared with the Ellipta® and the HandiHaler® inhalers. These results were similar irrespective of patients' COPD severity, age or gender.

Keywords: Peak inspiratory flow, Inspiratory effort, Dry powder inhalers, Pressure drop, Breezhaler®

* Correspondence: pablo.altman@novartis.com
[1]Novartis Pharmaceuticals Corporation, East Hanover, NJ, USA
Full list of author information is available at the end of the article

Background

The progressive nature of chronic obstructive pulmonary disease (COPD), characterised by persistent airflow obstruction, necessitates regular self-administration of inhaled medications that are delivered directly to the desired site to relieve symptoms while minimizing systemic side effects [1]. Clinical trial and real-world study data provide conclusive evidence enabling physicians to make informed decisions about choice of medication [1]; however, little consideration is given to attributes of the inhaler and patients' ability to use them [2], especially in elderly patients or those with severe disease [3]. The recently updated Global Initiative for Obstructive Lung Disease (GOLD) strategy document has taken a step towards reaching a consensus on considerations for ensuring effectiveness of the inhaled treatment [1]. However, there still seems to be a lack of agreement on considerations involved in choosing an appropriate inhaler.

A large variety of inhalers are currently available, each offering distinct advantages and disadvantages. Most metered-dose inhalers (MDIs) are not breath-actuated and use a pressurized propellant to deliver the drug, which means that less inspiratory effort is required. However, it is sometimes difficult for the patient to synchronize inhalation and actuation when using MDI devices [4, 5].

In contrast, breath-actuated dry powder inhalers (DPIs) [6] rely, amongst other factors, on the patient's ability to produce sufficient airflow [7]. Each DPI has an intrinsic resistance that affects the inspiratory effort needed to effectively inhale the drug from the device [8]. The inspiratory maneuver of the patient creates a pressure differential within a DPI (reflective of the patient's inspiratory effort), driving the airflow, which also depends on the intrinsic airflow resistance of the inhaler [9]. Inhalers with low airflow resistance allow air to flow through them more easily and are, therefore, more likely to allow the patients to inhale with a lower effort [10, 11] compared with higher resistance inhalers that require forceful inhalation [9]. An important

consideration when choosing an inhaler, therefore, should be the ease associated with the inhalation effort required to take the medication [10]. Inhalation effort assumes even greater importance for COPD patients with muscular weakness, since ability to generate higher flow rates comfortably might be compromised, especially in patients with severe and very severe airflow limitation [9].

The Breezhaler® inhaler is a unit-dose, capsule-based DPI that has low internal (airflow) resistance [12, 13] is easy to use correctly, delivers a consistent dose of inhaled medication across different inhalation flow rates [14–17] and was suggested previously, through in-vitro studies, to require lower inhalation effort [10].

The objective of this study was to compare the peak inspiratory flow rate (PIF) values generated by patients with COPD through three different types of DPIs, the Breezhaler®, the Ellipta® and the HandiHaler®. The effects of disease severity, age and gender on PIF values generated through these inhalers were also evaluated.

Methods

Study design

This was a multicenter, open-label, randomized, cross-over, Phase IV study conducted across five sites in Argentina from 16 December 2015 to 29 April 2016 in COPD patients with moderate, severe, or very severe airflow limitation (GOLD 2014) [18]. There were two visits in the study: one for screening and the second for testing procedures (Fig. 1). The three inhalers tested in this study were the Breezhaler® (B), Ellipta® (E) and HandiHaler® (H) inhalers. No active drug or placebo was administered to patients during the study; the Breezhaler® and HandiHaler® inhalers with closed empty clear hydroxypropyl methylcellulose capsules were provided to each site and pierced just before inhalation measurements. The drug containing blister strips of Ellipta® were replaced by empty strips during device preparation by the investigator (Novartis). The inhalers were modified using a pressure tap and transducer fitted at

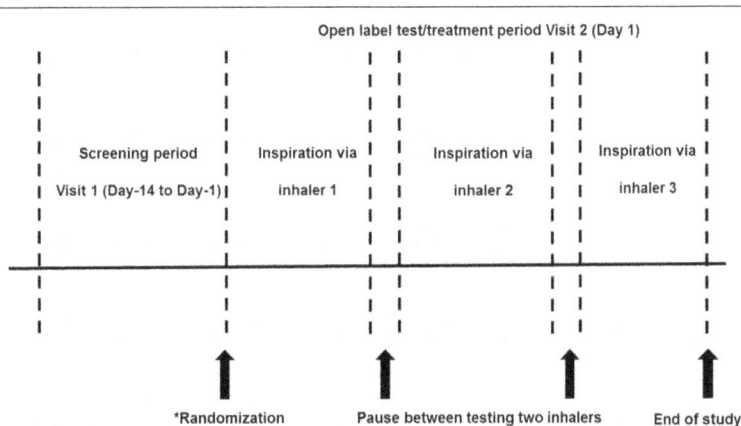

Fig. 1 Study design. *Sequence of testing via inhaler 1, 2 and 3 for each patient will depend on randomization

the wall of the mouthpiece. The inhalational measurement method has been tested and validated by measurement of the airflow resistance of each device before and after the modification with the pressure tap. The airflow resistance was confirmed as unchanged due to the modification.

Patients inhaled through the three DPIs following a randomized cross-over sequence (6 sequences used were: BEH, EHB, HBE, BHE, EBH and HEB). Before inhalation, patients were trained on use of each inhaler by the study personnel. A standard 'Investigator's Test Script' was used across all sites to standardize the inhalation maneuver. Each patient was required to record three inhalation profiles via each inhalation device. Patients were allowed to rest between successive inhalations from the same device, and between inhalations from two different devices. The highest PIF value, of the three replicate inhalations per device, was used for the analyses. A custom-built and calibrated inhalation profile recorder (IPR; The Technology Partnership, UK) was used to measure and record patients' inspiratory flow rates. Each inhaler was modified at the mouthpiece with a small stainless steel tube to connect to the IPR pressure transducer. The inhalers were characterized before the start of the study to ensure a specific pressure drop and the airflow through the device was comparable before and after attaching the instrumentation. Further, they were sanitized and packed for the study. Each device was given a unique identification number and label that were recorded in the case report form. During patient inhalation, the IPR measured the mouthpiece pressure drop, converted it into flow rate using inhaler resistance and plotted the results on the graphic–user interface (GUI) (Fig. 2). The PIF value was determined by the IPR software as the highest flow rate achieved by the patient and displayed on the GUI. The highest PIF value out of the three repeat runs per patient and per inhaler was used in the data analysis. Inhalation profiles were plotted using custom Matlab script according to the inhaler used and the subgroups: gender, age, and COPD severity, and manually reviewed.

Ethics approval and consent to participate

The study protocol was reviewed by the institutional review boards and ethics committees for each center (list included in Additional file 1). The study was conducted according to the ethical principles of the Declaration of Helsinki. Written informed consent was obtained from each patient prior to performing any study related assessment.

Participants

The study included men and women aged ≥40 years, diagnosed with moderate, severe, or very severe COPD, i.e. airflow limitation with post-bronchodilator forced expiratory volume in 1 s (FEV_1) < 80% of predicted normal and FEV_1/forced vital capacity < 0.70 at time of screening (GOLD 2014) [18]. Participants were current or ex-smokers with a smoking history of ≥10 pack years.

Patients were excluded if they experienced a COPD exacerbation that required treatment with antibiotics or oral corticosteroids or hospitalization within 6 weeks prior to screening, or had a respiratory tract infection within 4 weeks prior to screening, or had a history of asthma or onset of respiratory symptoms prior to the age of 40 years. Patients were also excluded if they were unable to use any of the three test inhalers due to cognitive impairment, neurological disorders, or any other condition affecting use of the DPIs.

Study objectives

The primary objective of the study was to compare the PIF values generated by patients with moderate, severe, or very severe airflow obstruction through the Breezhaler®, Ellipta® and HandiHaler® DPIs. Exploratory objectives included assessing the effect of age, gender and disease severity on the PIF values generated through the three DPIs. Additional analyses included comparison of the pressure drop at PIF (as a measure of inspiratory effort) across all devices as a function of COPD severity, age (40–64, 65–74 and ≥ 75) and gender.

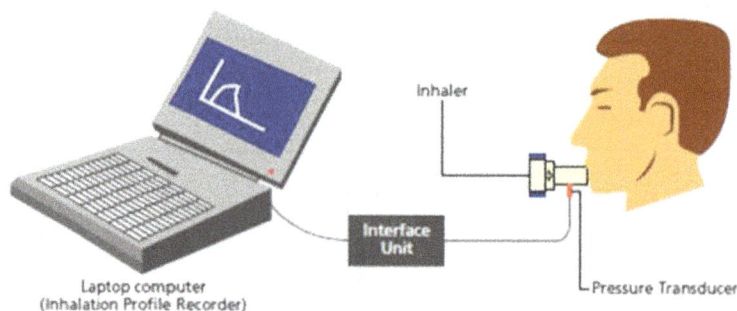

Fig. 2 Setup to record inhalation profile of patients

Assessments

Raw data included the pressure drop values, and flow rate was calculated using the equation:

$\sqrt{\Delta P} = Q * R$ where ΔP (kPa) is the pressure drop observed in the inhaler, Q (L/min) is the inhalation flow and R $(cmH_2O^{0.5}[L/min]^{-1})$ is the airflow resistance [9]. To convert pressure drop to flow rate, previously published 'measured internal resistance' values for Breezhaler®, Ellipta® and HandiHaler® inhalers (i.e. 0.060, 0.090 and 0.163 $cmH_2O^{0.5}[L/min]^{-1}$ [19, 20]) respectively, were used. Pressure drops at PIF were compared between the three inhalers as a function of COPD severity, age and gender. Safety was evaluated based on the incidence rate of adverse events (AEs), vital signs, and physical examination.

Statistical analysis

The full analysis set consisted of all 97 patients who conducted an inhalation maneuver through at least one inhaler. Profiles containing constant pressure values, termed 'flat lines', evaluated as incorrect profiles, were not considered in the final analysis. P-values were generated using a paired t-test with $P < 0.01$ indicating a significant difference which controls the familywise type 1 error rate at 3% under multiple testing for the primary PIF analysis on the FAS. P-values for subgroup analysis are exploratory in nature.

Sample size

A six-sequence Williams design was used to calculate the sample size. This design and an assumed standard deviation (SD) of 17.7 L/min (calculated according to previous findings) and a sample size of 96 patients (16 in each of the six possible sequences, i.e. $16 \times 6 = 96$) had > 90% power to detect a difference in PIF values between a pair of inhalers of 10 L/min (2-sided alpha 0.05).

Results

Participants

A total of 97 patients with a mean ± SD age of 69.0 ± 8.2 years enrolled and completed the study. Almost all patients were Caucasians and the majority of the population was male. The majority of patients had either moderate or severe COPD with mean ± SD time since diagnosis of 8.2 ± 4.2 years (Table 1). Overall, 15.5% of patients had experienced a COPD exacerbation in the previous year.

PIF values and pressure drop

In the overall population, patients produced the highest mean PIF values with the Breezhaler® inhaler followed by the Ellipta® and the HandiHaler® inhalers. The lowest mean pressure drop values were recorded with the Breezhaler® inhaler, again followed by the Ellipta® inhaler and the HandiHaler® inhaler (Table 2).

Table 1 Baseline demographics and clinical characteristics (Full analysis set)

Characteristic	Value (N = 97)
Age, years	69.0 ± 8.2
Male, n (%)	72 (74.2)
Race, n (%)	
Caucasian	96 (99.0)
Asian	1 (1.0)
BMI (kg/m²)	27.0 ± 5.3
Current smoker, n (%)	14 (14.4)
Severity of COPD, n (%)	
Moderate	49 (50.5)
Severe	38 (39.2)
Very severe	10 (10.3)
Number of COPD exacerbations in the previous year	0.2 ± 0.51
Post-bronchodilator FEV₁, % predicted	50.7 ± 15.5
Post-bronchodilator (%) FEV₁/FVC	48.3 ± 11.3

Data are presented as mean ± standard deviation, unless otherwise specified.
COPD severity is based on GOLD 2014 criteria
BMI body mass index, *FEV₁* forced expiratory volume in 1 s, *FVC* forced vital capacity, *GOLD* global initiative for chronic obstructive lung disease

Subgroup analysis by severity of COPD

The results observed across all COPD severities were in line with the overall population; i.e. patients of all subgroups produced highest mean PIF values with the Breezhaler® compared with the Ellipta® and the HandiHaler® inhalers. The lowest mean pressure drop values were observed for the Breezhaler® followed by the Ellipta® and the HandiHaler® inhalers (Table 3). For each inhaler, the mean PIF values were similar for patients with moderate and severe COPD, but lower for patients with very severe COPD (Table 3).

Subgroup analysis by age

Results observed across all age groups were also consistent with the overall results. Irrespective of age group, patients produced highest mean PIF values with the Breezhaler® versus the Ellipta® and the HandiHaler® inhalers, and the lowest mean pressure drop values were recorded for the Breezhaler® versus the Ellipta® and the HandiHaler® inhalers (Table 4). Across all inhalers, patients aged 40–64 years generated the highest mean PIF values, while patients aged ≥75 years generated mean PIF values comparable with those aged 65–74 years (Table 4).

Subgroup analysis by gender

Similar to the overall results, both male and female patient populations produced the highest mean PIF values with the Breezhaler® compared with the Ellipta® and the HandiHaler® inhalers. The lowest mean

Table 2 Comparison of mean PIF and pressure drop values in overall population

Variable	Breezhaler®	Ellipta®	HandiHaler®
n	97	91	97
R $(cmH_2O^{0.5}[L/min]^{-1})$[a]	0.060	0.090	0.163
PIF (L/min)	108 ± 23	78 ± 15	49 ± 9
Range (Min–Max)	54–156	45–109	22–70
Pressure drop at PIF (cmH_2O)	44 ± 18	51 ± 19	67 ± 23
ΔPIF vs Breezhaler® (L/min); 95% CI	–	30; 27 to 32	59; 56 to 62
P-value		< 0.0001	< 0.0001

Data are presented as mean ± standard deviation unless stated otherwise. P-values generated from a paired t-test on comparison of PIF values
Poor quality (flat-line) inhalational profiles with erroneous PIF values were not considered in the analysis
CI confidence interval, n number of patients, ΔPIF difference in mean PIF values, PIF peak inspiratory flow rate, R intrinsic airflow resistance of the inhaler
[a]Data published previously [19, 20]

pressure drop values were observed for the Breezhaler® versus the Ellipta® and the HandiHaler® inhalers, irrespective of gender (Table 5). Irrespective of the inhaler used, the PIF values observed for females were consistently lower than those observed for males (Table 5).

Safety

No AEs or serious AEs were reported in this study. No clinically significant observations were observed with regards to changes in vital signs.

Discussion

The clinical relevance of inhaled therapy relies on its ability to deliver drug directly to the intended site and avoiding systemic side effects [1]. While identifying the most appropriate treatment, health-care professionals are often more focused on pharmacological properties of a drug and tend to overlook, that inhaler characteristics may have an impact on the overall treatment benefit [21]. Patients' inhalation flow pattern can significantly influence the performance of an inhaler, thus impact effectiveness of the inhalation therapy [22]. However, there is limited data available comparing the inspiratory flow

Table 3 Comparison of mean PIF and pressure drop values based on severity of COPD

Severity	Variable	Breezhaler®	Ellipta®	HandiHaler®
	R $(cmH_2O^{0.5}[L/min]^{-1})$[a]	0.060	0.090	0.163
Moderate	n	49	44	49
	PIF (L/min)	109 ± 26	78 ± 15	50 ± 10
	Range (Min–Max)	54–152	45–102	22–68
	Pressure drop at PIF (cmH_2O)	45 ± 20	52 ± 19	68 ± 25
	ΔPIF vs Breezhaler® (L/min); 95% CI	–	31; 26 to 34	59; 54 to 64
	P-value	–	< 0.0001	< 0.0001
Severe	n	38	37	38
	PIF (L/min)	110 ± 22	79 ± 15	49 ± 8
	Range (Min–Max)	71–156	48–109	31–70
	Pressure drop at PIF (cmH_2O)	45 ± 17	53 ± 19	67 ± 22
	ΔPIF vs Breezhaler® (L/min); 95% CI	–	31; 26 to 33	61; 55 to 65
	P-value	–	< 0.0001	< 0.0001
Very severe	n	10	10	10
	PIF (L/min)	99 ± 14	71 ± 13	46 ± 7
	Range (Min–Max)	77–128	52–102	33–59
	Pressure drop at PIF (cmH_2O)	36 ± 10	42 ± 17	58 ± 17
	ΔPIF vs Breezhaler® (L/min); 95% CI	–	28; 24 to 32	53; 46 to 60
	P-value	–	< 0.0001	< 0.0001

Data are presented as mean ± standard deviation unless stated otherwise. P-values for subgroup analysis are exploratory in nature
Poor quality (flat-line) inhalational profiles with erroneous PIF values were not considered in the analysis
CI confidence interval, n number of patients, ΔPIF difference in mean PIF values, PIF peak inspiratory flow rate, R intrinsic airflow resistance of the inhaler
[a]Data published previously [19, 20]

Table 4 Comparison of mean PIF and pressure drop values based on age

Age (years)	Variable	Breezhaler®	Ellipta®	HandiHaler®
	R $(cmH_2O^{0.5}[L/min]^{-1})$[a]	0.060	0.090	0.163
40–64	n	27	27	27
	PIF (L/min)	123 ± 20	88 ± 13	53 ± 9
	Range (Min-Max)	77–156	57–109	32–70
	Pressure drop at PIF (cmH_2O)	56 ± 17	64 ± 18	76 ± 23
	ΔPIF vs Breezhaler® (L/min); 95% CI	–	35; 30 to 40	70; 65 to 76
	P-value	–	< 0.0001	< 0.0001
65–74	n	46	42	46
	PIF (L/min)	101 ± 22	73 ± 13	47 ± 9
	Range (Min-Max)	54–152	48–99	22–68
	Pressure drop at PIF (cmH_2O)	38 ± 16	45 ± 16	61 ± 23
	ΔPIF vs Breezhaler® (L/min); 95% CI	–	28; 23 to 30	54; 49 to 58
	P-value	–	< 0.0001	< 0.0001
≥75	n	24	22	24
	PIF (L/min)	105 ± 21	75 ± 16	50 ± 9
	Range (Min-Max)	65–151	45–102	29–66
	Pressure drop at PIF (cmH_2O)	41 ± 17	48 ± 18	67 ± 22
	ΔPIF vs Breezhaler® (L/min); 95% CI	–	30; 24 to 35	55; 49 to 62
	P-value	–	< 0.0001	< 0.0001

Data are presented as mean ± standard deviation unless stated otherwise. P-values for subgroup analysis are exploratory in nature
CI confidence interval, n number of patients, ΔPIF difference in mean PIF values, PIF peak inspiratory flow rate, R intrinsic airflow resistance of the inhaler
Poor quality (flat-line) inhalational profiles with erroneous PIF values were not considered in the analysis
[a]Data published previously [19, 20]

rates of the marketed products [17]. Our study provides direct comparison of inspiratory flows achieved by COPD patients between the three widely used dry powder inhalers i.e. the Breezhaler®, the Ellipta® and the HandiHaler® with varying internal resistance.

It is important to assess patients' characteristics when prescribing the medication. Patient characteristics such as age, gender and disease severity can affect the performance of the inhalers; studies have reported that increasing age [23] and COPD severity [24], may reduce patients'

Table 5 Comparison of mean PIF and pressure drop values based on gender

Gender		Breezhaler®	Ellipta®	HandiHaler®
	R $(cmH_2O^{0.5}[L/min]^{-1})$[a]	0.060	0.090	0.163
Male	n	72	68	72
	PIF (L/min)	111 ± 24	81 ± 16	51 ± 9
	Range (Min-Max)	54–156	45–109	22–70
	Pressure drop at PIF (cmH_2O)	47 ± 19	54 ± 20	71 ± 23
	ΔPIF vs Breezhaler® (L/min); 95% CI	–	30; 28 to 34	60; 57 to 65
	P-value	–	< 0.0001	< 0.0001
Female	n	25	23	25
	PIF (L/min)	98 ± 15	71 ± 11	45 ± 8
	Range (Min-Max)	71–121	49–89	32–57
	Pressure drop at PIF (cmH_2O)	36 ± 11	41 ± 12	56 ± 20
	ΔPIF vs Breezhaler® (L/min); 95% CI	–	27; 23 to 31	53; 49 to 57
	P-value	–	< 0.0001	< 0.0001

Data are presented as mean ± standard deviation unless stated otherwise. P-values for subgroup analysis are exploratory in nature
CI confidence interval, n number of patients, ΔPIF difference in mean PIF values, PIF peak inspiratory flow rate, R intrinsic airflow resistance of the inhaler
Poor quality (flat-line) inhalational profiles with erroneous PIF values were not considered in the analysis
[a]Data published previously [19, 20]

inhalation capability. Mahler et al. observed that suboptimal PIF values were predominantly exhibited by female patients when using DPI [25].

In this study, COPD patients produced the highest mean PIF rate when inhaling through the Breezhaler® inhaler compared with the Ellipta® and the HandiHaler® inhalers. Correspondingly, the lowest mean pressure drop was recorded when patients were using the Breezhaler® inhaler versus the Ellipta® or the HandiHaler® inhalers. This confirmed the prior knowledge that for a set inspiratory effort, the inhalation flows when using a low resistance DPI are expected be greater than when using a DPI with a higher resistance [26].

The mechanism of breath actuation in DPIs requires patients to generate airflow against the intrinsic airflow resistance of the inhaler. The reliance on patient-generated flow rate for effective inhalation can be minimized when using an inhaler with low intrinsic airflow resistance [11], so that patients need to exert lower inspiratory effort to generate sufficient and sustained airflow [8]. In this study, patients required least inspiratory effort when inhaling through the Breezhaler® compared with the Ellipta® and the HandiHaler® DPIs, suggesting that patients can inhale more comfortably though low resistance Breezhaler® inhaler. The results were similar irrespective of patients' age, gender or COPD severity.

Additionally, it has been previously shown that at pressure drop of up to 4 kPa (equivalent to 41 cmH$_2$O), patients are able to inhale comfortably through a DPI [27]. In this study, a pressure drop of 41 cmH$_2$O and 36 cmH$_2$O at PIF was achieved by patients of older age (≥75 years) and patients with very severe COPD, respectively, when using the Breezhaler® inhaler compared with either the Ellipta® or the HandiHaler® inhalers. The inspiratory effort determined for the Breezhaler® inhaler was less than 4 kPa at any estimated flow rate [28], indicating that patients inhaled most comfortably when using this device.

The inspiratory efforts required by patients' becomes an important consideration in treatment decisions, when a minimum inhalation flow through a specific DPI is critical for efficient de-aggregation of drug particles [26] which is not the case with the low resistance DPIs like Breezhaler® inhaler. Previously published studies for glycopyrronium and indacaterol via Breezhaler® demonstrated there was consistent dose delivery performance from Breezhaler® using airflow rates between 50 and 100 L/min. In our present study also in overall population and in the sub-groups, by COPD severity or age or gender, all patients were able to generate PIF rates of at least 54 L/min through Breezhaler, suggesting consistent dose delivery performance from Breezhaler® irrespective of patients' age, gender or COPD severity.

Some COPD patients may have difficulty with the effort required to generate sufficient inspiratory flow through a high-resistance inhaler because of loss of muscle mass and/or COPD severity [29, 30]. Therefore, when prescribing an inhalation treatment, it is important to establish whether patients can inhale comfortably through the inhaler device to be used to deliver that treatment. The ease with which patients are able to inhale through an inhaler is an important aspect of COPD management. Our results show that patients, irrespective of their COPD severity, age and gender, were able to inhale with least inspiratory effort (pressure drop) and generate highest PIF values when inhaling through the Breezhaler® inhaler compared with either the Ellipta® or the HandiHaler® inhalers. Although, we observed a slightly aberrant pattern with higher PIF values in patients aged ≥75 years (105 L/min) than that in patients aged 65–74 years (101 L/min), this could be due to comparatively less number of patients analyzed in ≥75 years age group ($n = 24$ versus $n = 46$ in 65–74 years) in the study.

The strengths of this study include minimization of inter-subject variability as measures like PIF or pressure drop are objective physical and mathematical measures, which may not be affected by prior use or experience of the patients unlike handling, preference or other measures. Furthermore random allocation and cross over design further minimizes any potential sequence bias. This study had certain limitations: the pharmacological effect of drug inhalation was not studied because this study design required multiple inhalations through the inhalers over short period of time and the PIF values may not reflect a non-research setting such as at home or during an exacerbation.

Information on the comparative inhalational flow rates and inhalation profiles from the studies DPIs and across the various studies COPD patients sub-groups would allow physicians to make informed decisions in selecting the right inhaler for the patient. Further studies would be useful to establish the generalizability of these results.

Conclusion

The results showed that mean PIF values increased and mean pressure drop values at the PIF decreased with decreasing airflow resistance of the inhalers. Patients with COPD were able to inhale with the least inspiratory effort and generate the highest mean PIF value through the Breezhaler® inhaler when compared with the Ellipta® inhaler and the HandiHaler® inhaler. The results were similar irrespective of patients' COPD severity, age or gender.

Abbreviations

AE: Adverse event; BMI: Body mass index; DPI: Dry-powder inhaler; FEV_1: Forced expiratory volume in 1 s; GOLD: Global initiative for obstructive lung disease; GUI: Graphic user interface; IPR: Inhalation profile recorder; MDI: Metered-dose inhaler; PIF: Peak inspiratory flow rate; SAE: Serious adverse event; SD: Standard deviation

Acknowledgements

The authors were assisted in the preparation of the manuscript by Praveen Kaul and Jisha John (Medical Writers, Novartis).
Breezhaler®, also referred to as Concept1 device (and known as the Neohaler™ device in the USA) is a registered trademark of Novartis AG. Ellipta® and HandiHaler® are registered trademarks of the GlaxoSmithKline and Boehringer Ingelheim International GmbH, respectively.

Funding

The study was sponsored by Novartis Pharma AG.

Authors' contributions

LW, PA, JD, TG, BA, MCM, AVP, PG have contributed towards data analysis, drafting and revising of the manuscript. All authors read and approved the final manuscript and agree to be accountable for all aspects of the work.

Competing interests

The authors declared that they have no competing interests.

Author details

[1]Novartis Pharmaceuticals Corporation, East Hanover, NJ, USA. [2]Instituto Ave Pulmo, Fundación Enfisema, Mar del Plata, Argentina. [3]Novartis Pharma AG, Basel, Switzerland. [4]Novartis Ireland Limited, Dublin, Ireland. [5]Novartis Pharmaceuticals Corporation, San Carlos, California, USA. [6]Novartis Argentina S.A, Buenos Aires, Argentina.

References

1. Global Strategy for the Diagnosis, Management and Prevention of COPD, Global Initiative for Chronic Obstructive Lung Disease (GOLD). 2017.
2. Bonini M, Usmani OS. The importance of inhaler devices in the treatment of COPD. COPD Res Prac. 2015;1:9.
3. Lavorini F, Mannini C, Chellini E, Fontana GA. Optimising inhaled pharmacotherapy for elderly patients with chronic obstructive pulmonary disease: the importance of delivery devices. Drugs Aging. 2016;33(7):461–73.
4. Dolovich MB, Ahrens RC, Hess DR, Anderson P, Dhand R, Rau JL, et al. Device selection and outcomes of aerosol therapy: evidence-based guidelines: American College of Chest Physicians/American College of Asthma, allergy, and immunology. Chest. 2005;127(1):335–71.
5. Lenney J, Innes JA, Crompton GK. Inappropriate inhaler use: assessment of use and patient preference of seven inhalation devices. EDICI Respir Med. 2000;94(5):496–500.
6. Atkins PJ. Dry powder inhalers: an overview. Respir Care. 2005;50(10):1304–12. discussion 1312
7. Pedersen S, Steffensen G. Fenoterol powder inhaler technique in children: influence of inspiratory flow rate and breath-holding. Eur J Respir Dis. 1986;68(3):207–14.
8. Labiris NR, Dolovich MB. Pulmonary drug delivery. Part II: the role of inhalant delivery devices and drug formulations in therapeutic effectiveness of aerosolized medications. Br J Clin Pharmacol. 2003;56(6):600–12.
9. Clark AR, Hollingworth AM. The relationship between powder inhaler resistance and peak inspiratory conditions in healthy volunteers-implications for in vitro testing. J Aerosol Med. 1993;6(2):99–110.
10. Dederichs JJ, Singh D, Pavkov R. Inspiratory flow profiles generated by patients with COPD through the Breezhaler® inhaler and other marketed dry powder inhalers. Poster presented at the Am J Respir Crit Care Med, American Thoracic Society International Conference, May 15–20, 2015, Denver, CO, USA, 2015. Vol. 191.
11. Colthorpe P, Voshaar T, Kieckbusch T, Cuoghi E, Jauernig J. Delivery characteristics of a low-resistance dry-powder inhaler used to deliver the long-acting muscarinic antagonist glycopyrronium. J Drug Assess. 2013;2(1):11–6.
12. Mueller S, Haeberlin B. S. E. Comparison of performance characteristics for Foradil Aerolizer® and Foradil Concept1 (a new single dose dry powder inhaler) at different test flow rates. Resp Drug Deliv. 2008;3:67–678.
13. Pavkov R, Singh D. Concept1 (a new single dose dry powder inhaler) peak inspiratory flow rate study with COPD patients. Resp Drug Deliv. 2008;3:683–6.
14. Kuttler A, Dimke T. A novel biophysical simulation model of drug deposition implemented to predict and optimize QVA149 delivery to the lungs., American Thoracic Society International Conference, San Diego, CA, US, 16 May–21 May., 2014. Vol Abstract A3038.
15. Pavkov R, Mueller S, Fiebich K, Singh D, Stowasser F, Pignatelli G, et al. Characteristics of a capsule based dry powder inhaler for the delivery of indacaterol. Curr Med Res Opin. 2010;26(11):2527–33.
16. Molimard M, Raherison C, Lignot S, Balestra A, Lamarque S, Chartier A, et al. Chronic obstructive pulmonary disease exacerbation and inhaler device handling: real-life assessment of 2935 patients. Eur Respir J. 2017;49(2)
17. Chapman KR, Fogarty CM, Peckitt C, Lassen C, Jadayel D, Dederichs J, et al. Delivery characteristics and patients' handling of two single-dose dry-powder inhalers used in COPD. Int J Chron Obstruct Pulmon Dis. 2011;6:353–63.
18. Global Strategy for the Diagnosis, Management and Prevention of COPD, Global Initiative for Chronic Obstructive Lung Disease (GOLD). 2014.
19. Chodosh S, Flanders JS, Kesten S, Serby CW, Hochrainer D, Witek TJ Jr. Effective delivery of particles with the HandiHaler dry powder inhalation system over a range of chronic obstructive pulmonary disease severity. J Aerosol Med. 2001;14(3):309–15.
20. Phillip Krüger BE, Zier M, Greguletz R. Inspiratory flow resistance of marketed dry powder inhalers (DPI). Eur Respir J. 2014;2014(44):4635.
21. Darba J, Ramirez G, Sicras A, Francoli P, Torvinen S, Sanchez-de la Rosa R. The importance of inhaler devices: the choice of inhaler device may lead to suboptimal adherence in COPD patients. Int J Chron Obstruct Pulmon Dis. 2015;10:2335–45.
22. Hira D, Koide H, Nakamura S, Okada T, Ishizeki K, Yamaguchi M, et al. Assessment of inhalation flow patterns of soft mist inhaler co-prescribed with dry powder inhaler using inspiratory flow meter for multi inhalation devices. PLoS One. 2018;13(2):e0193082.
23. Ibrahim M, Verma R, Garcia-Contreras L. Inhalation drug delivery devices: technology update. Med Devices (Auckl). 2015;8:131–9.
24. Prime D, de Backer W, Hamilton M, Cahn A, Preece A, Kelleher D, et al. Effect of disease severity in asthma and chronic obstructive pulmonary disease on inhaler-specific inhalation profiles through the ELLIPTA(R) dry powder inhaler. J Aerosol Med Pulm Drug Deliv. 2015;28(6):486–97.
25. Mahler DA, Waterman LA, Gifford AH. Prevalence and COPD phenotype for a suboptimal peak inspiratory flow rate against the simulated resistance of the Diskus(R) dry powder inhaler. J Aerosol Med Pulm Drug Deliv. 2013;26(3):174–9.
26. Price D, Chrystyn H. Concept review of dry powder inhalers: correct interpretation of published data. Multidiscip Respir Med. 2015;10:36.
27. Behara SR, Larson I, Kippax P, Stewart P, Morton DA. Insight into pressure drop dependent efficiencies of dry powder inhalers. Eur J Pharm Sci. 2012;46(3):142–8.
28. Ciciliani AM, Langguth P, Wachtel H. In vitro dose comparison of Respimat((R)) inhaler with dry powder inhalers for COPD maintenance therapy. Int J Chron Obstruct Pulmon Dis. 2017;12:1565-77.
29. Wieshammer S, Dreyhaupt J. Dry powder inhalers: which factors determine the frequency of handling errors? Respiration. 2008;75(1):18-25.
30. Brennan VK, Osman LM, Graham H, Critchlow A, Everard ML. True device compliance: the need to consider both competence and contrivance. Respir Med. 2005;99(1):97-102.

12

Mobile health applications in self-management of patients with chronic obstructive pulmonary disease

Fen Yang[1†], Yuncui Wang[1†], Chongming Yang[2], Hui Hu[1*] and Zhenfang Xiong[1*†]

Abstract

Background: Mobile health applications are increasingly used in patients with Chronic Obstructive Pulmonary Disease (COPD) to improve their self-management, nonetheless, without firm evidence of their efficacy. This meta-analysis was aimed to assess the efficacy of mobile health applications in supporting self-management as an intervention to reduce hospital admission rates and average days of hospitalization, etc.

Methods: PubMed, Web of Science (SCI), Cochrane Library, and Embase were searched for relevant articles published before November 14th, 2017. A total of 6 reports with randomized controlled trials (RCTs) were finally included in this meta-analysis.

Results: Patients using mobile phone applications may have a lower risk for hospital admissions than those in the usual care group (risk ratio (RR) = 0.73, 95% CI [0.52, 1.04]). However, there was no significant difference in reducing the average days of hospitalization.

Conclusion: Self-management with mobile phone applications could reduce hospital admissions of patients with COPD.

Keywords: Chronic obstructive pulmonary disease, Self-management, Hospital admissions, Mobile applications

Background

Chronic Obstructive Pulmonary Disease (COPD) is a major global chronic disease which affected millions of people worldwide [1], causing considerable hospital admissions. The World Health Organization (WHO) has estimated that COPD which causes considerable hospital admission will become the third cause of global deaths by 2020 [2–5]. These patients are heavy users of healthcare and social service resources [6, 7]. As there is currently no cure for COPD, appropriate self-care and management may play an important role in the patients' lifetime. Self-management techniques, such as adherence to medication, exercises, and prompt medical care, are crucial to improve the health status and have the potential to reduce hospital admissions [8–11].

Mobile health (mHealth), is now widely used for self-management of COPD, a term used to describe medical practice and healthcare in support of mobile computing and mobile devices (such as tablets, mobile phones, etc.). However, it is unclear whether these applications are beneficial to patients [12]. The deployment of eHealth applications is conducive to the availability of health care, which in turn enhances the patient's understanding of his illness, sense of control, and willingness to manage himself [13]. However, cheaper and widely available mobile phones are not other specialized medical devices. Mobile phones with applications to monitor, prompt, and record health behaviors have become a feasible and acceptable intervention [14]. Some reviews

* Correspondence: xiong_zhenfang@126.com; xiong_zhenfang@126.com
†Fen Yang, Yuncui Wang and Zhenfang Xiong contributed equally to this work.
1School of Nursing, Hubei University of Chinese Medicine, Wuhan, China
Full list of author information is available at the end of the article

reported that mHealth applications were effective in promoting disease self-management and daily lifestyle changes [15–17]. Several studies showed that mobile phones could deliver effective behavior change interventions and had many positive evidences [9, 18–20]. Mobile phones were also found effective in promoting COPD patients' physical activity and exercise capacity [21]. However, another study found that COPD patients with telephone-based care had greater mortality than usual care [22]. It is not clear how effectively mobile phone interventions could improve hospital admissions and lengths of hospitalization of COPD patients. Therefore, this study was aimed to compare the efficacy of mobile phone intervention with usual care in self-management, in terms of hospital admissions and the lengths of hospitalization.

Methods

Data sources and searches

A literature search without language restriction was performed using PubMed, Web of Science, the Cochrane Library, and Embase databases to identify potentially eligible studies published prior to November 14, 2017. All titles, keywords, and abstracts were examined in accordance with our search criteria. Full reports also were reviewed in case of uncertainty. In addition, references of retrieved studies and review articles were also manually checked to identify additional relevant studies. Some authors were even contacted for further information.

Study selection

Each study had to meet four criteria to be included in this study. First, studies were RCTs reported in full text with a title and abstract. Second, it included adults with a clinical diagnosis of COPD and compare mobile phone application interventions with the control group in usual care only (namely, routine or standard care). Third, tele-monitoring studies entailed a self-management by COPD patients with ≥1 month follow-up. Fourth, the trials evaluated at least one of the following primary or secondary outcomes. The primary outcome was a hospital admission. The secondary outcome was the length of hospitalization, activity level, and lung function (e.g., predicted FEV1 percentage). Inclusion of each study was evaluated and determined independently by two reviewers. Exclusion criteria included: (1) reports based on systematic reviews and meta-analyses; (2) mobile-based interventions only via phone calls or sending messages.

Data extraction and quality assessment

From the articles that met the inclusion criteria, two reviewers independently extracted descriptions of the objectives, design, participants, interventions, and follow-up time. Any disagreements in data extraction were resolved by a discussion among the reviewers, and a final decision was made by another reviewer. If it is difficult or unclear to extract data from an article, its author was directly contacted to request the original data. The Cochrane Group's predesigned table [23] was used to assess the quality of the studies, including randomization, allocation concealment, similarity of baseline, criteria of inclusion/exclusion, blinding of participants and researchers, blinding of assessors, attrition rates, reporting of lost participants, and other sources of biases. Studies were scored one point for each fulfilled criterion. The quality of the studies was divided into three levels: low (≤3 points), moderate (4–6 points), and high (7–9 points).

Data synthesis and analysis

Eight studies were selected for the systematic review [24–31] and six of that were included for the meta-analysis with a random-effects model [24–29]. The outcomes reported by similar multiple studies were combined for the analysis. Also, meta-analyzed were the RCTs that reported the number of readmissions and the average days of hospitalization of each group (usual care vs. eHealth).

Data were obtained from the original selected studies or calculated [32] from the raw data. Risk ratios (RRs) were calculated for hospital admissions and mortality rates. Statistical heterogeneity was measured with the chi-square (χ^2) and I^2 statistics whose values greater than 50% indicate a high heterogeneity for the latter [33]. Publication bias was depicted with Begg's plot. Standard Mean Differences (SMD) were estimated with random effects modeling. All analyses were performed using Stata 12.0.

Results

Basic characteristics of the studies

From the 4072 potentially relevant reports initially identified, 3350 publications were excluded. The remainder of 722 retrieved reports were selected for full-text assessments and detailed evaluations. Finally, eight articles fulfilled our inclusion criteria [24–31] and only six articles were included in our meta-analysis [24–29] because two didn't report the patients' hospital admission [30, 31]. Figure 1 shows the literature flow diagram. We also extracted some additional information, such as country, mean age, the sample size of each group, sex, FEV1, the intervention methods, the length of follow-up and BMI, as shown in Table 1. Most RCTs compared a continued care with a usual care. Six RCTs reported the primary outcome of hospital admissions [24–29]. Only one study was a multicenter RCTs, and the others were conducted in single centers. There were totally 391 participants with COPD,

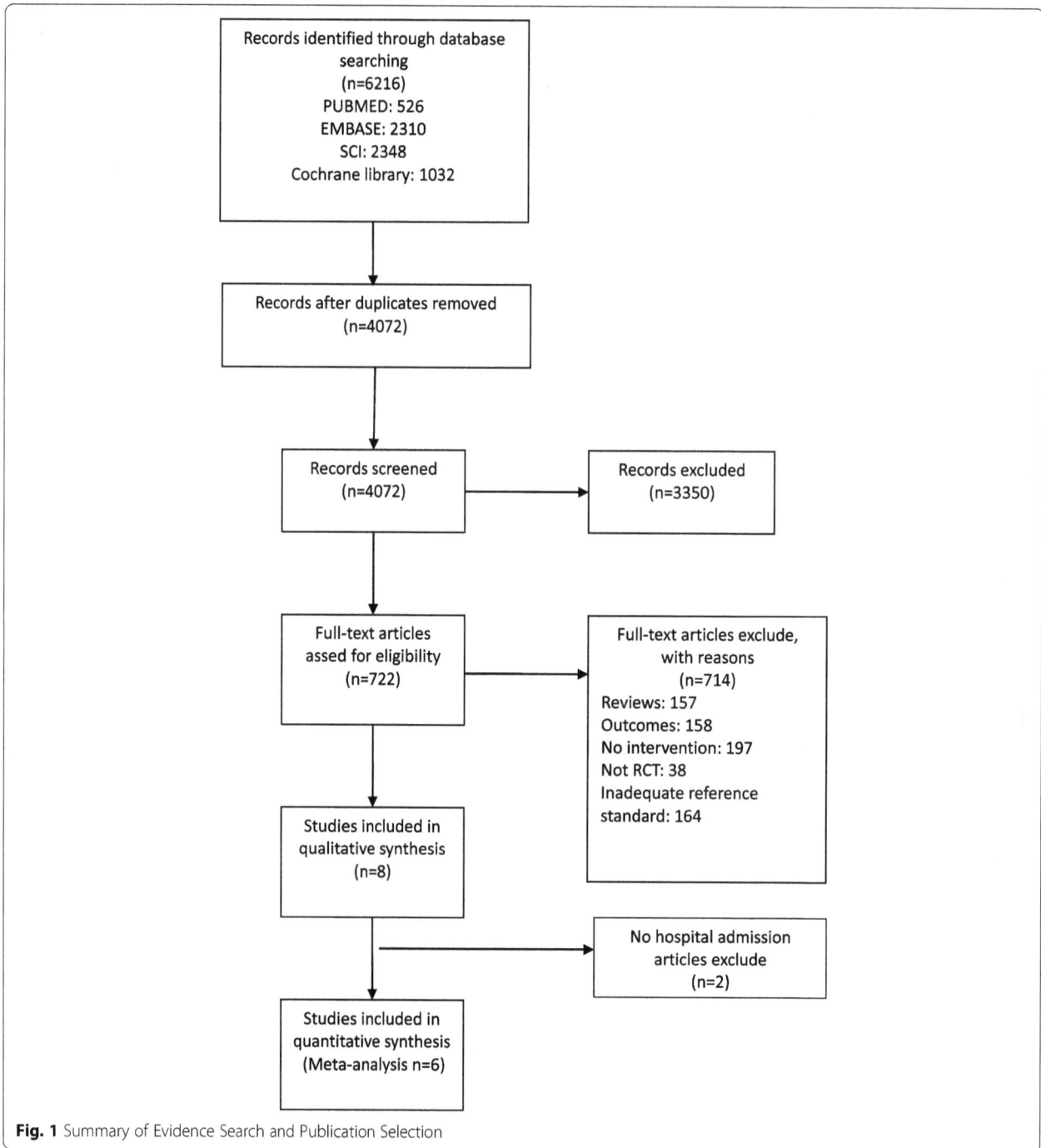

Fig. 1 Summary of Evidence Search and Publication Selection

293 (74.9%) of whom were men. The participants in one study had additional heart failures [27]. The sample sizes of subjects ranged from 24 to 99. There were six studies reporting the duration of the intervention equal or more than 6 months. The age of participants ranged from 63.5 to 81.0 years. The lung dysfunction was indicated by FEV1 (% predicted) that ranged from 37.9 to 58.9%. BMI ranged from 23.2 to 28.8 kg/m^2. Follow-ups were conducted for a range of 1 to 12 months and a mean of 6.9 months.

The intervention of the five studies included mobile/ smartphones with different software (Phone-personal digital assistant, MMA400, HTC P3600/3700, Sony Ericsson K600i, and HTC Desire S) and measuring devices. Applications were installed on smartphones to support patients in recording and monitoring their own physiological status, such as oxygen saturation levels, pulse rates, pedometers, or blood pressure monitors; or health behaviors, such as medications and dietary intake and exercise levels. Patients uploaded the data to their phones and sent

Table 1 Description of included trials

Source	Country	Mean (Age, y)	N	Setting	Male (%)	FEV1%	BMI (kg/m²)	Months of follow-up	Intervention
Liu WT et al., 2008 [26]	China	72.1	IG:24;CG:24	Single-center	48(100.0)	45.6	23.2	12	Patients were asked to complete respiratory symptoms by a cell phone using a Java application software, before they started daily endurance walking training.
Chau JP et al., 2012 [25]	China	72.9	IG:22;CG:18	single-center	39(97.5)	37.9	NR	2	The ASTRI telecare system (AST): a device kit which includes a mobile phone, a respiratory rate sensor and a pulse oximeter, an online network platform, a call center and a networking system. Participants in the intervention group measured their oxygen saturation, pulse rate and respiration rate at home and sent the results to the online network platform by mobile phone.
Jehn M et al., 2013 [24]	Germany	66.6	IG:32;CG:30	single-center	48(74.4)	51.4	27.3	9	Tele-monitoring: COPD Assessment Test (CAT), daily lung function and weekly 6-minute walk test (6MWT). The patients entered CAT by mobile phone (PDA system, MMA400).
Martin-Lesende I et al., 2013 [27]	Spain	81.0	IG:28;CG:30	Multicenter	34(58.6)	NA	NR	3, 6, 12	Tele-monitoring: daily transmissions from the patients' homes of the following self-measured clinical parameters (such as blood oxygen saturation, blood pressure, heart and respiratory rates, body weight and temperature) using a smart phone– personal digital assistant (PDA).
Pedone C et al., 2013 [28]	Italy	74.8	IG:50;CG:49	Single-center	67(67.7)	54.0	NR	9	"SweetAge" monitoring system: A commercial cellular telephone was equipped with a software that allowed the reception of the data(oxygen saturation, heart rate, near-body temperature, overall physical activity) transmitted by the wristband and sent the data to the monitoring system.
Tabak M et al., 2014 [29, 30]	the Netherlands	63.5	IG:12;CG:12	Single-center	12(50.0)	43.0	26.8	9	Condition Coach: teleconsultation (module for comments and asking questions of the patient's primary care physiotherapist and vice versa), Web-based exercising (including breathing exercises, relaxation, mobilization, resistance and endurance training, and mucus clearance), self-management and activity coach(A smartphone shows the measured activity cumulatively in a graph).
Tabak M et al., 2014 [29, 30]	the Netherlands	66.6	IG:14;CG:16	Single-center	19(63.3)	52.6	28.8	1	Tele-rehabilitation: (1) a smartphone (HTC P3600/3700) was used for activity coach; (2) web portal with a symptom diary for self-treatment of exacerbations and an overview of the measured activity levels.
Wang CH et al., 2014 [31]	China	71.7	IG:14;CG:16	Single-center	26(86.7)	58.9	23.5	6	Patients in the intervention group performed daily endurance exercise training under mobile phone guidance, and adherence was reported back to the central server.

NR not reported, *IG* Intervention Group, *CG* Control Group

the data to the networking/monitoring systems for health-care providers to follow up and personalize feedbacks. The aim of the intervention was to train patients and promote self-monitoring and healthy lifestyle behaviors. In three of all the trials, the mobile/smartphone was used to coach activities. The patients in control groups received usual care.

Study quality and publication Bias

The overall quality of the studies (Table 2) was moderate to high (4–7 scores). Five studies scored less than or equal to 6, and three studies scored less than 9. The most common reason for lower scores was the absence of a double–blind procedure, which was impossible due to the nature of the intervention. The assessors were not blinded to the outcomes in all the studies (100.0%) and researchers/participants were not blinded in 6 studies (75.0%). Only one study (12.5%) did not report the characteristics of participants lost for follow-ups. Begg's plot that was used to examine publication bias showed that there was no evident publication bias ($p = 1.00$).

Hospital admission rates

Figure 2 presented our meta-analyses and RR calculations of RCTs reported hospital admission. Six studies [24–29] assessed the effect of mobile health applications on hospital admission. As Martín-Lesende [27] reported the data of patients at the follow-up of 3 months, 6 months, and 12 months, we treated it as three separate experiments in our meta-analysis. We found that a lower risk for hospital admission among patients using mobile phone applications than that of the usual care group (RR = 0.73 [95% CI, 0.52 to 1.04]). The study by Jehn M [24] found that the hospital admission rates decreased significantly (RR, 0.30 [95% CI, 0.15 to 0.59]). But the heterogeneity in the overall pooled effect is 51.4% ($I^2 = 51.4\%$, $p = 0.04$), implying that effect sizes varied across studies.

Average days of hospitalization

As shown in Fig. 3, six studies reported the average days of hospital stays. No significant difference was found between the intervention group and control group (SMD -0.06 [95% CI, – 0.31 to 0.18]).

Other results

Five articles reported that phone-based system could significantly improve exercise capacity and activity levels [24, 26, 29–31]. One study showed a significant reduction (lower predicted FEV1 percentage) in lung function of tele-monitoring intervention groups [24]. However, there was no significant differences found in another study [26].

Sensitivity analysis

A sensitivity analysis was performed for the primary outcome to test an overall pooled effect. The results were no different between fixed and random statistical effects (RR = 0.73; $P = 0.000$). The effect of sequentially omitting a low-quality study [24] and recalculating the pooled estimates for the remaining studies did not significantly alter the effect on all cause readmission (RR = 0.73 vs. 0.83; $P = 0.000$).

Discussion

Our results showed that mobile phone-based health applications in self-management currently could reduce hospital admissions of patients with COPD and could improve exercise capacity and activity levels, but could not reduce the average days of hospitalization.

Our findings were slightly different from another telemonitoring study which used a touch screen telemonitoring equipment to record and transmit a daily questionnaire about symptoms and corresponding treatment, and did not provide any convincing evidence of effectiveness on hospital admission and the duration of admissions [34]. The inconsistence may be due to the difference between screen telemonitoring and mobile phone. Mobile phone-based applications were found easy to learn and use by the participants as well as the patients with COPD. Mobile phone-based health applications could be practically more feasible as an intervention. Some studies reported they were a simple, reliable, easy to perform, and cost-saving intervention in behavior-changes, with advantages like adherence and intensity of the interventions, and more willingness of patients to use than other electronic devices [35, 36]. In addition, the virtual link created by sending self-monitoring data to a research nurse provided patients with a sense of continuity of care [37].

Mobile-phone-based system provides a feasible, efficient exercise training in improving exercise capacity, which was similar with other studies [38, 39]. Patients with COPD have decreased exercise capacity in their daily activities and they may have an inactive lifestyle [40–43]. Mobile phone applications, as a feasible and acceptable method for patients with COPD, can increase the capacity of self-management and the exercise adherence [44]. This result was similar with another review which evaluated the effectiveness of interventions delivered by computer and by mobile technology versus face-to-face or hard copy/digital documentary-delivered interventions [45]. A recent systematic review reported that mobile-based exercise programs could improve exercise capacity in patients with COPD in short and long term [30].

There are several limitations of our study. First, most RCTs compared an intervention with "usual care" whose details were not reported. Second, we only selected studies that reported the proportion of hospital admitted

Table 2 Quality assessment of included studies

Study	Randomization	Concealing Allocation	Baseline Similarity	Inclusion/Exclusion Criteria	Blinded Researchers/ Participants	Blinded Assessors	Attrition Rate Reported	Describing Lost Participants	Intention-to-Treat Analysis	Power Analysis	Total
Liu WT et al., 2008 [26]	Yes	No	Yes	Yes	No	No	Yes	Yes	No	Yes	6
Chau JP et al., 2012 [25]	Yes	No	Yes	Yes	No	No	Yes	Yes	No	No	5
Jehn M et al., 2013 [24]	Yes	No	Yes	Yes	No	No	Yes	No	No	No	4
Martín-Lesende I et al., 2013 [27]	Yes	No	Yes	Yes	No	No	Yes	Yes	No	Yes	6
Pedone C et al., 2013 [28]	Yes	No	Yes	Yes	No	No	Yes	Yes	Yes	Yes	7
Tabak M et al., 2014 [29, 30]	Yes	Yes	Yes	Yes	Yes	No	Yes	Yes	No	No	7
Tabak M et al., 2014 [29, 30]	Yes	Yes	Yes	Yes	Yes	No	Yes	Yes	No	No	7
Wang CH et al., 2014 [31]	Yes	No	Yes	Yes	No	No	No	Yes	No	No	4

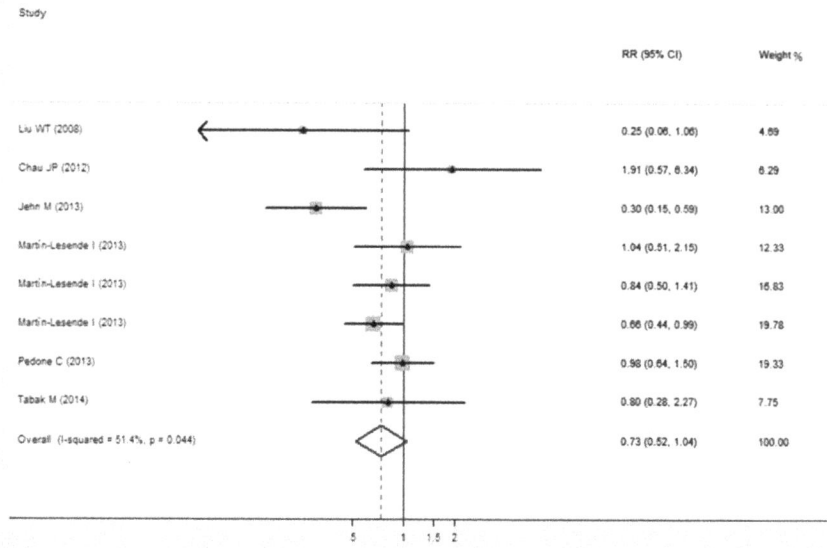

Fig. 2 Hospital admission for Intervention Group Compared with Control Group. Weights were from the random effects analysis

patients, but ignored information about secondary outcomes such as costs. Third, only eight studies were included in this systematic review and 6 studies in meta-analysis, most interventions were performed in short terms which could have influenced the results. Mobile phones will continue to evolve and are expected to be robust ubiquitous devices in the future, and researchers may think about how mobile phones can be used in future self-management of chronic disease. With the development of information technology and the expansion of mobile applications in medicine, we could improve the designs and clarify the effects of mobile health applications interventions for reducing hospital admission in patients with COPD in the future.

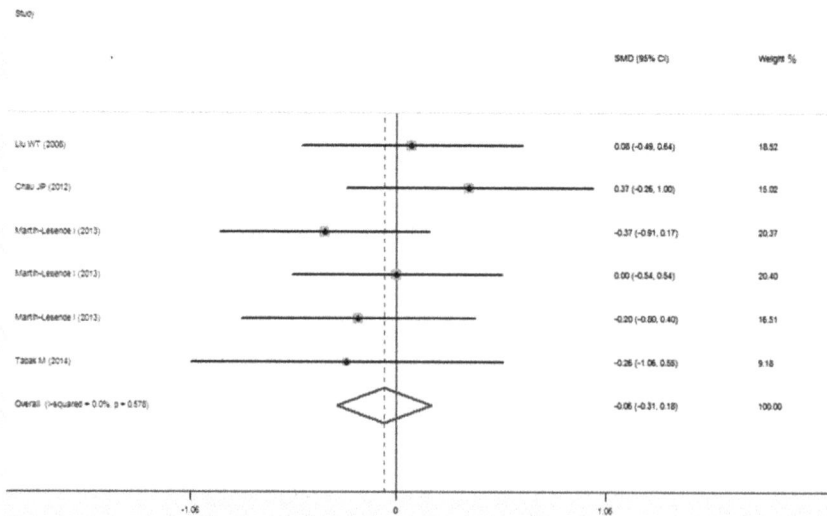

Fig. 3 Average hospital staying days for Intervention Group Compared with Control Group. Weights are from the random effects analysis

Conclusions

The effectiveness of self-management with mobile or smart phones may help to reduce hospital admissions or improve health status of patients with COPD. Mobile phone with convenient applications have a great potential to minimize health problems and improve healthcare delivery.

Abbreviations

COPD: Chronic obstructive pulmonary disease; mHealth: Mobile health; RCTs: Randomized controlled trials; RRs: Risk ratios; SCI: Web of science

Authors' contributions

YF preformed the work of design, acquisition of data and drafting the manuscript; WYC acquitted the data and wrote part of article; YCM and XZF analysed the data; HH conceived the report and wrote the manuscript. All the authors have read and approved the final manuscript.

Competing interests

The authors declare that they have no competing interests.

Author details

[1]School of Nursing, Hubei University of Chinese Medicine, Wuhan, China. [2]Research Support Center, Brigham Young University, Provo, UT, USA.

References

1. Global initial for chronic obstructive lung disease: Gloable strategy for the diagnosis, management, and prevention of chronic obstructive pulmonary disease (2017 report). Retrieved on August 1, 2018 at https://goldcopd.org/gold-2017-global-strategy-diagnosis-management-prevention-copd/.
2. Puhan MA, Scharplatz M, Troosters T, Steurer J. Respiratory rehabilitation after acute exacerbation of COPD may reduce risk for readmission and mortality - a systematic review. Respir Res. 2005;6(1):54.
3. Mannino DM, Buist AS. Global burden of COPD: risk factors, prevalence, and future trends. Lancet. 2007;370(9589):765–73.
4. Lopez AD, Shibuya K, Rao C, Mathers CD, Hansell AL, Held LS, et al. Chronic obstructive pulmonary disease: current burden and future projections. Eur Respir J. 2006;27(2):397–412.
5. Buist AS, McBurnie MA, Vollmer WM, Gillespie S, Burney P, Mannino DM, et al. International variation in the prevalence of COPD (the BOLD study): a population-based prevalence study. Lancet. 2007;370(9589):741–50.
6. Mapel DW, McMillan GP, Frost FJ, Hurley JS, Picchi MA, Lydick E, et al. Predicting the costs of managing patients with chronic obstructive pulmonary disease. Respir Med. 2005;99(10):1325–33.
7. Tynan AJ, Lane SJCOPD. Illness severity, resource utilization and cost. Ir Med J. 2005;98(2):41–2.
8. Efraimsson EO, Hillervik C, Ehrenberg A. Effects of COPD self-care management education at a nurse-led primary health care clinic. Scand J Caring Sci. 2008;22(2):178–85.
9. Bourbeau J, Julien M, Maltais F, Rouleau M, Beaupré A, Bégin R, et al. Reduction of hospital utilization in patients with chronic obstructive pulmonary disease: a disease-specific self-management intervention. Arch Intern Med. 2003;163(5):585–91.
10. Zwerink M, Brusse-Keizer M, Van PD ZGA, Monninkhof EM, van der Palen J, et al. Self-management for patients with chronic obstructive pulmonary disease. Cochrane Database Syst Rev. 2014;3(3):CD002990.
11. Warwick M, Gallagher R, Chenoweth L, Stein-Parbury J. Self-management and symptom monitoring among older adults with chronic obstructive pulmonary disease. J Adv Nurs. 2010;66(4):784–93.
12. Black AD, Car J, Pagliari C, Anandan C, Cresswell K, Bokun T, et al. The impact of eHealth on the quality and safety of health care: a systematic overview. PLoS Med. 2011;8(1):e1000387.
13. Boulos MN, Brewer AC, Karimkhani C, Buller DB, Dellavalle RP. Mobile medical and health apps: state of the art, concerns, regulatory control and certification. Online J Public Health Inform. 2014;5(3):229.
14. Nguyen HQ, Wolpin S, Chiang KC, Cuenco D, Carrieri-Kohlman V. Exercise and symptom monitoring with a mobile device. AMIA Annu Symp Proc. 2006;1047
15. Nour M, Chen J, Allman-Farinelli M. Efficacy and external validity of electronic and mobile phone-based interventions promoting vegetable intake in young adults: systematic review and meta-analysis. J Med Internet Res. 2016;18(4):e58.
16. Devi BR, Syed-Abdul S, Kumar A, Iqbal U, Nguyen PA, Li YC, et al. An updated systematic review with a focus on HIV/AIDS and tuberculosis long term management using mobile phones. Comput Methods Prog Biomed. 2015;122(2):257–65.
17. Cui M, Wu X, Mao J, Wang X, Nie M. T2DM self-management via smartphone applications: a systematic review and meta-analysis. PLoS One. 2016;11(11):e0166718.
18. Hurling R, Catt M, Boni MD, Fairley BW, Hurst T, Murray P, et al. Using internet and mobile phone technology to deliver an automated physical activity program: randomized controlled trial. J Med Internet Res. 2007;9(2):e7.
19. Brendryen H, Drozd F, Kraft P. A digital smoking cessation program delivered through internet and cell phone without nicotine replacement (happy ending): randomized controlled trial. J Med Internet Res. 2008;10(5):e51.
20. Wennberg DE, Marr A, Lang L, O'Malley S, Bennett G. A randomized trial of a telephone care-management strategy. N Engl J Med. 2010;363(13):1245–55.
21. Martínez-García MDM, Ruiz-Cárdenas JD, Rabinovich RA. Effectiveness of smartphone devices in promoting physical activity and exercise in patients with chronic obstructive pulmonary disease: a systematic review. COPD. 2017;14(5):543–51.
22. Polisena J, Tran K, Cimon K, Hutton B, McGill S, Palmer K, et al. Home telehealth for chronic obstructive pulmonary disease: a systematic review and meta-analysis. J Telemed Telecare. 2010;16(3):120–7.
23. Higgins J, Green S. Cochrane Handbook for Systematic Reviews of Interventions. Chichester: J Wiley; 2006.
24. Jehn M, Donaldson G, Kiran B, Liebers U, Mueller K, Scherer D, et al. Tele-monitoring reduces exacerbation of COPD in the context of climate change–a randomized controlled trial. Environ Health. 2013;12:99.
25. Chau JP, Lee DT, Yu DS, Chow AY, Yu WC, Chair SY, et al. A feasibility study to investigate the acceptability and potential effectiveness of a telecare service for older people with chronic obstructive pulmonary disease. Int J Med Inform. 2012;81(10):674–82.
26. Liu WT, Wang CH, Lin HC, Lin SM, Lee KY, Lo YL, et al. Efficacy of a cell phone-based exercise programme for COPD. Eur Respir J. 2008;32(3):651–9.
27. Martín-Lesende I, Orruño E, Bilbao A, Vergara I, Cairo MC, Bayón JC, et al. Impact of telemonitoring home care patients with heart failure or chronic lung disease from primary care on healthcare resource use (the TELBIL study randomised controlled trial). BMC Health Serv Res. 2013;13:118.
28. Pedone C, Chiurco D, Scarlata S, Incalzi RA. Efficacy of multiparametric telemonitoring on respiratory outcomes in elderly people with COPD: a randomized controlled trial. BMC Health Serv Res. 2013;13:82.
29. Tabak M, Brusse-Keizer M, van der Valk P, Hermens H, Vollenbroek-Hutten M. A telehealth program for self-management of COPD exacerbations and promotion of an active lifestyle: a pilot randomized controlled trial. Int J Chron Obstruct Pulmon Dis. 2014;9:935–44.
30. Tabak M, Vollenbroek-Hutten MM, van der Valk PD, van der Palen J, Hermens HJ. A telerehabilitation intervention for patients with chronic obstructive pulmonary disease: a randomized controlled pilot trial. Clin Rehabil. 2014;28(6):582–91.
31. Wang CH, Chou PC, Joa WC, Chen LF, Sheng TF, Ho SC, et al. Mobile-phone-based home exercise training program decreases systemic inflammation in COPD: a pilot study. BMC Pulm Med. 2014;14:142.
32. Borenstein M, Hedges LV, Higgins JP, Rothstein HR. A basic introduction to fixed-effect and random-effects models for meta-analysis. Res Synth Methods. 2010;1(2):97–111.
33. Higgins JP, Thompson SG, Deeks JJ, Altman DG. Measuring inconsistency in meta-analyses. BMJ. 2003;327(7414):557–60.
34. Pinnock H, Hanley J, McCloughan L, Todd A, Krishan A, Lewis S, et al. Effectiveness of telemonitoring integrated into existing clinical services on hospital admission for exacerbation of chronic obstructive pulmonary

disease: researcher blind, multicenter, randomized controlled trial. BMJ. 2013;347:f6070.

35. Kobayashi M, Hiyama A, Miura T, Asakawa C, Hirose M, Ifukube T. Elderly user evaluation of mobile touchscreen interactions. Springer Berlin Heidelberg. 2011;6946:83–99.

36. Velardo C, Shah SA, Gibson O, Clifford G, Heneghan C, Rutter H, et al. Digital health system for personalised COPD long-term management. BMC Med Inform Decis Mak. 2017;17(1):19.

37. Abaza H, Marschollek M. mHealth application areas and technology combinations. A comparison of literature from high and low/middle income countries. Methods Inf Med. 2017;56(7):e105–22.

38. Gosselink R, Langer D, Burtin C, Probst V, Hendriks HJM, van der Schans CP, et al. Clinical practice guideline for physical therapy in patients with COPD – practice guidelines. Dutch J Phys Ther. 2008;118(suppl):1–60.

39. Langer D, Hendriks E, Burtin C, Probst V, van der Schans C, Paterson W, et al. A clinical practice guideline for physiotherapists treating patients with chronic obstructive pulmonary disease based on a systematic review of available evidence. Clin Rehabil. 2009;23(5):445–62.

40. Sandland CJ, Singh SJ, Curcio A, Jones PM, Morgan MD. A profile of daily activity in chronic obstructive pulmonary disease. J Cardpulm Rehabil. 2005;25(3):181–3.

41. Pitta F, Troosters T, Spruit MA, Probst VS, Decramer M, Gosselink R. Characteristics of physical activities in daily life in chronic obstructive pulmonary disease. Am J Respir Crit Care Med. 2005;171(9):972–7.

42. Tabak M, Vollenbroek-Hutten M, van der Valk P, van der Palen J, Tönis T, Hermens H. Telemonitoring of daily activity and symptom behavior in patients with COPD. Int J Telemed Appl. 2012;2012:438736.

43. Lores V, Garcia-Rio F, Rojo B, Alcolea S, Mediano O. Recording the daily physical activity of COPD patients with an accelerometer: an analysis of agreement and repeatability. Arch Bronconeumol. 2006;42(12):627–32.

44. Dale J, Connor S, Tolley K. An evaluation of the west surrey telemedicine monitoring project. J Telemed Telecare. 2003;9(Suppl 1):S39–41.

45. McCabe C, McCann M, Brady AM. Computer and mobile technology interventions for self-management in chronic obstructive pulmonary disease. Cochrane Database Syst Rev. 2017;5:CD011425.

13

Pulmonary tumor thrombotic microangiopathy and pulmonary veno-occlusive disease in a woman with cervical cancer treated with cediranib and durvalumab

Dante A. Suffredini[1*], Jung-Min Lee[2], Cody J. Peer[3], Drew Pratt[4], David E. Kleiner[4], Jason M. Elinoff[1] and Michael A. Solomon[1,5]

Abstract

Background: Pulmonary tumor thrombotic microangiopathy (PTTM) is a rare cause of pulmonary hypertension that is associated with malignancies and is marked by the presence of non-occlusive tumor emboli and fibrocellular intimal proliferation of small pulmonary arteries leading to increased pulmonary vascular resistance and right heart failure. The diagnosis of PTTM is challenging to make pre-mortem and guidelines on treatment are lacking.

Case presentation: A 45-year-old woman with advanced squamous cell carcinoma of the cervix developed symptoms of dyspnea and evidence of right heart failure during a phase I clinical trial with cediranib and durvalumab. After an extensive evaluation, pre-capillary pulmonary hypertension was confirmed by right heart catheterization. Vasodilator therapy was initiated but resulted in the development of symptomatic hypoxemia and was discontinued. Despite continued supportive care, she continued to decline and was transitioned to hospice care. At autopsy, the cause of her right heart failure was found to be due to PTTM with features of pulmonary veno-occlusive disease (PVOD).

Conclusion: PTTM and PVOD are important diagnoses to consider in patients with a malignancy and the development of right heart failure and may be manifestations of a spectrum of similar disease processes.

Keywords: Pulmonary tumor thrombotic microangiopathy, Pulmonary hypertension, Cediranib, Durvalumab, Cervical cancer

Background

Pulmonary tumor thrombotic microangiopathy (PTTM) is a rare condition characterized by microscopic tumor cell emboli, which cause proliferative changes in the pulmonary microvasculature leading to a syndrome of hypoxemia, pulmonary hypertension, right heart failure and death [1]. In the initial report, unique pathologic changes in 21 patients were described with non-occluding microscopic tumor emboli limited to the small pulmonary arterial vessel wall, isolated or clumped in the vessel lumen and often with secondary thrombosis. The endothelial attachment of tumor cells was associated with fibrocellular intimal proliferation. The resultant obstruction of the small arteries and increase in pulmonary vascular resistance is thought to contribute to the clinical presentation of progressive cor pulmonale and death. It was notable that in nearly all the described cases lymphangiosis carcinomatosa was present, but the relationship to PTTM was unclear. Thus, PTTM is thought to be a unique clinical entity based on the presence of intimal proliferation, distinguishing it from obstructive pulmonary tumor emboli. In a larger case series, adenocarcinoma was

* Correspondence: dante.suffredini@nih.gov
[1]Critical Care Medicine Department, National Institutes of Health Clinical Center, Bethesda, MD, USA
Full list of author information is available at the end of the article

the most common underlying malignancy and in nearly all cases the tumor emboli were positive for vascular endothelial growth factor (VEGF), platelet derived growth factor and tissue factor by immunohistochemistry [2]. Over-expression of these growth factors on the surface of the embolized tumor cell may result in a trophic effect on the pulmonary vascular endothelium, leading to the described pathologic findings [3]. Here we describe a woman being treated with the combination of a VEGF receptor (VEGFR) inhibitor and a programmed death-ligand 1 (PD-L1) inhibitor who developed pulmonary hypertension and right heart failure and was subsequently found to have PTTM with features of pulmonary veno-occlusive disease (PVOD).

Case presentation

A 45-year-old woman with metastatic squamous cell carcinoma of the cervix refractory to standard of care chemotherapy was referred to the National Institutes of Health (NIH) for enrollment in a Phase I clinical trial (NCT02484404) of combination therapy with daily cediranib, a VEGFR tyrosine kinase inhibitor, and once every 2 weeks of durvalumab, a PD-L1 inhibitor. Her first four treatment cycles were well tolerated. Treatment related side effects included hypertension, subclinical hypothyroidism, non-nephrotic range proteinuria and mild diarrhea.

During a routine study clinic visit the patient was found to be in sinus tachycardia. Upon further questioning, the patient noted progressive dyspnea on exertion and fatigue over the previous month and was therefore admitted to the NIH Clinical Center for further evaluation. Vital signs revealed a temperature of 37°C, heart rate of 120 beats per minute, a manual blood pressure of 90/72 mmHg without orthostatic changes and oxygen saturation ranging from 93 to 97% on room air. Physical examination findings were notable for a normal jugular venous pressure, regular heart rate without a prominent P2, clear breath sounds, and warm extremities without edema. Intravenous fluid was administered for possible dehydration due to diarrhea, but symptoms did not improve. A portable chest x-ray revealed hazy bibasilar interstitial markings (Fig. 1). Laboratory studies revealed a hemoglobin of 9.8 g/dL (normal range 11.2-15.7 g/dl), a platelet count of 159 k/μL (normal range 173-369 k/μL), normal coagulation indices (PT 13.8 s; aPTT 35.5 s; thrombin time 15.8 s), a D-dimer of 0.98 μg/mL (normal range 0.00–0.50 μg/mL), a fibrinogen of 517 mg/dL (normal range 177–466 mg/dL), a pro-brain natriuretic peptide of 4541 pg/mL (normal range 0–124 pg/mL) and a troponin-T of 0.022 ng/mL (normal range 0.000–0.009 ng/mL). Echocardiography demonstrated a dilated right ventricle with decreased function (tricuspid annular plane systolic excursion (TAPSE) of 8 mm; normal ≥17 mm) and an

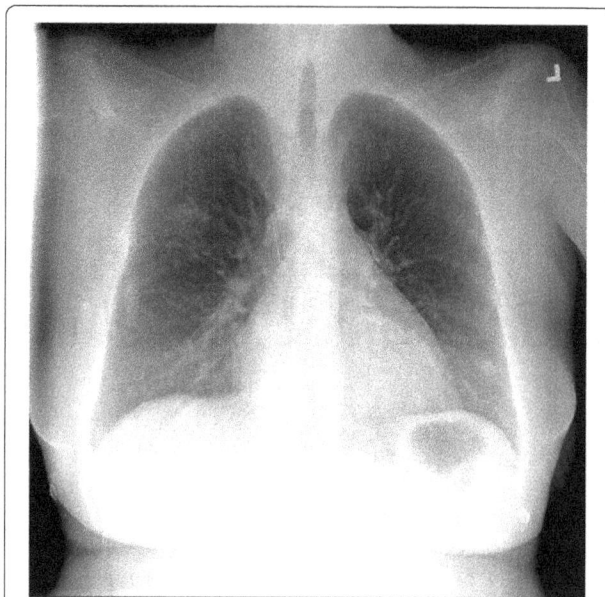

Fig. 1 An anteroposterior chest radiograph demonstrating hazy bibasilar interstitial infiltrates. A port is noted as well in the right upper chest with catheter ending at the cavoatrial junction

elevated right ventricular systolic pressure of 67 mmHg, new findings compared to her baseline echocardiogram completed just 4 months earlier. Cardiac MRI, performed to evaluate for possible treatment related myocarditis, demonstrated severely reduced right ventricular function (ejection fraction of 27%; normal 61±10%) with volume and pressure overload consistent with pulmonary hypertension, but no evidence of myocarditis. A CT angiogram showed no evidence of pulmonary emboli, however there was a prominence of interstitial markings (Fig. 2a, b), the main pulmonary artery was enlarged (Fig. 2c) and the right atrium and ventricle were both severely dilated (Fig. 2d). A ventilation (Fig. 3a) - perfusion (Fig. 3b) scan (VQ) demonstrated mismatched perfusion defects along the pleural margins that were interpreted as a high probability of pulmonary emboli. Doppler ultrasonography revealed no evidence of venous thrombosis in the lower extremities. Despite the equivocal findings, therapeutic anti-coagulation was started for possible pulmonary emboli.

Over the ensuing 10 days the patient's clinical course progressively deteriorated heralded by a syncopal event and the development of significant resting hypoxemia. The patient was referred for right and left heart catheterization which confirmed pre-capillary pulmonary hypertension with an associated low cardiac output state (Table 1). Vasodilator challenge with nitric oxide (40 ppm) plus 100% oxygen paradoxically increased pulmonary artery mean and occlusion pressure, but did not result in symptomatic pulmonary edema. Balloon occlusion pulmonary venous blood sampling did not reveal any circulating tumor cells. Aggressive therapy for right heart

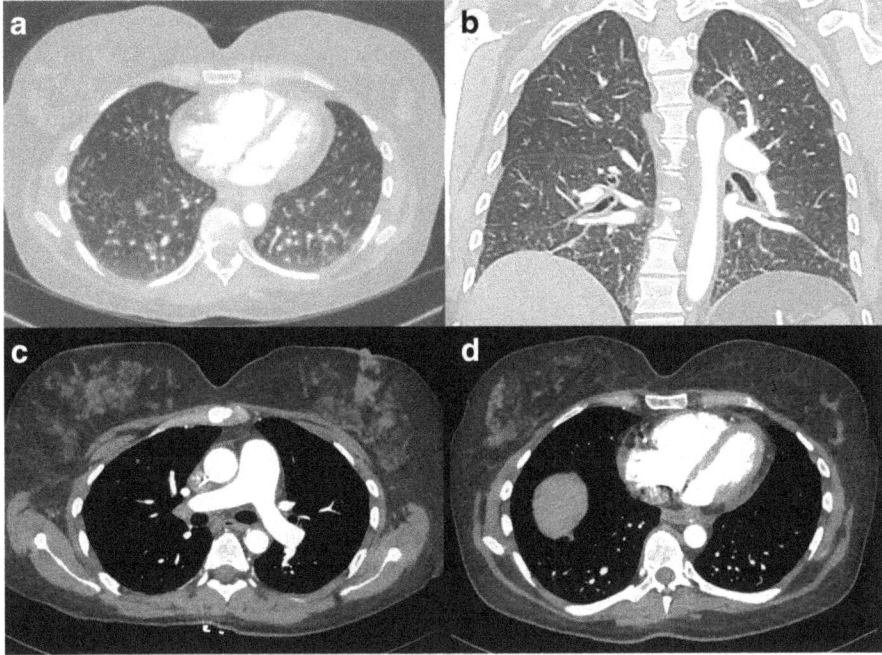

Fig. 2 Contrast enhanced CT image with axial (**a**) and coronal (**b**) sections demonstrating a prominence of interstitial markings predominantly in posterior and basilar lung fields. In mediastinal windowing accentuating the pulmonary vasculature (**c**) the pulmonary artery trunk is enlarged and (**d**) the right ventricle and right atria appear larger in area than their corresponding left sided chambers; findings suggestive of pulmonary hypertension

failure was initiated including intravenous diuresis, inotropic support and pulmonary vasodilator therapy. Riociguat was initiated due to the concern for possible chronic thromboembolic pulmonary hypertension (CTEPH). Ultimately, intravenous epoprostenol was added due to persistent symptoms of severe right heart failure. Soon after starting epoprostenol the patient became severely hypoxic. As a result, pulmonary vasodilator therapy was discontinued and she was treated with diuretics and high flow oxygen. Given her advanced disease and poor

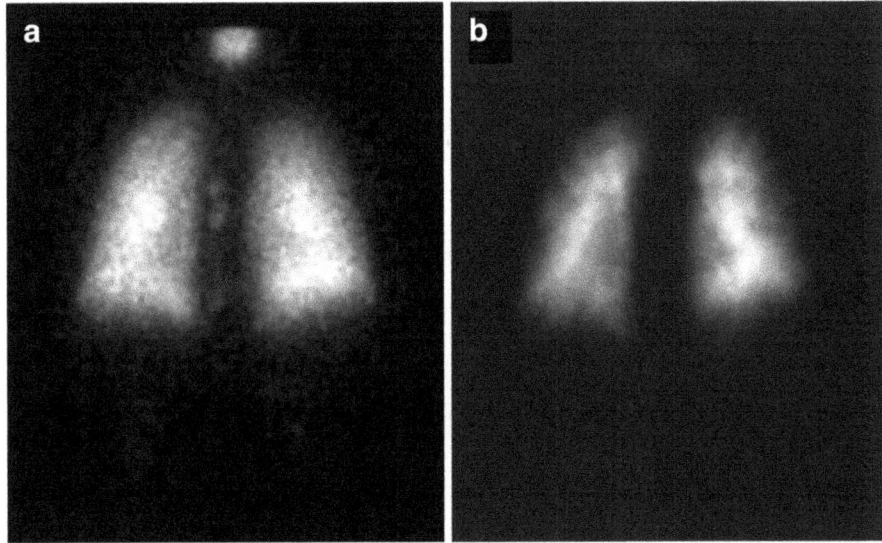

Fig. 3 A posterior view of a ventilation (**a**) and perfusion (**b**) nuclear medicine scan demonstrate significant perfusion defects along the pleural margin (dark rim surrounding lung) that are not matched with a ventilation defect

Table 1 Hemodynamic measures from left and right heart catheterization with vasodilator testing

	Room air	Nitric Oxide (40 ppm) plus 100% O_2
Heart rate, beats per minute	107	105
Mean right atrial pressure, mmHg	18	14
Pulmonary artery pressure (mean), mmHg	72/30 (44)	72/34 (47)
Mean pulmonary artery occlusion pressure, mmHg	11	15
Aortic pressure (mean), mmHg	92/61 (72)	108/64 (80)
Left ventricle end-diastolic pressure, mmHg	10	–
Arterial blood gas, pH/pCO$_2$/pO$_2$	7.45/32/66	7.42/39/344
Arterial oxygen saturation, %	92.1	99.1
Mixed venous oxygen saturation, %	43.4	59.6
Cardiac index[a], L/min/m^2	1.5	1.6
Pulmonary vascular resistance, Wood units	12.4	11.1

[a] Calculated by the Fick method using a measured hemoglobin of 11.1 g/dL and estimated VO$_2$ (mL/min/m^2)

functional status her protocol treatment was stopped and she was discharged home with hospice care. She died 1 day later and an autopsy was performed.

Gross examination of the lungs showed scattered white plaques, nodular and gritty on palpation, covering the pleural surface of the lower lobes. Microscopic sections of the lung showed metastatic carcinoma with lymphangitic spread (Fig. 4a) within the septa and sub-pleural spaces with associated congestion and fibrosis. These findings were associated with fibromuscular thickening of lymphatic vessels which may represent a type of desmoplastic response to lymphatic obstruction. Pulmonary arterioles (Fig. 4b, c) were occluded by organized thrombi, some with evidence of recanalization, as well as smooth muscle proliferation and ingrowth of fibroblasts. Some arteries showed fresh thrombi with metastatic tumor foci. Pulmonary venules were also occluded with ingrowth of fibroblasts. Some of these vessels showed evidence of chronic occlusion and recanalization, (Fig. 4d) while others were completely occluded. No tumor cells were identified in any venules. No evidence of infection or pneumonia was identified. Collectively, these findings were most consistent with a primary diagnosis of PTTM with features of PVOD [1, 4].

Discussion

We present a case of a woman with metastatic squamous cell carcinoma of the cervix who developed pulmonary hypertension and right heart failure during combination treatment with a VEGFR inhibitor and a PD-L1 inhibitor. At autopsy, she was found to have PTTM with features of PVOD.

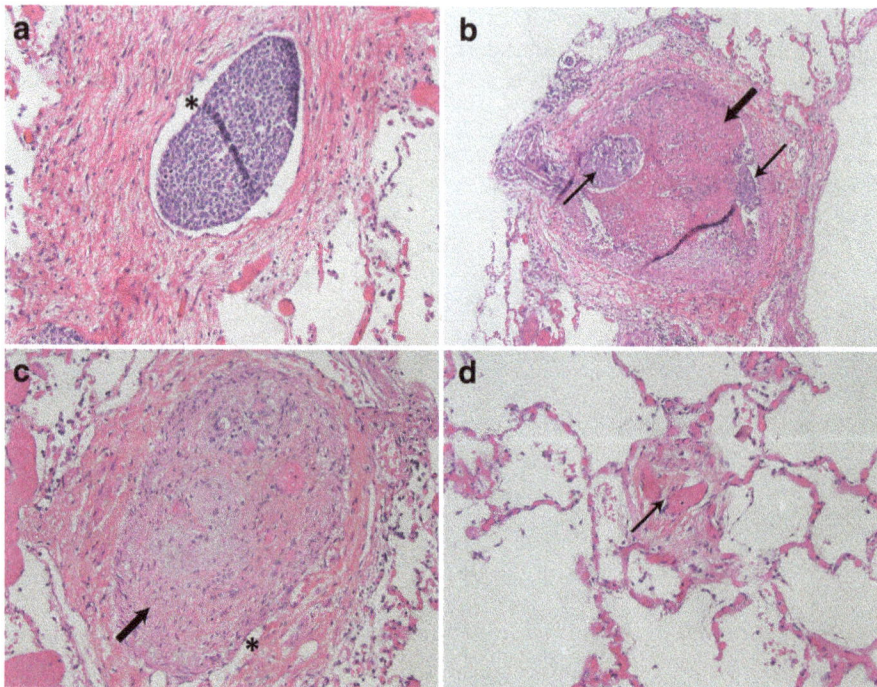

Fig. 4 Pulmonary vascular disease associated with metastases. **a** Dilated lymphatic space (asterisk) containing tumor (200×). **b** Pulmonary artery with small tumor embolus (thin arrows) and both fresh and partially organized thrombus (thick arrow) (100×). **c** Pulmonary artery showing occlusion (thick arrow) and recanalization (asterisk) (200×). **d** Small pulmonary vein with narrowing and recanalization (thin black arrow) (200×)

A definitive pre-mortem diagnosis of PTTM is challenging as a number of other causes of right heart failure have a similar clinical presentation [5]. For example, our patient's initial CT angiogram revealed prominent bibasilar septal lines, which may have represented lymphangitic spread of tumor, drug-induced pulmonary toxicity or PVOD [6]. Other non-specific radiographic findings in PTTM include multifocal beaded peripheral pulmonary arteries, diffuse thickening of the intralobular septa or peripheral wedge-shaped opacities suggestive of infarction [7]. A VQ scan can reveal peripheral unmatched perfusion defects in patients with tumor emboli [8]. However, this finding is also present in patients with acute pulmonary emboli or CTEPH and cannot be easily distinguished [9]. Pulmonary microvascular cytology has been used as a diagnostic tool to identify circulating tumor cells, however these cells can be mistaken as normal pulmonary megakaryocytes [10]. The presence of right ventricular hypertrophy by cardiac MRI suggested subacute or chronic pulmonary vascular disease in our patient and right and left heart catheterization confirmed the presence of pre-capillary pulmonary hypertension. Therefore other conditions in the differential included drug-induced pulmonary arterial hypertension (PAH) and CTEPH.

The development of hypoxia after the start of prostacyclin treatment raised suspicion for PVOD as the underlying cause of her pulmonary hypertension. Although histopathologically PVOD typically affects post-capillary venules, hemodynamically PVOD has a pre-capillary pattern on right heart catheterization similar to our patient [11]. In addition, the patient's regimen included multiple chemotherapeutic agents including cisplatin and docetaxel and radiation therapy, all of which are associated with development of PVOD [12, 13]. However, based on the original descriptions of PTTM, concurrent histological evidence of PVOD in our patient was unexpected [1]. Nevertheless, cases of PTTM with pulmonary venous involvement have been previously reported [4, 14].

Many cases of PTTM are treated in a similar manner to idiopathic PAH, although it is unclear such therapies are effective and as demonstrated by this case, they may be harmful. In patients with PVOD, pulmonary edema may develop with pulmonary vasodilator therapy due to increased pulmonary artery blood flow in the face of high post-capillary venule resistance. Alternatively, systemic administration of a potent pulmonary vasodilator may cause ventilation and perfusion mismatching leading to hypoxia. Based on the pulmonary histopathology, the hypoxemia seen in our patient was likely due to both pulmonary edema from venule obstruction and ventilation perfusion mismatch.

In contrast to a suspected role for angiogenic growth factors such as VEGF in the pathogenesis of PTTM, and anecdotal case reports of positive outcomes with imatinib

treatment [15] our patient not only developed, but also progressed to symptomatic PTTM during prolonged treatment with a VEGFR inhibitor. Importantly, pharmacokinetic studies done in our patient revealed that co-administration of durvalumab significantly decreased clearance of cediranib [16]. While the effect of VEGFR inhibition on the development or progression of PTTM is unknown, there is experimental evidence that exposure to a single dose of a VEGFR inhibitor, semaxanib (SU-5416), followed by chronic hypoxia leads to angioobliterative PAH in rats that mimics the histopathologic findings in patients with PAH, including hyperproliferative plexiform lesions [17]. In rodents, VEGFR blockade induces widespread pulmonary artery endothelial cell apoptosis which in the presence of chronic hypoxia is thought to result in the development of an apoptosis-resistant, hyperproliferative endothelial cell phenotype [18]. As a result of VEGFR blockade in this model, elevated levels of VEGFR ligands as well as other angiogenic factors (e.g. fibroblast growth factor and placental growth factor) may promote hyperproliferation and vascular remodeling [18]. In patients treated with VEGFR inhibitors, elevated circulating levels of fibroblast growth factor, placental growth factor and hepatocyte growth factor (HGF) have also been detected prior to disease progression [19, 20]. Similarly, in murine models of human non-small cell lung cancer, treatment with vandetanib and cediranib initially led to tumor regression followed by resistance to therapy and progression that was associated with upregulation of both HGF and its receptor, c-MET [21]. Studies of the tumor microvasculature in these murine models revealed HGF-dependent dysregulated angiogenesis with tortuous blood vessel formation. Interestingly, at autopsy immunohistochemical staining revealed lung metastatic foci that were VEGF negative but HGF positive. Thus, it is tempting to speculate that prolonged exposure to high levels of the VEGF receptor inhibitor could similarly provoke an abnormal response in the pulmonary vasculature that either induced or accelerated the development of PTTM in our patient. Moreover, levels of interferon and TNFα as well as other inflammatory cytokines closely linked to pulmonary vascular remodeling in PAH [22–24] may be elevated in the setting of PD-L1 blockade due to compensatory feedback mechanisms [25, 26]. Therefore, although PD1 and PD-L1 inhibitors have not been associated with the development of pulmonary hypertension [27], this ensuing pro-inflammatory state may act synergistically with VEGFR inhibition to disrupt angiogenesis and promote abnormal vessel formation [18]. In our patient, PD-L1 staining was performed on a lymph node taken prior to checkpoint inhibitor therapy and revealed positive staining on approximately 20% of tumor cells. Nevertheless, any association of VEGFR and PD-L1 inhibition to the development of PTTM and PVOD remains speculative.

Histopathology is necessary to definitively diagnose PTTM, yet a surgical lung biopsy is prohibitively risky in the presence of severe pulmonary hypertension and right heart failure. Thus, similar to our report, mechanistic studies of PTTM are lacking due to the difficulty in making a definitive pre-mortem diagnosis. Finally, as a single case report, there are many inherent limitations to our manuscript. The major limitation is the inability to establish causality between the patient's experimental therapy and her risk for the development of PTTM.

Conclusion

In the setting of malignancy, PTTM should be included in the differential diagnosis of a patient that presents with subacute to chronic pulmonary hypertension. Serial echocardiography may be useful for identifying evidence of pulmonary hypertension or right ventricular dysfunction prior to the onset of severe symptoms. However, these findings are non-specific and there are no established criteria for screening patients who are at higher risk for developing PTTM. This case report illustrates that a pre-mortem diagnosis of PTTM is difficult to confirm, treatment guidelines are lacking and the prognosis is poor. In addition, our case provides further support for the premise that both PTTM and PVOD share a common pathogenesis and may be manifestations of a spectrum of similar disease processes.

Abbreviations

CTEPH: chronic thromboembolic pulmonary hypertension; HGF: hepatocyte growth factor; NIH: National Institutes of Health; PAH: pulmonary arterial hypertension; PD-L1: programmed death-ligand 1; PTTM: pulmonary tumor thrombotic microangiopathy; PVOD: pulmonary veno-occlusive disease; TAPSE: tricuspid annular plane systolic excursion; TNFα: tumor necrosis factor alpha; VEGF: vascular endothelial growth factor; VEGFR: vascular endothelial growth factor receptor; VQ scan: ventilation perfusion scan

Acknowledgements

The authors would like to thank Kelly Byrne for her assistance in preparation of the manuscript.

Funding

This work was supported in part by the Intramural Research Program of the National Institutes of Health Clinical Center.

Authors' contributions

DAS, JME and MAS participated in the drafting of the manuscript. JML, JME and MAS were involved in the management of the case. DP and DEK interpreted the gross and histopathology. CJP performed the pharmacokinetic studies. All authors read and approved the final version of this manuscript.

Authors' information

The findings and conclusions in this report are those of the authors and do not necessarily represent the views of the National Institutes of Health.

Competing interests

The authors declare that they have no competing interests.

Author details

[1]Critical Care Medicine Department, National Institutes of Health Clinical Center, Bethesda, MD, USA. [2]Women's Malignancies Branch, Center for Cancer Research, National Cancer Institute, National Institutes of Health, Bethesda, USA. [3]Clinical Pharmacology Program, Center for Cancer Research, National Cancer Institute, National Institutes of Health, Bethesda, USA. [4]Laboratory of Pathology, Center for Cancer Research, National Cancer Institute, National Institutes of Health, Bethesda, USA. [5]Cardiovascular Branch, National Heart, Lung, and Blood Institute, National Institutes of Health, Bethesda, USA.

References

1. von Herbay A, Illes A, Waldherr R, Otto HF. Pulmonary tumor thrombotic microangiopathy with pulmonary hypertension. Cancer. 1990;66(3):587–92.
2. Uruga H, Fujii T, Kurosaki A, Hanada S, Takaya H, Miyamoto A, Morokawa N, Homma S, Kishi K. Pulmonary tumor thrombotic microangiopathy: a clinical analysis of 30 autopsy cases. Intern Med. 2013;52(12):1317–23.
3. Abe H, Hino R, Fukayama M. Platelet-derived growth factor-a and vascular endothelial growth factor-C contribute to the development of pulmonary tumor thrombotic microangiopathy in gastric cancer. Virchows Arch. 2013; 462(5):523–31.
4. Godbole R, Saggar R, Zider A, Betancourt J, Wallace WD, Suh RD, Kamangar N. Insights on pulmonary tumor thrombotic microangiopathy: a seven-patient case series. Pulm Circ. 2017;7(4):813–20.
5. Gavin MC, Morse D, Partridge AH, Levy BD, Loscalzo J. Clinical problem-solving. Breathless. N Engl J Med. 2012;366(1):75–81.
6. Frazier AA, Franks TJ, Mohammed TL, Ozbudak IH, Galvin JR. From the archives of the AFIP: pulmonary veno-occlusive disease and pulmonary capillary hemangiomatosis. Radiographics. 2007;27(3):867–82.
7. Restrepo CS, Betancourt SL, Martinez-Jimenez S, Gutierrez FR. Tumors of the pulmonary artery and veins. Semin Ultrasound CT MR. 2012;33(6):580–90.
8. Boudreau RJ, Lisbona R, Sheldon H. Ventilation-perfusion mismatch in tumor embolism. Clin Nucl Med. 1982;7(7):320–2.
9. Auger WR, Kerr KM, Kim NH, Fedullo PF. Evaluation of patients with chronic thromboembolic pulmonary hypertension for pulmonary endarterectomy. Pulm Circ. 2012;2(2):155–62.
10. Masson RG, Krikorian J, Lukl P, Evans GL, McGrath J. Pulmonary microvascular cytology in the diagnosis of lymphangitic carcinomatosis. N Engl J Med. 1989;321(2):71–6.
11. Rambihar VS, Fallen EL, Cairns JA. Pulmonary veno-occlusive disease: antemortem diagnosis from roentgenographic and hemodynamic findings. Can Med Assoc J. 1979;120(12):1519–22.
12. Ranchoux B, Gunther S, Quarck R, Chaumais MC, Dorfmuller P, Antigny F, Dumas SJ, Raymond N, Lau E, Savale L, et al. Chemotherapy-induced pulmonary hypertension: role of alkylating agents. Am J Pathol. 2015;185(2):356–71.
13. Kramer MR, Estenne M, Berkman N, Antoine M, de Francquen P, Lipski A, Jacobovitz D, Lafair J. Radiation-induced pulmonary veno-occlusive disease. Chest. 1993;104(4):1282–4.
14. Kumar N, Price LC, Montero MA, Dimopoulos K, Wells AU, Wort SJ. Pulmonary tumour thrombotic microangiopathy: unclassifiable pulmonary hypertension? Eur Respir J. 2015;46(4):1214–7.
15. Price LC, Wells AU, Wort SJ. Pulmonary tumour thrombotic microangiopathy. Curr Opin Pulm Med. 2016;22(5):421–8.
16. Lee JM, Cimino-Mathews A, Peer CJ, Zimmer A, Lipkowitz S, Annunziata CM, Cao L, Harrell MI, Swisher EM, Houston N, et al. Safety and Clinical Activity of the Programmed Death-Ligand 1 Inhibitor Durvalumab in Combination With Poly (ADP-Ribose) Polymerase Inhibitor Olaparib or Vascular Endothelial Growth Factor Receptor 1–3 Inhibitor Cediranib in Women's Cancers: A Dose-Escalation, Phase I Study. J Clin Oncol. 2017;35(19):2193–202.
17. Tuder RM, Chacon M, Alger L, Wang J, Taraseviciene-Stewart L, Kasahara Y, Cool CD, Bishop AE, Geraci M, Semenza GL, et al. Expression of angiogenesis-related molecules in plexiform lesions in severe pulmonary hypertension: evidence for a process of disordered angiogenesis. J Pathol. 2001;195(3):367–74.
18. Voelkel NF, Gomez-Arroyo J. The role of vascular endothelial growth factor in pulmonary arterial hypertension. The angiogenesis paradox. Am J Respir Cell Mol Biol. 2014;51(4):474–84.

19. Kopetz S, Hoff PM, Morris JS, Wolff RA, Eng C, Glover KY, Adinin R, Overman MJ, Valero V, Wen S, et al. Phase II trial of infusional fluorouracil, irinotecan, and bevacizumab for metastatic colorectal cancer: efficacy and circulating angiogenic biomarkers associated with therapeutic resistance. J Clin Oncol. 2010;28(3):453–9.

20. Welti J, Loges S, Dimmeler S, Carmeliet P. Recent molecular discoveries in angiogenesis and antiangiogenic therapies in cancer. J Clin Invest. 2013; 123(8):3190–200.

21. Cascone T, Xu L, Lin HY, Liu W, Tran HT, Liu Y, Howells K, Haddad V, Hanrahan E, Nilsson MB, et al. The HGF/c-MET pathway is a driver and biomarker of VEGFR-inhibitor resistance and vascular remodeling in non-small cell lung Cancer. Clin Cancer Res. 2017;23(18):5489–501.

22. George PM, Oliver E, Dorfmuller P, Dubois OD, Reed DM, Kirkby NS, Mohamed NA, Perros F, Antigny F, Fadel E, et al. Evidence for the involvement of type I interferon in pulmonary arterial hypertension. Circ Res. 2014;114(4):677–88.

23. Hurst LA, Dunmore BJ, Long L, Crosby A, Al-Lamki R, Deighton J, Southwood M, Yang X, Nikolic MZ, Herrera B, et al. TNFalpha drives pulmonary arterial hypertension by suppressing the BMP type-II receptor and altering NOTCH signalling. Nat Commun. 2017;8:14079.

24. Rabinovitch M, Guignabert C, Humbert M, Nicolls MR. Inflammation and immunity in the pathogenesis of pulmonary arterial hypertension. Circ Res. 2014;115(1):165–75.

25. Kondo A, Yamashita T, Tamura H, Zhao W, Tsuji T, Shimizu M, Shinya E, Takahashi H, Tamada K, Chen L, et al. Interferon-gamma and tumor necrosis factor-alpha induce an immunoinhibitory molecule, B7-H1, via nuclear factor-kappaB activation in blasts in myelodysplastic syndromes. Blood. 2010;116(7):1124–31.

26. Cunningham CR, Champhekar A, Tullius MV, Dillon BJ, Zhen A, de la Fuente JR, Herskovitz J, Elsaesser H, Snell LM, Wilson EB, et al. Type I and type II interferon coordinately regulate suppressive dendritic cell fate and function during viral persistence. PLoS Pathog. 2016;12(1):e1005356.

27. Postow MA, Sidlow R, Hellmann MD. Immune-related adverse events associated with immune checkpoint blockade. N Engl J Med. 2018;378(2):158–68.

Outcomes of community-based and home-based pulmonary rehabilitation for pneumoconiosis patients

Eric W. Tsang[1,2], Henry Kwok[2], Aidan K. Y. Chan[3], Kah Lin Choo[4], Kin Sang Chan[5], Kam Shing Lau[6] and Chetwyn C. H. Chan[2*] (iD)

Abstract

Background: Pneumoconiosis patients receive community-based or home-based pulmonary rehabilitation (PR) for symptom management and enhancement of physical and mental well-being. This study aimed to review the clinical benefits of community-based rehabilitation programmes (CBRP) and home-based rehabilitation programmes (HBRP) for PR of pneumoconiosis patients.

Methods: Archival data of pneumoconiosis patients who participated in CBRP and HBRP between 2008 and 2011 was analysed. There were 155 and 26 patients in the CBRP and HBRP respectively. The outcome measures used in the pre- and post-tests were Knowledge, Health Survey Short Form-12 (SF-12), Hospital Anxiety and Depression Scale (HADS), 6-Min Walk Test (6MWT), and Chronic Respiratory Questionnaire (CRQ). Paired t-tests and the Analysis of Covariance (ANCOVA) using the patients' baseline lung functions as the covariates were performed to examine the changes in the outcomes after completing the programmes. Hierarchical multiple regression analyses were used to examine the relationships between patient's programme participation factors and different scores of the outcome measures.

Results: After controlling for patients' baseline lung capacities, significant improvements were revealed among patients participated in CBRP in the scores of the 6MWT, Knowledge, HADS, SF-12 PCS, and CRQ emotion and mastery. The different scores in the Knowledge and HADS were correlated with the patients' levels of programme participation. In contrast, significant improvements were only found in the scores of the Knowledge and 6MWT among patients who participated in HBRP. The gain scores of the 6MWT were correlated with the patients' levels of programme participation.

Conclusions: Both CBRP and HBRP benefited patients' levels of exercise tolerance and knowledge about the disease. CBRP provided greater benefits to patients' mental and psychosocial needs. In contrast, HBRP was found to improve patients' physical function, but did not have significant impacts on patients' mental health and health-related quality of life. The attendance of patients and the participation of their relatives in treatment sessions were important factors in enhancing the positive effects of CBRP and HBRP. These positive outcomes confirm the value of pulmonary rehabilitation programmes for community-dwelling pneumoconiosis patients.

Keywords: Pneumoconiosis, Physical exercise, Mental health, Health-related quality of life, Community-based pulmonary rehabilitation, Home-based pulmonary rehabilitation

* Correspondence: Chetwyn.Chan@polyu.edu.hk
[2]Department of Rehabilitation Sciences, The Hong Kong Polytechnic University, Hung Hom, Kowloon, Hong Kong, China
Full list of author information is available at the end of the article

Background

Pneumoconiosis is an occupational disease of the lungs caused by inhaling organic or non-organic dust retained in the lungs [1, 2]. Patients with pneumoconiosis typically suffer from reduced lung functions [3–5], different mood and respiratory symptoms [6], and decreased tolerance for physical exercise [5]. Together, they contribute towards the deterioration of health-related quality of life (HRQOL) [4, 7]. Patients with chronic obstructive pulmonary diseases (COPD), including pneumoconiosis, are frequently referred to pulmonary rehabilitation (PR) programmes [8]. These programmes aim to relieve symptoms and to improve capacity for exercise, emotional function, sense of control, and HRQOL [8]. The content and settings of different PR programmes, their model of delivery, and personnel involved in the delivery may vary according to local health care systems and resources [9, 10]. Most PR programmes for COPD patients include either low or high-intensity exercise training, endurance-training and strength training [9–11]. Apart from rehabilitating the physical aspect of patients, these programmes may include health education, psychosocial support, and/or nutritional counseling [10, 11]. The common settings in which PR programmes are delivered include hospital-based [12], community-based [4, 13], or patient's home [14–18]. Different settings cater for the different needs of the patients. The common duration of PR programme is 8 weeks [19]. A recent meta-analysis reviewed 65 studies on PR programmes. It was reported that PR programmes led to significant benefits in relieving dyspnoea and fatigue, and on improving exercise capacity and HRQOL, among COPD patients [8].

In Hong Kong, PR services for patients with pneumoconiosis were funded by the Pneumoconiosis Compensation Fund Board. It is a statutory body established by the local government. Three public hospitals and 2 nongovernmental organisations (NGOs) were responsible for conducting PR services [1, 20]. PR services included two core programmes: Community-Based Rehabilitation Programme (CBRP) and Home-Based Rehabilitation Programme (HBRP).

CBRP was the standard programme consisting of protocol-based classes delivered by healthcare professionals at community centres. Typical classes include breathing re-training, exercise re-conditioning, health education, teaching energy conservation techniques and panic control skills (see Additional file 1). The duration was four to 6 weeks with a frequency of twice per week.

HBRP was designed to cater for patients unable to access community-based services due to profound incapacities. The content of the programme was customised according to the needs of the patients during home visits. Unlike the typical PR services offered by CBRP, HBRP provided additional psychological support to the patients and their family. Examples of tailored services included home modification, carer-training, and living skills-training (see Additional file 1). HBRP was delivered by healthcare professionals offering eight home visits, each lasting at least 1 hour. CBRP and HBRP were complemented by adjunctive programmes that helped pneumoconiosis patients better manage their illnesses. Detailed description of each of the programmes as aforementioned can be found in the Additional file 1.

Several systematic reviews have reported positive effects of PR programmes on patients with COPD. They include minimizing COPD symptoms, improving exercise capacities, as well as improving health-related quality of life [8, 21–25]. Previous studies as well as expert opinions have consistently shown that PR programmes did not bring about improvement in the lung functions of patients with COPD [23–26]. Nevertheless, lung function had been identified as an important factor influencing HRQOL in pneumoconiosis patients [4]. It is worthwhile to explore whether the physical and psychological benefits brought about by the PR [8, 21, 22] are independent of the patients' initial lung functions. Ascertaining this is essential for a greater understanding of the precise benefits of PR programmes for patients with pneumoconiosis.

Moreover, the majority of previous studies had not recruited pneumoconiosis patients. This calls for an investigation on the effect of PR programmes on patients who suffered from pneumoconiosis. This study aims to examine the outcomes of both the CBRP and HBRP for pneumoconiosis patients based on archived data from 2008 to 2011 by the Hong Kong Hospital Authority. Moreover, we performed covariance analyses to examine the outcomes of CBRP and HBRP independent from patients' baseline lung functions. The relationships among patients' characteristics, types of program participations, and clinical outcomes were examined. The findings will pave the way for contents of future PR programmes to be enhanced for pneumoconiosis patients.

Methods

Subjects

From 2008 to 2011, 685 pneumoconiosis patients enrolled in the CBRP or HBRP programmes offered by three hospitals in Hong Kong. The outcomes of the programmes were captured by a voluntary assessment scheme. It covered the physical and psychosocial functions of the patients before and shortly after the rehabilitation programmes. A review of the database identified 181 patients who had complete records of all physical, mental, and HRQOL outcome measures (Table 1). These cases included 155 patients from the CBRP and 26 from the HBRP. On average, patients who completed the HBRP were older. They had lower baseline forced-expiratory volume (FEV_1) values and higher percentages of

Table 1 Demographic characteristics of the 181 pneumoconiosis patients

Type of Program	CBRP	HBRP
Number of cases	155	26
Gender (male/female)	153/2	26/ 0
Age (SD) in years	70.74 (8)	74.54 (8.3)
Baseline FEV$_1$ (SD) in L/min	1.64 (0.58)	1.17 (0.58)
%DOI (SD)	18.52 (15.84)	34.81 (25.51)
Smoking (nonsmoker, former smoker, current smoker)	44/97/14	0/23/3

SD standard deviation, %DOI percent of degree of incapacity

degree of impairment (%DOIs), relative to the patients who completed the CBRP. Due to the retrospective nature of the study, ethics approval was granted on the basis of not requiring the consent from the patients for participating in the study from the Institutional Review Boards of each of the three hospitals.

Data collection

A number of patients included in the study had participated in CBRP or HBRP programme more than once within the study period. These cases were identified, and only the latest available set of assessments, reflecting the collective treatment effects over the period studied, was analysed.

There are two categories of data fields. The first category consists of demographic characteristics, disease-specific information and programme participation. They include age, sex, %DOI, Body Mass Index (BMI) score, smoking history, CBRP or HBRP enrolment, number of adjunctive programmes involved, and baseline lung function (FEV$_1$). The second category focuses on the outcome measures used to assess the benefits of the PR programme. They are Chronic Respiratory Questionnaire (CRQ) [27], Hospital Anxiety and Depression Scale (HADS) [28], physical (PCS) and mental (MCS) health scales of Short Form-12 (SF-12) [29], Knowledge (Additional file 2), and the 6-Min Walk Test (6MWT) [30]. As PR had not been shown to improve lung function [23–26], it was not recommended as an outcome of the PR programme according to the Quality Standards for Pulmonary Rehabilitation in Adults of British Thoracic Society [11]. Post-treatment FEV$_1$ was therefore not included as an outcome for CBRP or HBRP. Baseline FEV$_1$ only served as a covariate variable in this study.

Data analyses

To ensure the relevance of the analysis, the records kept by each of the participating hospitals were pooled. Analyses of patients in the CBRP and the HBRP were conducted respectively. Paired t-tests were first used to compare the scores of the outcome measures before and

after the treatment. Repeated measure analyses of covariance (rmANCOVA) were then conducted to ascertain the effects of the treatments. The patients' baseline FEV$_1$ values were the covariate. Hierarchical multiple regression analyses (stepwise) were performed to examine the relationships among the patients' characteristics, programme participation levels, and clinical outcomes. The dependent variables were the clinical outcomes (different score between post- and pre-treatment): CRQ, HADS, SF-12, Knowledge, and 6MWT. The three blocks of independent variables were: 1) the patient's demographic including age, gender, %DOI, smoking history, baseline FEV$_1$ value, and BMI score; 2) the total number of programme participation (TOTAL) and the number of the CBRP or HBRP participation; and 3) the number of adjunctive programmes they participated in, including the CPDP, LTOT, CHCP, SMP, SMP relative, RHP, RHP relative, HLP, and HLP relative. These three blocks of variables were sequentially entered into the regression analysis. The data files used for the analyses are provided in Additional files 3 and 4.

Results

Differences between the pre- and post-test after CBRP and HBRP participation

Among the patients in the CBRP, pair t-tests revealed significant differences in the pre- and post-test scores on all the outcome measures except the BMI (Table 2). Significant increases in scores were found in the CRQ dyspnoea [t (154) = 4.32, $P < 0.0001$], CRQ fatigue [t (154) = 3.8, $P < 0.0001$], CRQ emotion [t (154) = 5.75, $P < 0.0001$], CRQ mastery [t (154) = 4.83, $P < 0.0001$] and Knowledge [t (154) = 10.61, $P < 0.0001$], the SF-12 PCS [t (154) = 4.39, $P < 0.0001$] and MCS [t (154) = 2.62, $P = 0.01$], and the 6MWT [t (154) = 12.88, $P < 0.0001$]. CBRP patients also showed significant decreases in HADS scores of the anxiety [t (154) = − 6.27, $P < 0.0001$] and depression [t (154) = − 7.42, $P < 0.0001$]. The results were re-examined using rmANCOVAs with the baseline FEV$_1$ as the covariate.

Similarly, significant increases were found in scores of CRQ emotion [F (1) = 4.91, $P = 0.04$], CRQ mastery [F (1) = 4.69, $P = 0.04$], Knowledge [F (1) = 18.91, $P < 0.0001$], 6MWT [F (1) = 19.22, $P < 0.0001$,] and SF-12's PCS [F (1) = 4.01, $P = 0.047$], and significant decreases in scores were found in the HADS anxiety [F (1) = 5.72, $P = 0.02$] and depression [F (1) = 6.41, $P = 0.01$]. However, no significant differences were revealed in the CRQ dyspnoea and the SF-12 MCS.

Among the patients in the HBRP, paired t-tests revealed significant increases in scores of Knowledge [t (25) = 3.78, $P < 0.0001$], SF-12 PCS [t (25) = 2.3, $P = 0.03$] and MCS [t (25) = 2.44, $P = 0.02$], and the 6MWT [t (25) = 4, $P < 0.0001$]. Moreover, there was a significant decrease in HAD anxiety [t (25) = − 2.95, $P = 0.007$] (Table 3). No significant

Table 2 Comparisons of scores of outcome measures before and after patients participated in CBRP

Variables	Mean (SD)			P values		
	Before	After	95%CI	Paired t-tests	ANCOVA	Partial η^2
CRQ Dyspnea	4.51 (1.28)	4.85 (1.33)	0.19, 0.51	$< 0.0001^b$	$= 0.1$	0.018
CRQ Fatigue	4.41 (1.17)	4.72 (1.14)	0.15, 0.47	$< 0.0001^b$	$= 0.73$	0.001
CRQ Emotion	5.03 (1.09)	6.45 (1.09)	0.24, 0.5	$< 0.0001^b$	$= 0.04^a$	0.07
CRQ Mastery	4.95 (1.4)	6.25 (1.2)	0.23, 0.55	$< 0.0001^b$	$= 0.04^a$	0.04
HAD Anxiety	4.75 (2.35)	2.48 (2.1)	−2.45, − 1.28	$< 0.0001^b$	$= 0.02^a$	0.05
HAD Depression	4.94 (4.22)	2.71 (3.39)	−2.82, − 1.63	$< 0.0001^b$	$= 0.01^a$	0.08
Knowledge	19.34 (2.9)	21.82 (2.33)	2, 2.94	$< 0.0001^b$	$< 0.0001^b$	0.11
SF-12 PCS	41.65 (7.95)	44.11 (8.14)	1.35, 3.56	$< 0.0001^b$	$= 0.047^a$	0.03
SF-12 MCS	46.4 (10.05)	48.32 (9.78)	0.47, 3.36	$=0.01^a$	$= 3.99$	0.005
6MWT	383.61 (91.33)	443.08 (89.41)	50.35, 68.58	$< 0.0001^b$	$< 0.0001^b$	0.12
BMI	24.66 (18.85)	23.08 (3.38)	−4.49, 1.33	$= 0.29$	$= 0.54$	0.01

$N = 155$; 95%CI, 95% Confidence Interval of difference in means; $^aP < 0.05$; $^bP < 0.01$

changes in scores were revealed in the CRQ scales, HAD depression, and BMI. After controlled for the baseline FEV_1, the rmANCOVA indicated significant increases only in the gain scores of Knowledge [F (1) = 6.19, P = 0.02] and the 6MWT [F (1) = 11, P = 0.003].

Factors influencing the outcomes of pulmonary rehabilitation Programmes

For patients in the CBRP, the different scores in HAD depression were predicted by the TOTAL, CHCP, and HLP relative (Multiple $R = 0.37$, $R^2 = 0.14$). Based on this model, a 1.0-episode increase in the number of family members participating in the HLP was associated with a 1.76-point decrease in the HAD depression score; a 1.0-unit increase in patients' CHCP participation was associated with a 1.15-point decrease in HAD depression score; and a 1.0-unit increase in TOTAL was associated with a 0.31-point decrease in HAD depression score

(Table 4A and Fig. 1a). The different scores in Knowledge were predicted by the number of participations in CBRP and RHP relative (Multiple $R = 0.29$, $R^2 = 0.09$). The model illustrated that a 1.0-episode increase in the RHP relative was associated with a 1.54-point increase in the Knowledge score; and a 1.0-unit increase in the CBRP participation was associated with a 1.23-point increase in the Knowledge score (Table 4b and Fig. 1b). No other significant regression model was found.

For patients in the HBRP, the 6MWT was the only outcome variable that was predicted by the TOTAL and the number of participation in HBRP and RHP (Multiple $R = 0.68$, $R^2 = 0.47$). Based on this model, a 1.0-unit increase in the RHP participation was associated with a 52.23-m increase in the 6MWT. This is followed by a 1.0-unit increase in the HBRP participation, which was associated with a 41.96- m increase in the 6MWT. Furthermore, a 1.0-unit increase in

Table 3 Comparisons of scores on the outcome measures before and after patients participated in HBRP

Variables	Mean (SD)			P values		
	Before	After	95%CI	Paired t-tests	ANCOVA	Partial η^2
CRQ Dyspnea	3.95 (1.49)	4.09 (1.48)	−0.34, 0.61	$= 0.55$	$= 0.79$	0.003
CRQ Fatigue	4.06 (1.18)	4.3 (0.93)	−0.17, 0.64	$= 0.24$	$= 0.82$	0.002
CRQ Emotion	5.13 (1.16)	5.23 (1.14)	−0.3, 0.49	$= 0.63$	$= 0.3$	0.05
CRQ Mastery	4.87 (1.25)	5.01 (1.24)	−0.25, 0.53	$= 0.46$	$= 0.74$	0.005
HAD Anxiety	4.38 (4.02)	2.81 (3.74)	−2.68, −0.47	$= 0.007^b$	$= 0.31$	0.042
HAD Depression	4.15 (4.67)	4.27 (5.17)	−1.07, 1.3	$= 0.84$	$= 0.57$	0.014
Knowledge	20.08 (2.47)	21.92 (1.57)	0.84, 2.85	$= 0.001^b$	$= 0.02^a$	0.21
SF-12 PCS	40.8 (7.24)	44.01 (8.48)	0.34, 6.08	$= 0.03^a$	$= 0.93$	0.0001
SF-12 MCS	43.18 (10.9)	47.85 (9.57)	0.73, 8.62	$= 0.02^a$	$= 0.37$	0.03
6MWT	256.27 (110.37)	303.88 (125.98)	23.08, 72.15	$< 0.0001^b$	$= 0.003^b$	0.31
BMI	22.16 (3.64)	22.08 (3.4)	−0.32, 0.17	$= 0.54$	$= 0.7$	0.01

$N = 26$; 95%CI, 95% Confidence Interval of difference in means; $^aP < 0.05$; $^bP < 0.01$

Table 4 Results of hierarchical multiple regression analyses

	CBRP	(N = 155)					
	Predictor	B	β	R	R^2	ΔR^2	ΔF
A.							
	DV: Different score in HAD depression						
Model 1	TOTAL	−0.21	−0.28	0.28	0.08	0.08	12.63[b]
Model 2	TOTAL	−0.28	−0.37	0.34	0.12	0.04	6.97[b]
	CHCP	−1.05	−0.22				
Model 3	TOTAL	−0.31	−0.4	0.37	0.14	0.02	4.02[a]
	CHCP	−1.15	−0.24				
	HLP relative	−1.76	−0.16				
B.							
	DV: Different score in knowledge						
Model 1	CBRP	1.14	0.21	0.21	0.04	0.05	7.08[b]
Model 2	CBRP	1.23	0.23	0.29	0.09	0.04	6.77[a]
	RHP relative	1.54	0.2				
	HBRP	(N = 26)					
C.							
	DV: Different score in 6MWT						
Model 1	TOTAL	2.77	0.41	0.41	0.17	0.17	4.92[a]
Model 2	TOTAL	3.05	0.45	0.59	0.35	0.18	6.07[b]
	HBRP	38.53	0.42				
Model 3	TOTAL	2.38	0.36	0.68	0.47	0.12	6.39**
	HBRP	41.96	0.46				
	RHP	52.23	0.36				

DV, dependent variable; B, unstandardized coefficient; β, standardized coefficient
[a] $P < 0.05$; [b] $P < 0.01$

TOTAL was associated with a 2.38-m increase in the 6MWT (Table 4c and Fig. 1c).

Discussion

To our knowledge, this study is the first to report the outcomes of community-based and home-based pulmonary rehabilitation programmes provided by the same teams of rehabilitation professionals from three separate hospitals. Therefore, the treatment outcomes of the two types of programmes are very comparable. This reveals specific strengths and weaknesses associated with each programme. This is also the first report of pulmonary rehabilitation treatment outcomes independent of patients' baseline lung functions, particularly regarding the importance of patients' participation in influencing the physical and psycho-social aspects of the treatment outcomes on pneumoconiosis patients.

The results suggested that the CBRP had positive effects in enhancing the patients' HRQOL (CRQ fatigue, emotion, and mastery) and reducing their psychological symptoms (HADS anxiety and depression). Patients who participated in the CBRP were found to show improvement in their knowledge about the disease as well as the exercise capacity (6MWT). The findings on the improvement in the patients' quality of life are consistent with those of previous studies [13, 31]. However, the finding that the CBRP did not improve the CRQ dyspnoea score is inconsistent with findings reported in previous studies [32, 33]. A plausible reason for this discrepancy is that this study incorporated patients' baseline lung function as a covariate, which was not the case in previous studies. Future studies should further explore how a patient's lung function, particularly different levels of initial lung capacities, would influence the treatment outcomes of PR programmes.

Several studies proposed that social support [31, 34–36] embedded in community-based PR programmes contributes towards the improvement in patient's psychological symptoms [31, 36, 37]. The results of this study further substantiate this proposition. A higher number of home visits (CHCP) made to the patients, as well as their relatives having attended educational talks more frequently (in HLP) were factors found to be significantly associated with the reduction of depression symptoms among patients who completed the CBRP. The CHCP consisted of home visits by healthcare professionals to monitor the health and psycho-social statuses of patients (see content in Additional file 1). The HLP involved educational talks to patients and their relatives on self-maintenance and healthy lifestyles. The RHP provided lectures on pneumoconiosis and respiratory hygiene. Open to both patients and their relatives, the talks were arranged by NGOs but conducted by healthcare professionals. These classes were useful for enhancing patient's knowledge on the disease. This postulation is supported by findings on the significant relationships among the relatives' participation in the CBRP and RHP and patient's gain in the knowledge (Fig. 1b).

Apart from learning about the disease, the patients showed improvements in mobility function after participating in the CBRP. A mean improvement of 59.5 m in 6MWT was found to exceed the clinical threshold of 54 m set in other studies [38, 39]. Our findings on mobility, as general exercise capability, are consistent with those reported in other studies on community-based programmes, which considered mobility as an important outcome to patients with pneumoconiosis [13, 33].

In general, the effects of the HBRP were more modest than those of the CBRP. After controlling for patients' baseline lung capacities, significant improvements were found in patients' knowledge about the disease and in exercise capacity after completing the HBRP. The improvements in exercise capacity after completing the HBRP were consistent with previous findings [14, 15, 17, 40]. Patients who completed the HBRP showed a mean increase of 47.6 m on the 6MWT, which is below the clinical threshold of improvements suggested in other studies [38, 39]. This is perhaps because patients in the HBRP were of older age, had

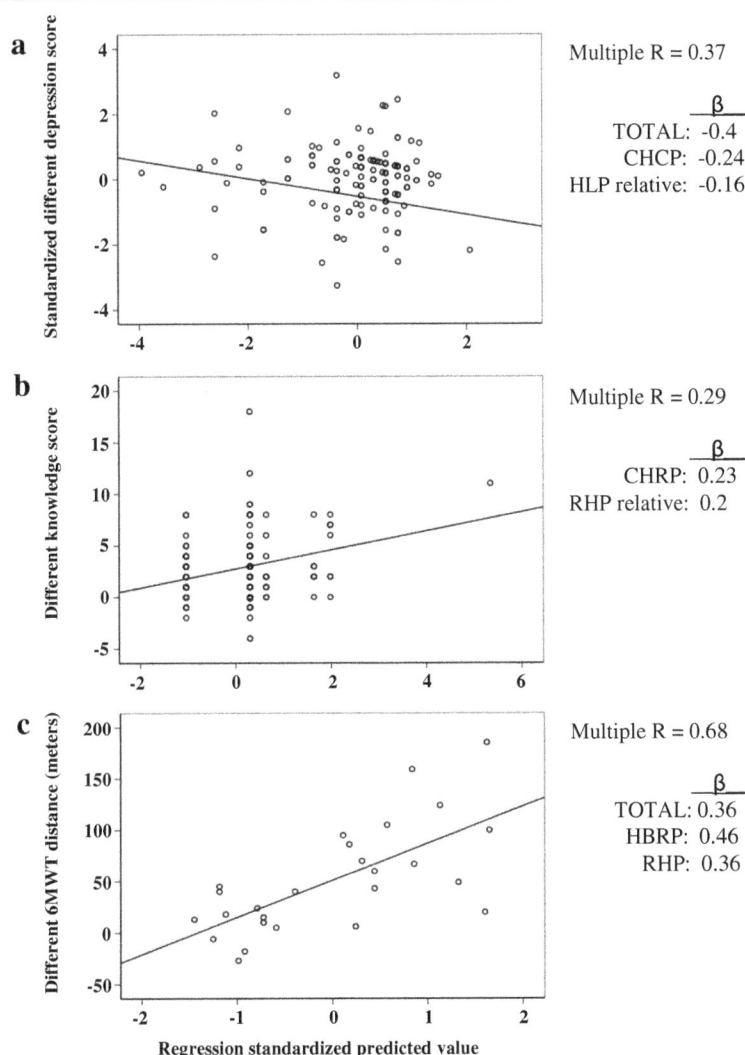

Fig. 1 Scatterplots illustrating the relationships between outcome variables and program participations. **a** The y-axis represents the standardized different HAD depression scores in CBRP patients and the x-axis represents the standardized predicted values of program participations including TOTAL, CHCP, and HLP relative. **b** The y-axis represents different knowledge scores in CBRP patients and the x-axis represents standardized predicted values of CBRP and RHP relative program participations. **c** The y-axis represents the different distance of 6MWT in meters in HBRP patients and the x-axis represents the standardized predicted values of program participations including TOTAL, HBRP, and RHP. Multiple R, correlation coefficient for multiple regression; β, standardized coefficient of each independent variable

greater baseline %DOIs, and lower lung capacities than those in the CBRP. Of note, the HBRP did not appear to produce significant positive effects in improving patients' health-related quality of life and psychological symptoms. These findings are inconsistent with those reported in previous studies on home-based programmes [14, 15, 40, 41]. This inconsistency could have been due to the small sample size of the HBRP group. Previous studies indicated that patients of home-based programmes valued social support from and interactions with professionals, families, and peers [42–44]. A recent study suggested that home-based programmes should aim at improving physical capacities in order for patients to progress and participate in

community-based programmes, which bring stronger psychosocial benefits [17].

The improvement of the 6MWT in HBRP patients was related to the total number of programmes of HBRP and RHP that the patients had participated in (Table 4c and Fig. 1c). Pulmonary rehabilitation consists of many programmes that help improve patients' physical functions (Additional file 1). It is likely for patients who had participated in more PR programmes to gain more benefits, thus performing better in the 6MWT. The HBRP involved physical and respiratory training, which improved patients' exercise tolerance levels [14]. A longer training period was found to be more effective in enhancing the physical functions [31]. In the RHP, therapists taught patients about pneumoconiosis, respiratory hygiene, the use of inhalers, and energy conservation. These resulted in better health management [45] and the ability to achieve greater exercise tolerance levels for those who participated more frequently.

Limitations

The data obtained for this study was based on convenient sampling, hence, the findings should be interpreted with caution. Generalization of results to other groups of patients with pneumoconiosis would therefore be limited. The study was not a randomized controlled trial. Thus, the treatment effects reported showed, at best, trends in improvements.

No information on the medications taken by the patients was included in the data. Nevertheless, the common practices of all the case medical officers who referred the patients for enrolment in the community- or home-based rehabilitation programmes were: 1) patient was referred when the medications were deemed optimized for the symptom control; and 2) the medications typically prescribed to the patients included various types of inhaled bronchodilators. Despite taking a relatively unified approach to the medication prescriptions, the possibility that the differences in the outcomes among the patients between the two programmes due to the differences in the medications taken by the patients cannot be completely excluded.

Another drawback is that the patients' data was under-reported. This is rather common in studying outcomes of pulmonary rehabilitation among patients with COPD [14, 46]. The 181 completed cases out of the 685 total cases may not fully represent the typical patients receiving the services. Many of the patients had repeatedly participated in the CBRP or HBRP, so the treatment effects could have been inflated. Further studies should generate evidence on the efficacy of these programmes by employing a more stringent research design and larger sample size.

Conclusion

Patients with pneumoconiosis require long-term rehabilitation services. To best fulfil their needs, rehabilitation programmes are offered in the community or at home. The patients were found to show positive gains in areas of knowledge, exercise tolerance, quality of life, and psychological symptoms after attending community-based programmes. Some of these gains were related to patients' attendance frequency levels of adjunctive programs and the involvement levels of their relatives in the treatment processes. Home-based programmes, in contrast, produced less obvious treatment effects, particularly regarding quality of life and psychological symptoms. The findings suggest the importance of strengthening psycho-social intervention for patients who take part in home-based rehabilitation programmes.

Abbreviations
%DOI: Percentage of the degree of impairment; 6MWT: 6-Min Walk Test; BMI: Body Mass Index; CBRP: Community-based rehabilitation programmes with maintenance pulmonary rehabilitation programmes; CHCP: Comprehensive Home Care Program; CPDP: Comprehensive Post Discharge Program; CRQ: Chronic Respiratory Questionnaire; FEV₁: Baseline forced-expiratory volume; HADS: Hospital Anxiety and Depression Scale; HBRP: Home-Based Rehabilitation Program; HLP relative: HLP participated by patients' relatives; HLP: Healthy Lifestyle Program; HRQOL: Health-related quality of life; LTOT: Long Term Oxygen Therapy; MRP: Maintenance Rehabilitation Program; NGO: Nongovernmental organization; PR: Pulmonary rehabilitation; RHP relative: RHP participated by patients' relatives; RHP: Respiratory Hygiene Program; SF-12's PCS and MCS: Health survey Short Form-12's physical and mental components; SMP relative: SMP participated in by the patients' relatives; SMP: Self-Management Program; TOTAL: Total number of programme participation (core plus adjunctive programmes)

Acknowledgements
We thank Chiu Sin Man RN, Yee Ping Vong PT and Ching Han Leung OT of *North District Hospital*, Ki Tsing Ko RN of Haven of Hope Hospital, and Elsie Ong for their assistances in data collection.

Funding
This study was supported by the Pneumoconiosis Compensation Fund Board, Hong Kong.

Authors' contributions
EWT Data collection, Data Analysis, Manuscript writing and revision; HK Conceptualization of study, Data Analysis Manuscript review and revision; AKYC Manuscript review and revision; KLC Data collection, Manuscript review; KSC Data collection, Manuscript review, KSL Data collection, Manuscript review, CCHC Conceptualization of study, Data Analysis, Manuscript review and revision.

Competing interests
The authors declare that they have no competing interests.

Author details
[1]The Laboratory of Neuroscience for Education, Faculty of Education, The University of Hong Kong, Hong Kong, China. [2]Department of Rehabilitation Sciences, The Hong Kong Polytechnic University, Hung Hom, Kowloon, Hong Kong, China. [3]Department of Life Science, Imperial College of London, London, UK. [4]Department of Medicine, North District Hospital, Hong Kong, China. [5]Department of Medicine, Haven of Hope Hospital, Hong Kong, China. [6]Department of Medicine, Ruttonjee Hospital, Hong Kong, China.

References
1. Chan CCH, Tsang EW, Kwok H, Siu A, Cheng A. Independent review: Current rehabilitation programs in Hong Kong funded by the PCFB; 2014.
2. Law YW, Leung MC, Leung CC, Yu TS, Tam CM. Characteristics of workers attending the pneumoconiosis clinic for silicosis assessment in Hong Kong: retrospective study. Hong Kong Med J. 2001;7:343–349.
3. Sirajuddin A, Kanne JP. Occupational lung disease. J Thorac Imaging. 2009; 24;310–320.
4. Tang WK, Lum CM, Ungvari GS, Chiu HF. Health-related quality of life in community-dwelling men with pneumoconiosis. Respiration. 2006;73:203 208.

5. Spielmanns M, Boeselt T, Nell C, Eckhoff J, Koczulla RA, Magnet FS, Storre JH, Windisch W, Baum K. Effect of pulmonary rehabilitation on inspiratory capacity during 6-min walk test in patients with COPD: a prospective controlled study. J Cardiopulm Rehabil Prev. 2017;38:264–268.

6. Jones PW, Quirk FH, Baveystock CM, Littlejohns P. A self-complete measure of health status for chronic airflow limitation. The St George's Respiratory Questionnaire. Am Rev Respir Dis. 1992;145:1321–7.

7. Engstrom CP, Persson LO, Larsson S, Sullivan M. Health-related quality of life in Copd: why both disease-specific and generic measures should be used. Eur Respir J. 2001;18:69–76.

8. McCarthy B, Casey D, Devane D, Murphy K, Murphy E, Lacasse Y. Pulmonary Rehabilitation For Chronic Obstructive Pulmonary Disease. Cochrane Database Syst Rev. 2015;2:Cd003793.

9. Nici L, Donner C, Wouters E, Zuwallack R, Ambrosino N, Bourbeau J, Carone M, Celli B, Engelen M, Fahy B, et al. American Thoracic Society/European Respiratory Society statement on pulmonary rehabilitation. Am J Respir Crit Care Med. 2006;173:1390–413.

10. Spruit MA, Singh SJ, Garvey C, ZuWallack R, Nici L, Rochester C, Hill K, Holland AE, Lareau SC, Man WD, et al. An official American Thoracic Society/ European Respiratory Society statement: key concepts and advances in pulmonary rehabilitation. Am J Respir Crit Care Med. 2013;188:E13–64.

11. Quality Standards For Pulmonary Rehabilitation In Adults. Retrieved May 26, 2018, from [https://www.Brit-Thoracic.Org.Uk/Document-Library/Clinical-Information/Pulmonary-Rehabilitation/Bts-Quality-Standards-For-Pulmonary-Rehabilitation-In-Adults/].

12. Bourbeau J. Making pulmonary rehabilitation a success in Copd. Swiss Med Wkly. 2010;140:W13067.

13. Cambach W, Chadwick Straver RV, Wagenaar RC, van Keimpema AR, Kemper HC. The effects of a community-based pulmonary rehabilitation Programme on exercise tolerance and quality of life: a randomized controlled trial. Eur Respir J. 1997;10:104–13.

14. Ghanem M, Elaal EA, Mehany M, Tolba K. Home-based pulmonary rehabilitation program: effect on exercise tolerance and quality of life in chronic obstructive pulmonary disease patients. Ann Thorac Med. 2010;5: 18–25.

15. Grosbois JM, Gicquello A, Langlois C, Le Rouzic O, Bart F, Wallaert B, Chenivesse C. Long-term evaluation of home-based pulmonary rehabilitation in patients with Copd. Int J Chron Obstruct Pulmon Dis. 2015; 10:2037–44.

16. Holland AE, Mahal A, Hill CJ, Lee AL, Burge AT, Moore R, Nicolson C, O'Halloran P, Cox NS, Lahham A, et al. Benefits And Costs Of Home-Based Pulmonary Rehabilitation In Chronic Obstructive Pulmonary Disease - A Multi-Centre Randomised Controlled Equivalence Trial. Bmc Pulm Med. 2013;13:57.

17. McNamara RJ, Elkins MR. Home-based rehabilitation improves exercise capacity and reduces respiratory symptoms in people with COPD (PEDro synthesis). Br J Sports Med. 2016;51:206–207.

18. Nikoletou D, Man WD, Mustfa N, Moore J, Rafferty G, Grant RL, Johnson L, Moxham J. Evaluation of the effectiveness of a home-based inspiratory muscle training Programme in patients with chronic obstructive pulmonary disease using multiple inspiratory muscle tests. Disabil Rehabil. 2016;38:250–9.

19. Beauchamp MK, Janaudis-Ferreira T, Goldstein RS, Brooks D. Optimal duration of pulmonary rehabilitation for individuals with chronic obstructive pulmonary disease - a systematic review. Chron Respir Dis. 2011;8:129–40.

20. PCFB. Pneumoconiosis Compensation Fund Board. Annual Report. 2013.

21. Jacome C, Marques A. Pulmonary rehabilitation for mild Copd: a systematic review. Respir Care. 2014;59:588–94.

22. Rugbjerg M, Iepsen UW, Jorgensen KJ, Lange P. Effectiveness of pulmonary rehabilitation in COPD with mild symptoms: a systematic review with meta-analyses. Int J Chron Obstruct Pulmon Dis. 2015;10:791–801.

23. The European Respiratory Society. Pulmonary Rehabilitation. In: Gibson J, Loddenkemper R, Sibille Y, Lundbäck B, editors. The European Lung White Book; 2018. p. 340–7.

24. Spruit MA, Gosselink R, Troosters T, De Paepe K, Decramer M. Resistance versus endurance training in patients with COPD and peripheral muscle weakness. Eur Respir J. 2002;19:1072–8.

25. Franssen FM, Broekhuizen R, Janssen PP, Wouters EF, Schols AM. Effects of whole-body exercise training on body composition and functional capacity in normal-weight patients with Copd. Chest. 2004;125:2021–8.

26. Liu XD, Jin HZ, Ng BHP, Gu YH, Wu YC, Lu G. Therapeutic effects of qigong in patients with Copd: a randomized controlled trial. Hong Kong Journal Of Occupational Therapy. 2012;22:38–46.

27. Guyatt GH, Berman LB, Townsend M, Pugsley SO, Chambers LW. A measure of quality of life for clinical trials in chronic lung disease. Thorax. 1987;42:773–8.

28. Zigmond AS, Snaith RP. The hospital anxiety and depression scale. Acta Psychiatr Scand. 1983;67:361–70.

29. Gandek B, Ware JE, Aaronson NK, Apolone G, Bjorner JB, Brazier JE, Bullinger M, Kaasa S, Leplege A, Prieto L, Sullivan M. Cross-validation of item selection and scoring for the SF-12 health survey in nine countries: results from the IQOLA project. International quality of life assessment. J Clin Epidemiol. 1998;51:1171–8.

30. ATS Committee on Proficiency Standards for Clinical Pulmonary Function Laboratories. ATS statement: guidelines for the six-minute walk test. Am J Respir Crit Care Med. 2002;166:111–7.

31. Roman M, Larraz C, Gomez A, Ripoll J, Mir I, Miranda EZ, Macho A, Thomas V, Esteva M. Efficacy Of Pulmonary Rehabilitation In Patients With Moderate Chronic Obstructive Pulmonary Disease: A Randomized Controlled Trial. BMC Fam Pract. 2013;14:21.

32. Casey D, Murphy K, Devane D, Cooney A, McCarthy B, Mee L, Newell J, O'Shea E, Scarrott C, Gillespie P, et al. The effectiveness of a structured education pulmonary rehabilitation Programme for improving the health status of people with moderate and severe chronic obstructive pulmonary disease in primary care: the prince cluster randomised trial. Thorax. 2013; 68(10):922–8.

33. Lacasse Y, Goldstein R, Lasserson TJ, Martin S. Pulmonary Rehabilitation For Chronic Obstructive Pulmonary Disease. Cochrane Database Syst Rev. 2006: CD003793.

34. Griffiths TL, Burr ML, Campbell IA, Lewis-Jenkins V, Mullins J, Shiels K, Turner-Lawlor PJ, Payne N, Newcombe RG, Ionescu AA, et al. Results at 1 year of outpatient multidisciplinary pulmonary rehabilitation: a randomized controlled trial. Lancet. 2000;355:362–8.

35. Ketelaars CA, Abu-Saad HH, Schlosser MA, Mostert R, Wouters EF. Long-term outcome of pulmonary rehabilitation in patients with Copd. Chest. 1997; 112:363–9.

36. Moullec G, Ninot G. An integrated Programme after pulmonary rehabilitation in patients with chronic obstructive pulmonary disease: effect on emotional and functional dimensions of quality of life. Clin Rehabil. 2010;24:122–36.

37. Chavannes NH, Grijsen M, van den AM, Schepers H, Nijdam M, Tiep B, Muris J. Integrated disease management improves one-year quality of life in primary care Copd patients: a controlled clinical trial. Prim Care Respir J. 2009;18:171–6.

38. Guell R, Casan P, Belda J, Sangenis M, Morante F, Guyatt G, Sanchis J. Long-term effects of outpatient rehabilitation of COPD: a randomized trial. Chest. 2000;117:976–83.

39. Redelmeier DA, Bayoumi AM, Goldstein RS, Guyatt GH. Interpreting small differences in functional status: the six-minute walk test in chronic lung disease patients. Am J Respir Crit Care Med. 1997;155:1278–82.

40. Engstrom CP, Persson LO, Larsson S, Sullivan M. Long-term effects of a pulmonary rehabilitation Programme in outpatients with chronic obstructive pulmonary disease: a randomized controlled study. Scand J Rehabil Med. 1999;31:207–13.

41. Benzo R, Flume PA, Turner D, Tempest M. Effect of pulmonary rehabilitation on quality of life in patients with Copd: the use of SF-36 summary scores as outcomes measures. J Cardpulm Rehabil. 2000;20:231–4.

42. Burkow TM, Vognild LK, Johnsen E, Risberg MJ, Bratvold A, Breivik E, Krogstad T, Hjalmarsen A. Comprehensive Pulmonary Rehabilitation In Home-Based Online Groups: A Mixed Method Pilot Study In COPD. BMC Res Notes. 2015;8:766.

43. Hogg L, Grant A, Garrod R, Fiddler H. People with COPD perceive ongoing, structured and socially supportive exercise opportunities to be important for maintaining an active lifestyle following pulmonary rehabilitation: a qualitative study. J Physiother. 2012;58:189–95.

44. Lahham A, McDonald CF, Mahal A, Lee AL, Hill CJ, Burge AT, Cox NS, Moore R, Nicolson C, O'Halloran P, et al. Home-based pulmonary rehabilitation for

people with Copd: a qualitative study reporting the patient perspective. Chron Respir Dis. 2018;15:123–130.

45. Khoshkesht S, Zakerimoghadam M, Ghiyasvandian S, Kazemnejad A, Hashemian M. The effect of home-based pulmonary rehabilitation on self-efficacy in chronic obstructive pulmonary disease patients. J Pak Med Assoc. 2015;65:1041–6.

46. Puhan MA, Behnke M, Frey M, Grueter T, Brandli O, Lichtenschopf A, Guyatt GH, Schunemann HJ. Self-Administration And Interviewer-Administration Of The German Chronic Respiratory Questionnaire: Instrument Development And Assessment Of Validity And Reliability In Two Randomised Studies. Health Qual Life Outcomes. 2004;2:1.

15

Oxygen versus air-driven nebulisers for exacerbations of chronic obstructive pulmonary disease

George Bardsley[1,2] (iD), Janine Pilcher[1,2,3] (iD), Steven McKinstry[1,2,3] (iD), Philippa Shirtcliffe[1,2] (iD), James Berry[2,4] (iD), James Fingleton[1,2] (iD), Mark Weatherall[4] (iD) and Richard Beasley[1,2,3*] (iD)

Abstract

Background: In exacerbations of chronic obstructive pulmonary disease, administration of high concentrations of oxygen may cause hypercapnia and increase mortality compared with oxygen titrated, if required, to achieve an oxygen saturation of 88–92%. Optimally titrated oxygen regimens require two components: titrated supplemental oxygen to achieve the target oxygen saturation and, if required, bronchodilators delivered by air-driven nebulisation. The effect of repeated air vs oxygen-driven bronchodilator nebulisation in acute exacerbations of chronic obstructive pulmonary disease is unknown. We aimed to compare the effects of air versus oxygen-driven bronchodilator nebulisation on arterial carbon dioxide tension in exacerbations of chronic obstructive pulmonary disease.

Methods: A parallel group double-blind randomised controlled trial in 90 hospital in-patients with an acute exacerbation of COPD. Participants were randomised to receive two 2.5 mg salbutamol nebulisers, both driven by air or oxygen at 8 L/min, each delivered over 15 min with a 5 min interval in-between. The primary outcome measure was the transcutaneous partial pressure of carbon dioxide at the end of the second nebulisation (35 min). The primary analysis used a mixed linear model with fixed effects of the baseline $PtCO_2$, time, the randomised intervention, and a time by intervention interaction term; to estimate the difference between randomised treatments at 35 min. Analysis was by intention-to-treat.

Results: Oxygen-driven nebulisation was terminated in one participant after 27 min when the $PtCO_2$ rose by > 10 mmHg, a predefined safety criterion. The mean (standard deviation) change in $PtCO_2$ at 35 min was 3.4 (1.9) mmHg and 0.1 (1.4) mmHg in the oxygen and air groups respectively, difference (95% confidence interval) 3.3 mmHg (2.7 to 3.9), $p < 0.001$. The proportion of patients with a $PtCO_2$ change ≥4 mmHg during the intervention was 18/45 (40%) and 0/44 (0%) for oxygen and air groups respectively.

Conclusions: Oxygen-driven nebulisation leads to an increase in $PtCO_2$ in exacerbations of COPD. We propose that air-driven bronchodilator nebulisation is preferable to oxygen-driven nebulisation in exacerbations of COPD.

Keywords: Air, Bronchodilator agents, Hypercapnia, Nebulisation, Oxygen

* Correspondence: richard.beasley@mrinz.ac.nz
[1]Capital and Coast District Health Board, Wellington, New Zealand
[2]Medical Research Institute of New Zealand, Box 7902, Wellington, PO 6242, New Zealand
Full list of author information is available at the end of the article

Background

In acute exacerbations of chronic obstructive pulmonary disease (AECOPD), administration of high concentration oxygen may cause profound hypercapnia and increase mortality, compared with oxygen titrated to achieve an oxygen saturation of between 88 to 92% [1, 2]. Titrated oxygen regimens require two components: titrated supplemental oxygen to achieve a particular target arterial oxygen saturation measured by pulse oximetry (SpO_2), and bronchodilators delivered by either air-driven nebulisation or metered-dose inhalers with a spacer. Oxygen-driven nebulisation inadvertently exposes patients to high concentrations of inspired oxygen, particularly with prolonged or repeated use as may occur in patients with severe exacerbations during long pre-hospital transfers or if the mask is inadvertently left in place.

We have shown that air-driven bronchodilator nebulisation prevents the increase in arterial partial pressure of carbon dioxide ($PaCO_2$) that results from use of oxygen-driven nebulisers in patients with stable COPD [3]. However, there are only two small non-blinded randomised controlled trials of air compared to oxygen-driven nebulisation in patients admitted to hospital with AECOPD [4, 5]. These trials reported that administration of a single bronchodilator dose using oxygen-driven nebulisation increases the $PaCO_2$ in COPD patients who have baseline hypercapnia.

Robust determination of the risks of oxygen-driven nebulisation in AECOPD could identify whether widespread implementation of air-driven nebulisers, or use of metered-dose inhalers through a spacer, are required to ensure safe delivery of bronchodilators to this high-risk patient group. The objective of this study was to compare the effects on $PaCO_2$ of air- and oxygen-driven bronchodilator nebulisation in AECOPD. Our hypothesis was that two doses of oxygen-driven bronchodilator nebulisation would increase the $PaCO_2$ compared with air-driven nebulisation in patients hospitalised with an AECOPD.

Methods

Trial design and patients

This was a parallel-group double-blind randomised controlled trial at Wellington Regional Hospital, New Zealand. The full study protocol is available in the online supplement.

Participants were hospital inpatients, ≥40 years of age, with an admission diagnosis of AECOPD. Exclusion criteria included requirement for ≥4 L/min of oxygen via nasal cannulae to maintain SpO_2 between 88 to 92%; current requirement for non-invasive ventilation (NIV); baseline transcutaneous partial pressure of carbon dioxide ($PtCO_2$) > 60 mmHg; inability to provide written informed consent; and any other condition which at the Investigator's discretion, was believed may present a safety risk or impact on the feasibility of the study

results. Written informed consent was obtained before any study-specific procedures. The study was undertaken on the ward during the hospital admission. Ethics approval was obtained from the Health and Disability Ethics Committee, New Zealand (Reference 14/NTB/200). The full study protocol (original and updated version) can be found on the OLS (see Additional file 1 and 2).

Intervention

After written consent, participants had continuous $PtCO_2$ and heart rate monitoring using the SenTec® (SenTec AG, Switzerland) device and oxygen saturation (SpO_2) measured by pulse oximetry (Novametrix 512, Respironics, Carlsbad, USA). Participants were randomised to receive two nebulisations, both driven either by air or oxygen, at 8 L/min, each delivered over 15 min with a five minute break in-between. Randomisation was 1:1 by a block randomised computer generated sequence (block size six), provided in sealed opaque envelopes by the study statistician who was independent of recruitment and assessment of participants.

The participants and blinded investigator, who recorded heart rate and $PtCO_2$ were masked to the randomised treatments. If both oxygen and air ports were available in hospital on the wall behind the participant, these were used for driving nebulisation. If only oxygen ports were available, identical portable oxygen and air cylinders were placed behind the participant's bed prior to randomisation and used instead. Both the participant and blinded investigator faced forward for the full duration of the study. In addition, the blinded investigator sat towards the end of the bed - ahead of the participant, such that they could not see the participant's interventions. Likewise, the blinded investigator and patient could not view the SpO_2 on the Sentec device, as this was covered during the interventions, or the pulse oximeter which could only be viewed by the unblinded investigator. Interaction between blinded and unblinded investigators would only occur if a rise in $PtCO_2$ of ≥10 mmHg was demonstrated (a predefined safety criterion to abort intervention).

An initial 15 min wash-in and titration period was administered by the unblinded investigator using nasal cannulae, if required, to ensure that participant's SpO_2 were within 88 to 92%. If saturations were ≥ 88% on room air, no supplemental oxygen was required. Randomisation was performed after the 15 min wash-in period, when both patient and blinded investigator were already in a forward-facing position to maintain blinding. The unblinded investigator recorded SpO_2 on a separate pulse-oximeter from then onwards.

Immediately before the first nebulisation, denoted by the baseline reading at time-point zero, $PtCO_2$, SpO_2 and heart rate were recorded. Participants then received two administrations of 2.5 mg salbutamol by nebulisation, delivered by either air or oxygen - each for 15 min duration at a flow rate of 8 L/min. Hudson RCI Micro Mist Nebuliser Masks (Hudson RCI, Durham, North Carolina, USA) were used. The nebulisations were delivered by the unblinded investigator at time zero and at 20 min, allowing for a five minute interval between nebulisations. Recordings were continued for 45 min after completion of the last nebulisation (80 min after baseline). Measurements of $PtCO_2$, SpO_2 and heart rate were recorded at five minute intervals, and at six minutes after the start of each nebulisation, in view of the British Thoracic Society (BTS) guideline's recommendation for limiting oxygen-driven nebulisation to six-minutes in ambulance care, if air-driven nebulisation is unavailable [6].

Immediately before the first nebulisation and just before completion of the second nebulisation, at 35 min, a capillary blood gas sample was taken from the fingertip for measurement of $PcapCO_2$ and pH.

Oxygen delivery

During the wash-in and between the nebulisations oxygen was titrated, if required, via nasal prongs to maintain oxygen saturations between 88 to 92%. Participants in the air-driven group who were receiving oxygen at the start of nebulisation continued to receive titrated supplemental oxygen via nasal prongs underneath the nebuliser mask. Those in the oxygen-driven group had the prongs removed at the start, and reapplied after the completion of each nebulisation. At 35 min, oxygen was delivered via nasal prongs to participants at the flow rate they last received during titration (i.e. at 35 min and 20 min in the air-driven and oxygen-driven groups, respectively). From 35 min until 80 min, the oxygen flow rate was only increased (or initiated) if a participant's SpO_2 fell below 85%.

Outcomes

The primary outcome was originally planned to be $PcapCO_2$ at 35 min, at completion of the second nebulisation. However, after the first 14 participants had been studied, it was evident that obtaining adequate amounts of blood to fill the capillary tubes from some participants was difficult. At this stage of recruitment 4/14 (29%) of participants had missing data. The primary outcome variable was therefore changed to $PtCO_2$ at 35 min, with $PcapCO_2$ at 35 min reverting to a secondary outcome variable. Other secondary outcomes were the individual $PtCO_2$ measurements at each time point; the proportion of participants who had a rise in $PtCO_2$ or $PcapCO_2$ of ≥ 4 and ≥ 8 mmHg; capillary pH at 35 min, and heart rate and SpO_2 measurements at each time point.

Sample size calculation and statistical analysis

A rise in $PtCO_2$ from baseline of ≥ 4 mmHg is considered a physiologically significant change and ≥ 8 mmHg

a clinically significant change, based on previous criteria [7, 8]. In our study of oxygen versus air-driven nebulisers in stable COPD patients, the standard deviation (SD) of baseline $PtCO_2$ was 5.5 mmHg [3]. With 90% power and alpha of 5%, 82 patients were required to detect a 4 mmHg difference. Assuming a drop-out rate of 10% our target recruitment was 90 patients.

The primary analysis used a mixed linear model with fixed effects of the baseline $PtCO_2$, time, the randomised intervention, and a time by intervention interaction term; to estimate the difference between randomised treatments at 35 min. A power exponential in time correlation structure was used for the repeated measurements. The secondary outcome variables of $PtCO_2$ at the other time points, SpO_2 and heart rate used similar mixed linear models. $PcapCO_2$ and pH were compared by Analysis of Covariance with the baseline measurement as a continuous co-variate. As a post-hoc analysis we compared the difference in $PtCO_2$ between the 15 and 6 min, and the 35 and 26 min time points.

Comparison of categorical variables, $PtCO_2$ or $PcapCO_2$ change of ≥ 4 and 8 mmHg, was by estimation of a risk difference, and Fishers' exact test. As a post-hoc analysis we also compared the difference in paired proportions for those with $PtCO_2$ change of ≥ 4 mmHg in the oxygen arm only using McNemar's test and an appropriate estimate for the difference in paired proportions. The time for $PtCO_2$ to return to baseline during the observation period (defined as the time until the $PtCO_2$ was first equal to or below the baseline value, between 40 and 80 min), was compared using Kaplan-Meier survival curves and a Cox Proportional Hazards model. A simple t-test was used to compare the lowest value of the SpO_2 between 40 and 80 min, compared to baseline. SAS version 9.4 was used.

Results

Patients

The trial recruited between May 14th 2015 and June 29th 2016. The CONSORT diagram of the flow of the 90 recruited participants through the trial is shown in Fig. 1. One participant withdrew after 18 min of air-driven nebulisation because of feeling flushed, and so complete data was available for $PtCO_2$ for 89 participants. The baseline $PtCO_2$ for this participant was 34.3 mmHg and at the time of withdrawal it was 34.6 mmHg. Oxygen-driven nebulisation was stopped in another participant at 27 min when the $PtCO_2$ rose by > 10 mmHg from baseline, a pre-defined safety criterion. The baseline $PtCO_2$ for this participant was 43.4 mmHg and at the time of withdrawal it was 54.1 mmHg. This participant had study measurements continued after this for the full duration of the study. No clinical adverse events were noted during the intervention periods.

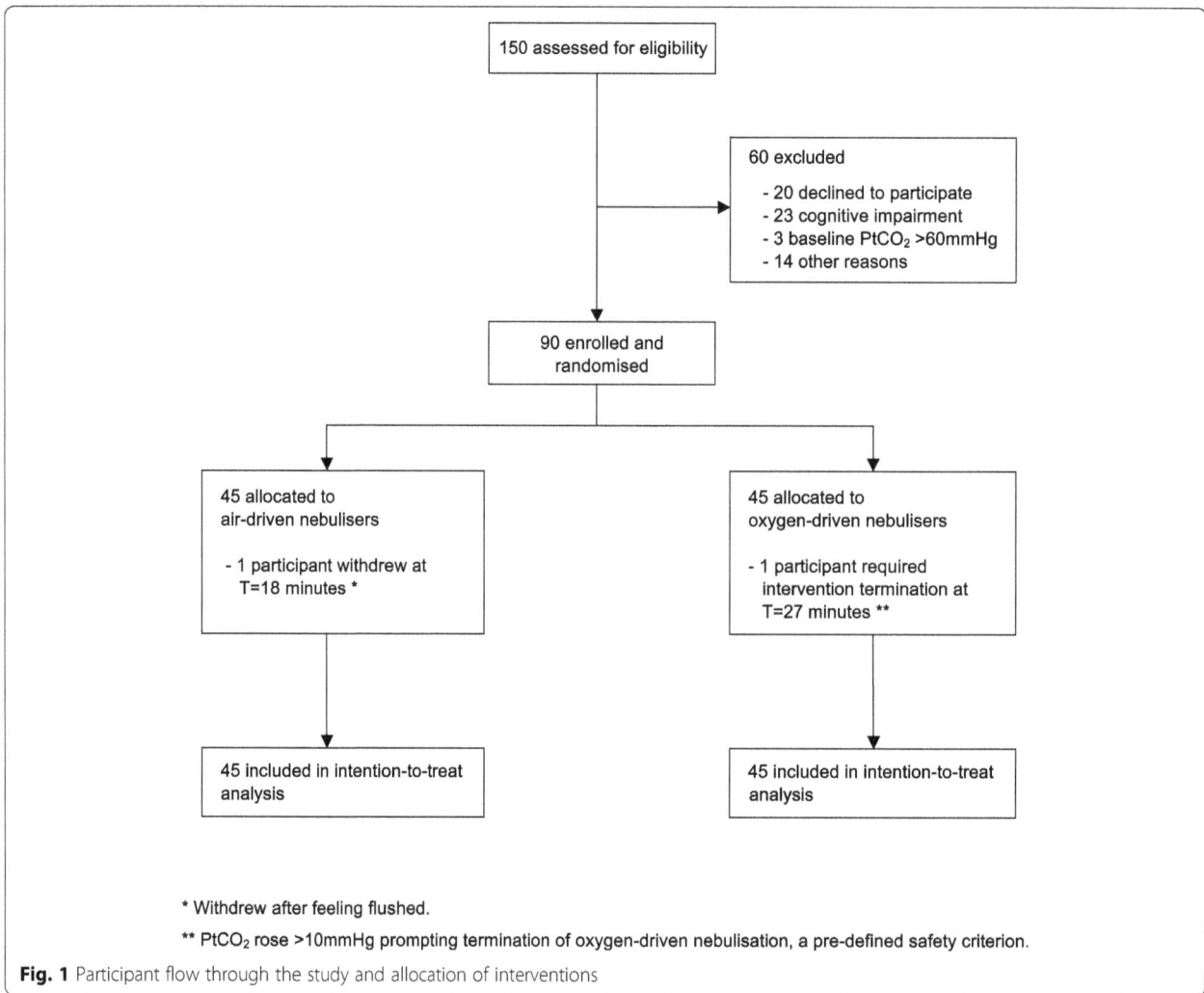

* Withdrew after feeling flushed.

** PtCO₂ rose >10mmHg prompting termination of oxygen-driven nebulisation, a pre-defined safety criterion.

Fig. 1 Participant flow through the study and allocation of interventions

A summary of baseline participant characteristics are shown in Table 1. Participants predominantly had severe airflow obstruction with a mean FEV_1 of 34.5% predicted. The mean (range) baseline $PtCO_2$ was 37.6 mmHg (24.3 to 58.5 mmHg), and mean SpO_2 was 93%. Patients randomised to the oxygen group were more likely to have required assisted ventilation previously. The mean (SD) time for the nebulised salbutamol to dissipate from the chamber was 5.2 (1.2) minutes.

PtCO₂

The mean (SD) change in $PtCO_2$ after 35 min was 3.4 (1.9) mmHg in the oxygen group ($n = 45$), compared to 0.1 (1.4) mmHg in the air group ($n = 44$). The difference (95% CI) in $PtCO_2$ for oxygen compared to air-driven nebulisations after 35 min was 3.3 mmHg (2.7 to 3.9), $p < 0.001$. (Table 2 and Fig. 2). After adjustment for baseline $PtCO_2$, a history of assisted ventilation, previous hypercapnia and baseline SpO_2, were not associated with the $PtCO_2$ at 35 min in either randomised group.

In 18/45 (40%) participants receiving oxygen-driven nebulisation, $PtCO_2$ increased from baseline by ≥4 mmHg at some stage during the intervention compared to none of the participants receiving air-driven nebulisation, risk difference (95% CI) 40% (25.7 to 54.3), $p < 0.001$. The full data description and comparisons at each time point are shown in the OLS. Two participants receiving oxygen-driven nebulisation had a rise in $PtCO_2 \geq 8$ mmHg, one of whom required intervention termination, exceeding the predefined safety criterion of a rise ≥10 mmHg from baseline.

The estimate (95% CI) of the time-related difference, 15 min minus six minutes, for oxygen compared to air, was 0.73 mmHg (0.11 to 1.35), $P = 0.021$; and for 35 min minus 26 min, 0.43 mmHg (-0.19 to 1.06), $P = 0.17$. In the oxygen treatment arm the proportion of patients in whom the $PtCO_2$ increased from baseline by ≥4 mmHg at 6 min was less than the proportion at 15 min: 6/45 (13.3%) and 13/45 (28.9%) respectively, paired difference in proportions (95% CI) 15.6% (3.3 to 27.8), $P = 0.013$

Table 1 Participant Characteristics

	Mean (SD)		P
	Oxygen N=45[a]	Air N=45[a]	
Age (years)	70·4 (10·3)	72·3 (8·3)	0.34
Age at diagnosis of COPD (years)	58·6 (12·1) N = 40	58·8 (12·2) N = 44	0.92
BMI (kg/m²)	27·2 (7·7)	25·5 (8·9)	0.33
Smoking pack years	39·3 (31·1)	51·2 (39·2)	0.11
FEV_1 (L)	0·81 (0·33) N = 35	0·85 (0·31) N = 37	0.69
FEV_1% predicted	35·0 (11·5) N = 35	34·0 (11·8) N = 37	0.73
mMRC	2·38 (1·09)	2·33 (1·04)	0.84
Baseline Transcutaneous Data			
$PtCO_2$ (mmHg)	38·0 (7·7)	37·2 (6·8)	0.59
SpO_2 (%)	92·6 (2·4)	92·6 (2·3)	0.93
Heart Rate (per minute)	89·6 (15·7)	87·0 (16·0)	0.89
Baseline capillary blood gas			
pH	7·42 (0·04) N = 43	7·44 (0·03) N = 41	0.11
$PcapCO_2$ (mmHg)	40·2 (7·0) N = 43	38·5 (5·9) N = 41	0.23
	N/45 (%)		P
	Oxygen	Air	
Male	17 (38)	24 (53)	0.20
Ethnicity			0.49
European	24 (53)	31 (69)	
Māori	7 (16)	4 (9)	
Pacific	5 (11)	4 (9)	
Other	9 (20)	6 (13)	
Previous Ventilation (ever)	12 (27)	3 (7)	0.02
Previous Ventilation Type			0.03
NIV	10 (22)	3 (7)	
Intubation	2 (4)	0 (0)	
Previous hypercapnia	23 (51)	17 (38)	0.29
Home Oxygen	2 (4)	1 (2)	0.99
Home Nebulisers	5 (11)	12 (27)	0.10
Comorbidities			
Heart Failure	8 (18)	3 (7)	0.20
Asthma	6 (13)	2 (4)	0.27
Bronchiectasis	3 (7)	4 (9)	0.99

COPD Chronic Obstructive Pulmonary Disease, *BMI* Body Mass Index, *FEV₁* Forced Expiratory Volume in 1 s at time of randomisation, *mMRC* Modified Medical Research Council dyspnea scale, *PtCO₂* Transcutaneous partial pressure of carbon dioxide, *SpO₂* peripheral oxygen saturation, *PcapCO₂* Capillary partial pressure of carbon dioxide, *NIV* non-invasive ventilation
[a]Unless indicated

(Additional file 1: Table S1). The proportion of patients in whom the $PtCO_2$ increased from baseline by ≥4 mmHg at 26 min (6 min into the second oxygen-driven nebulisation) was also less than the proportion at 35 min (completion of the second oxygen-driven nebulisation), although this difference was not statistically significant: 10/45 (22%)

and 14/45 (31%) respectively, paired difference in proportions (95% CI) 8.9% (− 3.3 to 20.9), P = 0.15.

The median (25th to 75th percentile) time taken for $PtCO_2$ to return to baseline after cessation of the second nebulisation was 40 (40 to 45) minutes in the air group compared to 50 (45 to 50) minutes in the oxygen group, hazard ratio (95% CI) 1.59 (1.01 to 2.52), P = 0.047.

$PcapCO_2$ and pH
Data summaries for capillary blood gas sampling are shown in Table 3. The difference (95% CI) between oxygen and air for $PcapCO_2$ after 35 min was 2.0 mmHg (1.1 to 2.8), p < 0.001. Thirteen (31.7%) participants receiving oxygen had a rise in $PcapCO_2$ of ≥4 mmHg compared with three (7.7%) receiving air; risk difference (95% CI) 24% (7.5 to 40.5), p = 0.01. In addition to the two participants in whom the $PtCO_2$ increased by ≥8 mmHg, there were two additional participants with capillary data receiving oxygen who had a rise in $PcapCO_2$ of ≥8 mmHg and none from the air group. The mean (95% CI) difference in pH after 35 min was 0.015 units (0.008 to 0.024, p < 0.001) lower for oxygen nebulisation compared to air. One participant experienced a reduction in pH of 0.06 units (from 7.38 to 7.32) in association with a rise in $PcapCO_2$ of 9 mmHg (55 to 64 mmHg).

SpO_2 and heart rate
The SpO_2 was higher throughout both the nebulisation and initial washout periods in the oxygen compared with the air group (see Additional file 3: Table S2). Figure 3 shows the trend for the SpO_2 in the oxygen group to fall below that of the air group after cessation of the second nebulisation. At the end of the observation period (80 min), the SpO_2 was lower in the oxygen group (difference − 1.22%, 95% CI -2.04 to − 0.39, p = 0.004). The maximum reduction in SpO_2 from baseline was 0·8% (95% CI -0.2 to 1.7, P = 0.10) lower after oxygen compared with air nebulisation. The heart rate was slower in the oxygen group at 35 min by 3.3 bpm (95% CI 0.31 to 6.25), p = 0.031 (see Additional file 1: Table S3).

Methods of PCO_2 measurement
Due to the requirement to change the primary outcome measure, a post-hoc analysis was undertaken to compare the two methods of measuring $PaCO_2$. Based on data for 80 paired $PtCO_2$ and $PcapCO_2$ measurements at baseline and 35 min, the mean (SD) change in $PtCO_2$ was 1.7 mmHg (2.2) with a range of − 2.5 to 8.0 mmHg, and the mean (SD) change in $PcapCO_2$ was 1.7 mmHg (2.3), with a range − 3.0 to 9.0 mmHg. The estimate of bias for change in $PcapCO_2$ minus $PtCO_2$ was − 0.03 mmHg (95% CI -0.44 to 0.38), P = 0.89. The limits of agreement between $PtCO_2$ and $PcapCO_2$ were +/− 3.8 mmHg for each individual measurement obtained.

Table 2 PtCO$_2$ by time and randomised group

Action	Time	PtCO$_2$ Mean (SD) [N = 45 for each unless specified]		Oxygen minus air (95% CI)	P
		Oxygen	Air		
Baseline	0	38·0 (7·7)	37·2 (6·8)		
1st nebulisation	5	39·9 (8·3)	37·0 (7·1)	2·10 (1·49 to 2·71)	< 0·001
	6	40·1 (8·4)	37·0 (7·1)	2·24 (1·63 to 2·86)	< 0·001
	10	40·8 (8·6)	37·2 (6·9)	2·76 (2·15 to 3·37)	< 0·001
	15	41·1 (8·8)	37·3 (6·9)	2·97 (2·36 to 3·59)	< 0·001
	20	38·6 (7·8)	37·0 (6·4)[a]	0·86 (0·25 to 1·48)	0·006
2nd nebulisation	25	40·5 (8·3)	36·8 (6·8)[b]	2·77 (2·15 to 3·39)	< 0·001
	26	40·6 (8·4)	36·8 (6·8)[b]	2·88 (2·26 to 3·50)	< 0·001
	30	41·1 (8·5)	37·1 (6·6)[a]	3·20 (2·59 to 3·82)	< 0·001
	35	41·3 (8·6)	37·3 (6·5)[a]	3·31 (2·70 to 3·93)	< 0·001
Observation period	40	39·0 (8·1)[a]	37·0 (6·7)[a]	1·14 (0·52 to 1·76)	< 0·001
	45	38·1 (7·5)	36·7 (6·3)[a]	0·61 (− 0·01 to 1·22)	0·053
	50	37·9 (7·4)	36·6 (6·2)[a]	0·59 (− 0·02 to 1·21)	0·059
	55	37·9 (7·3)	36·6 (6·0)[a]	0·51 (− 0·10 to 1·13)	0·1
	60	37·9 (7·3)	36·7 (6·1)[a]	0·51 (− 0·10 to 1·13)	0·1
	65	38·1 (7·2)	36·7 (6·1)[a]	0·63 (0·01 to 1·25)	0·045
	70	37·5 (6·5)[a]	36·7 (6·1)[a]	0·60 (− 0·02 to 1·21)	0·059
	75	37·8 (6·8)	36·7 (6·1)[a]	0·42 (− 0·20 to 1·03)	0·18
	80	37·9 (6·9)	36·7 (6·3)[a]	0·40 (− 0·21 to 1·02)	0·2

Air Air-driven nebuliser group, *Oxygen* Oxygen-driven nebuliser group, *PtCO$_2$* Transcutaneous partial pressure of carbon dioxide
[a]N = 44
[b]N = 43

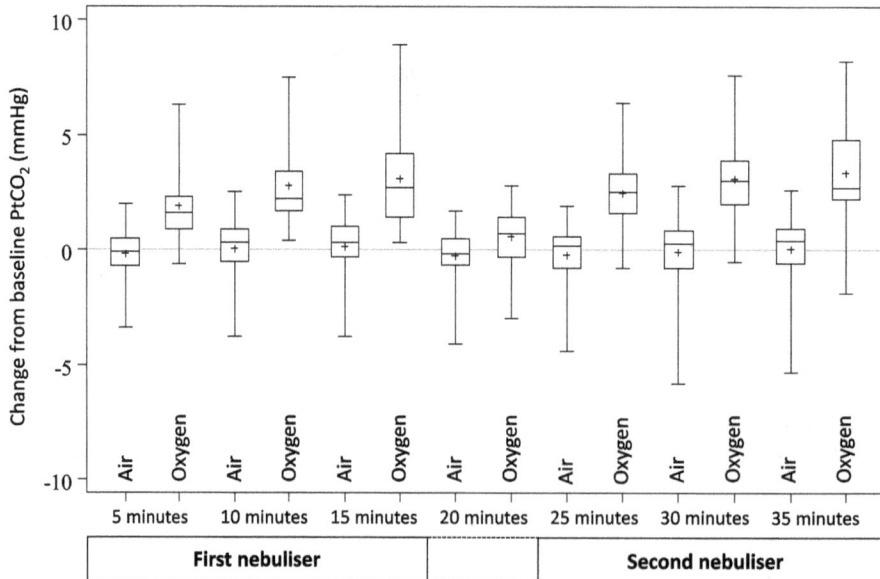

Air: Air-driven nebuliser group;   Oxygen: Oxygen-driven nebuliser group;

PtCO$_2$: Transcutaneous carbon dioxide tension

Fig. 2 PtCO$_2$ change from baseline (T = 0) to T = 35 min. Mean PtCO$_2$ with error bars showing one SD, by time and intervention

Table 3 Capillary blood gas measurements according to randomised treatment

Time (mins)	$P_{cap}CO_2$ Mean (SD)		Difference[a] (95% CI)	P
	Oxygen	Air		
0	40·2 (7·0) N = 43	38·5 (5·9) N = 41	–	–
35	42·6 (8·3) N = 41	39·0 (6·4) N = 39	2·0 (1·1 to 2·8)	< 0·001
Time (mins)	pH Mean (SD)		Difference[b] (95% CI)	P
	Oxygen	Air		
0	7·42 (0·04) N = 43	7·44 (0·03) N = 41	–	–
35	7·41 (0·04) N = 41	7·43 (0·04) N = 39	-0·015 (− 0·024 to − 0·008)	< 0·001

$P_{cap}CO_2$ Capillary partial pressure of carbon dioxide
[a]$P_{cap}CO_2$ at 35 min, adjusted for baseline
[b]pH at 35 min, adjusted for baseline

Discussion

In this study, oxygen-driven nebulisation increased the $PtCO_2$ in hospital in-patients with an AECOPD compared with air-driven nebulisation. Despite the small mean increase in $PtCO_2$ of 3.4 mmHg, the physiological relevance of this response is suggested by the increase in $PtCO_2$ of at least 4 mmHg in 18/45 (40%) of participants receiving oxygen-driven nebulisation, whereas no patient had an increase of 4 mmHg or more following air-driven nebulisation. The clinical relevance of this physiological response is suggested by the requirement to withdraw one participant during the second oxygen-driven nebulisation due to the $PtCO_2$ increasing by > 10 mmHg, and the increase of $PtCO_2$ or $PcapCO_2$ of at least 8 mmHg in 4/45 (9%) patients receiving oxygen-driven nebulisation, one of

whom had a fall in pH of 0.06 into the acidotic range (7.32). These findings suggest that air-driven nebulised bronchodilator therapy represents an important component of the conservative titrated oxygen regimen which has been shown to reduce the risk of hypercapnia, acidosis and mortality in AECOPD [1].

There are a number of methodological issues relevant to the interpretation of the study findings. Both the randomised controlled design and double-blinding of this study allow for robust and reliable data capture. The length of the nebuliser regimen was chosen to ensure adequate time for complete nebulisation to occur, and to replicate 'real-world' back to back treatments in the acute setting, by using two nebulisations separated by five minutes. It is possible that the magnitude of the

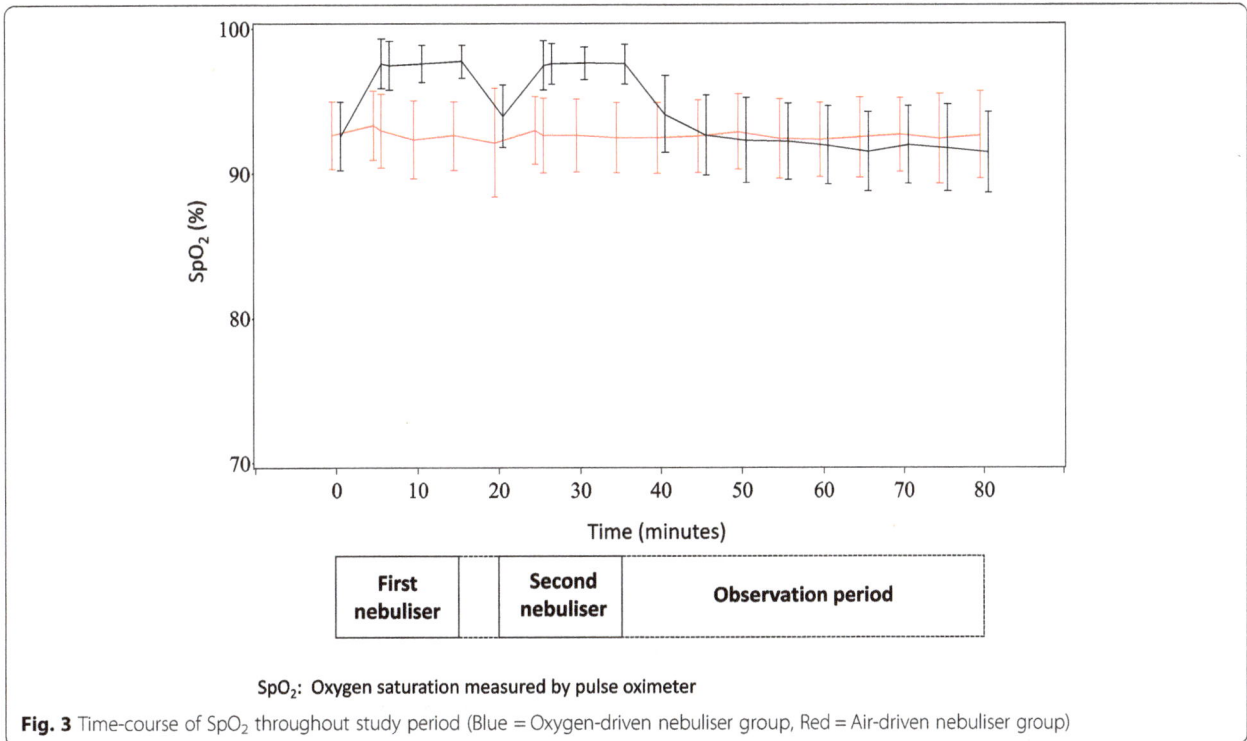

Fig. 3 Time-course of SpO_2 throughout study period (Blue = Oxygen-driven nebuliser group, Red = Air-driven nebuliser group)

differences in PCO_2 and pH may be even larger with continuous nebulisation which may occur in patients with severe exacerbations not responding to initial treatment or if the nebuliser is inadvertently left in place. The safety-based exclusion criteria of a baseline $PtCO_2 >$ 60 mmHg and an oxygen requirement of ≥ 4 L/minute (to maintain target SpO_2 of 88 to 92%), effectively excluded patients with the most severe exacerbations of COPD.

Whilst respiratory rate and neurological symptoms were not formally assessed as outcome measures, no adverse events were identified during the interventions. However, we acknowledge that if changes in PCO_2 and pH of this magnitude occurred in more severe patients at the time of their presentation, they would have been at risk of symptoms of hypercapnia and respiratory acidosis, and the requirement to escalate treatment.

The original primary outcome measure and time of measurement was $PcapCO_2$ after 35 min. Following the first 14 study participants, it was evident that obtaining adequate amounts of blood to fill the capillary tubes from some participants was difficult or impossible to the extent that 4 out of 14 participants had one or more missed samples. For this reason, the primary outcome was changed to $PtCO_2$ after 35 min. In other words, the method of capturing the change in PCO_2 was revised, rather than the outcome itself. $PtCO_2$ monitoring enabled continuous assessment to be undertaken, and is accurate in AECOPD, [9] and other acute settings [10–12]. The validity of this method was confirmed by the post hoc analysis of 80-paired samples, where each capillary blood gas sample obtained had a corresponding $PtCO_2$ measurement at the same time-point. This showed that the difference between the $PcapCO_2$ and $PtCO_2$ in the mean change from baseline was -0.03 mmHg with 95% confidence intervals of -0.44 to 0.38 mmHg. This data suggests that the use of $PtCO_2$ measurements did not adversely affect our ability to determine change in $PcapCO_2$ from baseline.

We did not investigate the potential mechanisms by which oxygen driven nebulisation increases $PtCO_2$. However as demonstrated in mechanistic studies of oxygen therapy in COPD, it is likely to be due to the combination of a reduction in respiratory drive, release of hypoxic pulmonary vasoconstriction, absorption atelectasis, and the Haldane effect [13, 14]. Furthermore, the study was not designed to assess costs related to each regimen, however it is reasonable to assume that improved clinical outcomes seen by avoiding a rise in $PtCO_2$ and associated acidosis, would lead to a reduction in healthcare costs.

The findings from our study complement those of our previous randomised controlled trial of a similar design in stable COPD patients in the clinic setting, in which there was a mean $PtCO_2$ difference between the oxygen- and air-driven nebulisation treatment arms of 3.1 mmHg (95% CI 1·6 to 4·5), $p < 0·001$, after 35 min. [3] In that study one of the 24 subjects was withdrawn due to an increase in $PtCO_2$ of 10 mmHg after 15 min of the first oxygen-driven nebulisation. As with the previous study, an increase in $PtCO_2$ occurred within 5 min, indicating the rapid time course of this physiological response. We had anticipated a greater effect in this current study as the patients had acute rather than stable COPD however the magnitude of the effect was similar, probably reflecting the similar severity of airflow obstruction, with a mean predicted FEV_1 of 35% and 27% in this and the previous study respectively.

The two previous open crossover studies of inpatients with AECOPD both showed oxygen-driven nebulisation worsened hypercapnia in patients with Type 2 respiratory failure [4, 5]. Gunawardena et al. [4] studied 16 patients with COPD and reported that only those with carbon dioxide retention at baseline ($n = 9$) demonstrated a rise in $PaCO_2$ after 15 min (mean of 7·7 mmHg), and one patient had a rise of 22 mmHg. Similarly, O'Donnell et al [5] reported that 6/10 patients, all with carbon dioxide retention at baseline, showed a rise in $PaCO_2$ after 10 min (mean of 12.5 mmHg).

The current BTS guidelines recommend air-driven nebulisation and, if this is not available in the ambulance service, the maximum use of 6 min for an oxygen-driven nebuliser. This is based on the rationale that most of the nebulised medication will have been delivered, and is categorised as grade D evidence [6]. We observed the mean time for dissipation of salbutamol solution from the nebuliser chamber of 5.2 min confirming that 6 min is adequate for salbutamol delivery. The proportion of participants with a $PtCO_2$ increase ≥ 4 mmHg was lower after 6 min than 15 min, suggesting some amelioration of risk with the shorter nebulisation treatment. Alternative methods of bronchodilator delivery include air-driven nebulisers or multiple metered dose inhaler actuations via a spacer [15].

The potential for rebound hypoxia after abrupt cessation of oxygen therapy has been observed both in the treatment of asthma and COPD [9, 16, 17]. We identified some evidence consistent with this phenomenon which is a potentially important yet poorly recognised clinical issue.

Conclusions

In summary, air-driven nebulisation avoids the potential risk of increasing the $PaCO_2$ associated with oxygen-driven bronchodilator administration in AECOPD. We propose that air-driven bronchodilator nebulisation is preferable to oxygen-driven nebulisation in AECOPD, and that when the use of oxygen-driven nebulisation is unavoidable, $PtCO_2$ is monitored if possible.

Abbreviations

AECOPD: Acute exacerbation of chronic obstructive pulmonary disease; BTS: British thoracic society; COPD: Chronic obstructive pulmonary disease; FEV_1: Forced expiratory volume over 1 s; FVC: Forced vital capacity; MRINZ: Medical research institute of new zealand; $PaCO_2$: Partial pressure of arterial carbon dioxide; $PcapCO_2$: Partial pressure of capillary carbon dioxide; PIS: Participant information sheet; $PtCO_2$: Partial pressure of transcutaneous carbon dioxide; SD: Standard deviation; Sentec: Transcutaneous monitor brand; SpO_2: Oxygen saturation measured by oximetry; StO_2: Oxygen saturation measured by transcutaneous monitor

Acknowledgements

We would like to give special thanks to all of the participants for their involvement in our study.

Presentation of findings

The preliminary results of this study were submitted as an abstract to the ERS 2017 Congress, and presented as a poster [18].

Funding

This study was funded by the Health Research Council of New Zealand. The funder of the study had no role in the study design, data collection, data analysis, data interpretation, or writing of the manuscript. The corresponding author had full access to all the data in the study and had final responsibility for the decision to submit for publication.

Authors' contributions

RB was the principal investigator for the study, is guarantor for the study, and affirms that this manuscript is an honest, accurate, and transparent account of the study being reported; that no important aspects of the study have been omitted; and that any discrepancies from the study as planned (and, if relevant, registered) have been explained. GB, JP, SM and JB were investigators on the study and collected the data. MW performed the statistical analysis. GB wrote the first draft of the manuscript. RB and PS conceived the study and wrote the first draft of the protocol with JP. GB, JP, SM, PS, JB, JF, MW and RB all contributed to study design, interpretation of results, manuscript writing, and reviewed the final manuscript prior to submission. All authors had full access to all of the data (including statistical reports and tables) in the study and can take responsibility for the integrity of the data and the accuracy of the data analysis. No writing assistance was received. All authors read and approved the final manuscript.

Competing interests

All authors have completed the ICMJE uniform disclosure form at www.icmje.org/coi_disclosure.pdf. All authors have no competing interests to declare, other than the MRINZ receiving research funding from Health Research Council of New Zealand.

Author details

[1]Capital and Coast District Health Board, Wellington, New Zealand. [2]Medical Research Institute of New Zealand, Box 7902, Wellington, PO 6242, New Zealand. [3]Victoria University Wellington, Wellington, New Zealand. [4]Wellington School of Medicine & Health Sciences, University of Otago Wellington, Wellington, New Zealand.

References

1. M a A, Wills KE, Blizzard L, et al. Effect of high flow oxygen on mortality in chronic obstructive pulmonary disease patients in prehospital setting: randomised controlled trial. BMJ. 2010;341:c5462.
2. Murphy R, Driscoll P, O'Driscoll R. Emergency oxygen therapy for the COPD patient. Emerg Med J. 2001;18:333–9.
3. Edwards L, Perrin K, Williams M, et al. Randomised controlled crossover trial of the effect on PtCO2 of oxygen-driven versus air-driven nebulisers in severe chronic obstructive pulmonary disease. Emerg Med J. 2012;29:894–8.
4. Gunawardena KA, Patel B, Campbell IA, et al. Oxygen as a driving gas for nebulisers: safe or dangerous? Br Med J (Clin Res Ed). 1984;288:272–4.
5. O'Donnell D, Kelly CP, Cotter P, Clancy L. Use of oxygen driven nebuliser delivery systems for beta-2 agonists in chronic bronchitis. Ir J Med Sci. 1985; 154:198–200.
6. British Thoracic Society Emergency Oxygen Guideline Group. BTS guidelines for oxygen use in adults in healthcare and emergency settings. Br Thorac Soc. 2017;72:1–214.
7. Wijesinghe M, Williams M, Perrin K, et al. The effect of supplemental oxygen on hypercapnia in subjects with obesity-associated hypoventilation: a randomised, crossover, clinical study. Chest. 2011;139:1018–24.
8. Perrin K, Wijesinghe M, Healy B, et al. Randomised controlled trial of high concentration versus titrated oxygen therapy in severe exacerbations of asthma. Thorax. 2011;66:937–41.
9. Rudolf M, Turner JA, Harrison BD, et al. Changes in arterial blood gases during and after a period of oxygen breathing in patients with chronic hypercapnic respiratory failure and in patients with asthma. Clin Sci. 1979; 57:389–96.
10. Senn O, Clarenbach CF, Kaplan V, et al. Monitoring carbon dioxide tension and arterial oxygen saturation by a single earlobe sensor in patients with critical illness or sleep apnea. Chest. 2005;128:1291–6.
11. Rodriguez P, Lellouche F, Aboab J, et al. Transcutaneous arterial carbon dioxide pressure monitoring in critically ill adult patients. Intensive Care Med. 2006;32:309–12.
12. McVicar J, Eager R. Validation study of a transcutaneous carbon dioxide monitor in patients in the emergency department. Emerg Med J. 2009;26:344–6.
13. Aubier M, Murciano D, Milic-Emili J, et al. Effects of the administartion of O2 on ventilation and blood gases in patients with chronic obstructive pulmonary disease during acute respiratory failure. Am Rev Resp Dis. 1980; 122:747–54.
14. Robinson TD, Freiberg DB, Regnis JA, Young IH. The role of hypoventilation and ventilation-perfusion redistribution in oxygen-induced hypercapnia during acute exacerbations of chronic obstructive pulmonary disease. Am J Respir Crit Care Med. 2000;161:1524–9.
15. van Geffen WH, Douma WR, Siebos DJ, Kerstjens HA. Bronchodilators delivered by nebuliser versus pMDI with spacer or DPI for eaxcerbations of COPD. Cochrane Database Syst Rev 2016 (8): CD011826, Epub 2016 Aug 29.
16. Auerbach D, Hill C, Baughman R, et al. Routine nebulised ipratropium and albuterol together are better than either alone in COPD. Chest. 1997;112:1514–21.
17. Kane B, Turkington PM, Howard LS, et al. Rebound hypoxaemia after administration of oxygen in an acute exacerbation of chronic obstructive pulmonary disease. BMJ. 2011;342:d1557.
18. Bardsley G, McKinstry S, Pilcher J, et al. Oxygen compared to air driven nebulisers for acute exacerbations of COPD: a randomised controlled trial. ERJ. 2017;50:PA684.

16

Pirfenidone improves survival in IPF: results from a real-life study

George A. Margaritopoulos[1,2†], Athina Trachalaki[1†] (ID), Athol U. Wells[2], Eirini Vasarmidi[1], Eleni Bibaki[1], George Papastratigakis[1], Stathis Detorakis[3], Nikos Tzanakis[1†] and Katerina M. Antoniou[1*†]

Abstract

Background: Pirfenidone is an antifibrotic compound approved for the treatment of idiopathic pulmonary fibrosis (IPF). We present our real-world experience in terms of Pirfenidone's effect on mortality and adverse events profile outside the restrictions of a clinical trial.

Methods: This is a retrospective observational intention to treat study of 82 consecutive IPF patients (UHH cohort).

Results: We observed a high 3-years survival rate of 73% without excluding patients who discontinued treatment for different reasons. The survival was compared to the survival of an IPF cohort from a tertiary referral center (RBH cohort). After exclusion of severe cases (DLco< 30%), in unadjusted analysis, the survival in the UHH cohort was better than in the RBH cohort (HR:0.32, 95% CI: 0.19–0.53, $p < 0.0001$). After adjustment for age, gender and FVC, the survival remained higher in the UHH cohort (HR:0.28, 95% CI: 0.16–0.48, $p < 0.0001$). We observed a similar safety profile compared to previously published data and a lower rate of drug discontinuation due to photosensitivity reactions. Conclusion: Pirfenidone provides a survival benefit in a real-life IPF cohort compared to previously used medications. Counselling patients and proactively managing possible adverse effects can reduce the necessity to discontinue pirfenidone.

Keywords: IPF, Survival, Pirfenidone, Real-life

Background

Idiopathic pulmonary fibrosis (IPF) is a rare disease of unknown etiology, characterized by progressive and irreversible fibrosis of the interstitium of the lung [1, 2]. The prevalence of IPF in Europe and North America has been estimated to be from 3 to 9 cases per 100,000 [3].

Pirfenidone is an orally administered drug with antifibrotic, anti-inflammatory and antioxidant effects that was approved in Europe in 2011 and in USA in 2014 for the treatment of IPF [4]. Together with nintedanib, the second antifibrotic compound, pirfenidone has received the label of "conditional recommendation for IPF treatment" in the recent update of the ATS/ERS/JRS/ALAT 2015 statement [5].

Three multinational, randomised, placebo-controlled phase III trials showed that pirfenidone can reduce the rate of IPF progression by 50% on average in 1 year as judged by serial changes in forced vital capacity (FVC) [6]. These trials were not powered to explore the effect of pirfenidone on mortality. However, a prespecified pooled analysis showed that pirfenidone reduced the risk of death at 1 year by 48% and the risk of treatment-emergent death due to IPF at 1 year by 68%. More recently, a pooled analysis of these trials and a meta-analysis including also a Japanese phase 2 trial, SP2 (trial duration 9 months), and a Japanese phase 3 trial, SP3 (trial duration 52 weeks) confirmed that pirfenidone is associated with a reduced risk of death compared to placebo and moreover the survival benefit of pirfenidone extended beyond 52 weeks and seemed to persist at 120 weeks [7].

The use of this type of analysis to study the effect of pirfenidone on mortality is justified by the fact that it is impossible to design a single trial, powered enough to provide a significant effect on mortality. Clinical

* Correspondence: kantoniou@med.uoc.gr
†George A. Margaritopoulos, Athina Trachalaki, Nikos Tzanakis and Katerina M. Antoniou contributed equally to this work.
[1]Respiratory Medicine Department, University Hospital of Heraklion, Crete, Greece
Full list of author information is available at the end of the article

trials adequate for evaluation of mortality as an end-point should include an extremely high number of patients and would require a much longer follow-up time in order to reach statistical significance [8].

In the recently published RECAP study, an open-label extension study evaluating the long-term safety of pirfenidone in patients with IPF who completed the phase III trials, the median on-treatment survival from the first dose of 2403 mg/day pirfenidone was 77.2 months confirming a survival benefit compared to historical data [9, 10]. However, this result should be interpreted cautiously because only patients who remained under observation for the whole study period were included in the survival analysis whereas patients who withdrew at different time-points for different reasons were excluded. This might have shifted the results towards a better survival. Furthermore, there is a doubt regarding the applicability of these observations obtained from pharmaceutical cohorts to the general IPF population. Patients with advanced disease and comorbidities were excluded. It is well recognised that baseline disease severity and presence of comorbidities have a significant impact on survival [11, 12]. Therefore, longitudinal real-world data from cohorts in which patients with advanced disease and comorbidities are included, are needed to shed light to the mortality benefit of pirfenidone in the general IPF population.

The aim of our study was to investigate the efficacy of Pirfenidone in newly diagnosed IPF patients presented in a referral centre. To strengthen our results, we compared the survival in our cohort with the survival in a historic IPF cohort studied in the pre-pirfenidone era [13]. We also investigated the safety profile of pirfenidone in comparison with the data obtained from the clinical trials.

Methods

This is a retrospective observational study aiming to assess the efficacy and safety of pirfenidone in IPF patients. Ninety consecutive IPF patients referred to the Interstitial Lung Diseases outpatient clinic of the University Hospital of Heraklion from July 2011 (when the manufacturer funded Named Patient Programme was initiated) to December 2016 were included in the study (herein referred to as the UHH cohort). All the patients were treatment naïve and completed at least 3 months of treatment with pirfenidone (2403 mg/day). We excluded 8 patients because the gap between diagnosis and treatment introduction was greater than 12 months and therefore the final UHH cohort included 82 patients. The patients remained under follow-up at UHH and their follow-up was complete at the specified cut-off date of 3 years. The diagnosis of IPF was based on ATS/ERS/JRS/ALAT criteria [10]. In case of

absence of a definite usual interstitial pneumonia (UIP) pattern on high resolution computed tomography (HRCT) and of inability to obtain a biopsy sample, a multidisciplinary team discussion confirmed the diagnosis using the inclusion criteria applied in the INPLULSIS trial [14]. The clinical behavior of IPF patients included in the placebo arm of the INPULSIS trial was similar regardless the presence of a definite or possible UIP pattern on HRCT [15]. The HRCT scans were reported by the same radiologist to avoid interobserver variations in the characterization of the radiologic pattern. Pirfenidone was prescribed either under the manufacturer funded Named Patient Programme (NPP) or as a standard treatment approved by the Greek NHS.

Patients underwent pulmonary function tests (PFTs) including body plethysmography, spirometry and single breath test for determination of diffusing capacity of the lung for carbon monoxide (DLCO), at the time of IPF diagnosis and thereafter at 3, 6, 12, 24 and 36 months after the introduction of treatment. Blood tests for full blood count and liver and renal function obtained at the time of diagnosis and then once monthly for the first 6 months and subsequently once every 3 months. The clinical records of the patients were reviewed to assess the presence of comorbidities, treatment-related side-effects, compliance with the treatment and survival.

The survival in the UHH cohort was compared with the survival of a historic IPF cohort which included 212 patients referred to the Royal Brompton Hospital, London, UK (herein referred to as the RBH cohort) between December 1990 and December 1996 and has been previously described [13]. Acknowledging that the inclusion and diagnostic criteria for IPF differ between the UHH and the RBH cohort, we applied the criteria used in the UHH cohort to the RBH cohort. The HRCT scans and the biopsy samples were reviewed again in the RBH MDT meeting. To avoid biases due to inclusion of more severe cases in the RBH cohort, we excluded severe cases defined as having a DLco< 30%. This threshold is the same that was used for patient's recruitment in the ASCEND trial [6].

In order to address the possibility of an interaction between treatment effect and age (given the major age difference between the cohorts), a sub-analysis was performed in which there was 1:1 age matching between the cohorts, with 64 patient couples. Eleven elderly patients from the UHH cohort could not be age-matched with RBH patients.

In order to minimise outcome differences due to the shorter duration of follow-up in the UHH cohort, a sub-analysis was performed in which follow-up was ended at 40 months.

Informed consent was obtained from all patients included in the UHH cohort. The study was approved by the Ethics Committees of the University Hospital of Herakleion (IRB number: 17030). Due to the retrospective nature of the analysis of the RBH cohort[13], ethics committee approval was not required.

Statistical analysis

Results were analyzed using STATA. Data were presented as mean values ± standard deviation for continuous and frequency (percentage) for nominal variables. Kaplan-Meier analysis and Cox proportional Hazards regression were used for survival analysis. A value of $p < 0.05$ was considered as statistically significant.

Results

Demographic characteristics of the UHH cohort

The demographic characteristics of the UHH cohort are shown in Table 1. The mean age was 74.9. Fifty-three patients (64.7%) were current or ex-smokers with a smoking history of 43.5 pack years. Mean FVC was 81.5% and mean DLco was 54.4% predicted. Seven patients (8.5%) had advanced disease. The radiologic pattern of definite UIP on HRCT was seen in 47 patients (57.3%) and the pattern of possible UIP was seen in 35 (42.7%). Thirteen patients underwent a surgical lung biopsy and the multidisciplinary team (MDT) discussion confirmed the diagnosis of IPF in the rest of the cases. Fifteen patients died during the study period. The main comorbidities are shown in Table 2. Comorbidities were either reported by the patient during the initial assessment as a new case or were diagnosed during the initial diagnostic work-up. Systemic hypertension was the most common comorbidity (64%), followed by gastroesophageal

Table 1 Demographic characteristics of the UHH cohort ($n = 82$)

Age	74.9 ± 11^a
Never smokers	29 (35.3%)
Smokers	53 (64.7%)
Pack Years	43.5 ± 32.1^a
Radiological pattern (Definite UIP/Possible UIP)	47(57.3%)/35(42.7%)
Advanced disease (DLco< 30%)	7(8.5%)
Surgical lung biopsy	13 (15.9%)
FEV_1%	87.4 ± 22.7^a
FVC %	81.5 ± 19.5^a
DLco %	54.4 ± 17.9^a
Median follow-up time (IQR)	17.4 months (9.5–30.9).
Deaths	15 (18.3%)

UIP usual interstitial pneumonia, FEV_1 forced expiratory volume in 1 s, FVC forced vital capacity, DLco diffusing capacity of the lung for carbon monoxide
[a]The values are expressed as mean ± SD

Table 2 Comorbidities in the UHH cohort

Comorbidities	$N = 82$
Systemic Hypertension	58 (64%)
Gastroesophageal Reflux Disease	42 (47%)
Ischemic Heart Disease	27 (30%)
Heart Failure	25 (28%)
Diabetes Mellitus	24 (27%)
Obstructive Sleep Apnea-Hypopnea Syndrome	23 (26%)
Depression	21 (23%)
Emphysema	19 (21%)
Pulmonary Hypertension	12 (13%)
Lung Cancer	2 (2%)
Venous Thromboembolism	1 (1%)

reflux disease (47%), ischemic heart disease (30%), heart failure (28%), combined pulmonary fibrosis and emphysema (21%), pulmonary hypertension (13%) and lung cancer (2%).

Pirfenidone efficacy

Survival

Survival analysis with Kaplan Meier curve is shown in Fig. 1. In this intention to treat study, the 3-years survival in the UHH cohort was 73%. When we excluded the patients who discontinued the treatment ($n = 22$) because of side-effects or lack of adherence to treatment as it happens in the treatment arms of the phase III trials, the result did not change.

In order to better understand the effect of Pirfenidone on survival, we compared the survival data from the UHH cohort to those obtained from a well characterized IPF cohort from a tertiary referral center in UK (Royal Brompton Hospital). To avoid biases due to the inclusion of more severe cases in the RBH cohort, we excluded cases with a DLco< 30%. The final analysis included 136 patients from the RBH cohort and 75 patients from the UHH cohort. In order to avoid using two cohorts in which different criteria for the diagnosis of IPF were used, we applied the same criteria used in UHH cohort [10, 14] to the RBH cohort. The characteristics of both cohorts are shown in Table 3. In unadjusted analysis, the survival in the UHH cohort was better than in the RBH cohort (HR:0.32, 95% CI: 0.19–0.53, $p < 0.0001$). After adjustment for FVC, age and gender the result did not change (HR:0.28, 95% CI: 0.16–0.48, $p < 0.0001$ (Table 4 and Fig. 2).

In an age-matched model comparing survival between cohorts in 64 age-matched patient couples, mortality was reduced in the pirfenidone treated cohort (HR 0.30, 95% CI 0.15, 0.59; $p < 0.001$. This finding was robust in a proportional hazards model, also containing FVC, age and gender as covariates (Table 5).

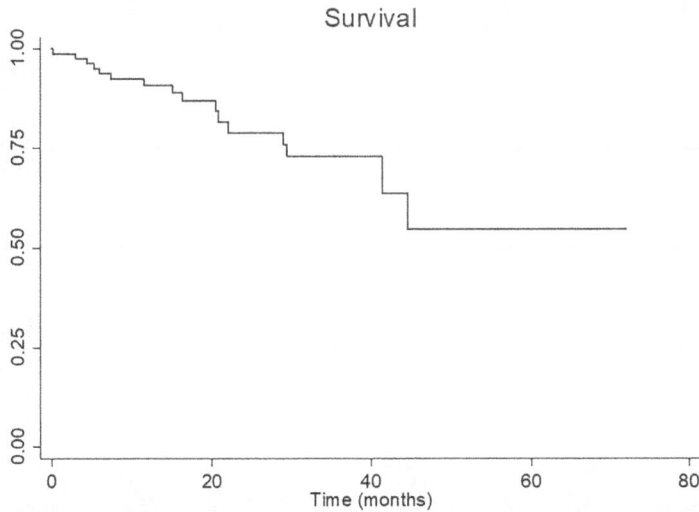

Fig. 1 Kaplan Meier survival curve for the whole UHH cohort

In a sub-analysis in which follow-up was terminated at 40 months, mortality was reduced in the pirfenidone-treated cohort (HR 0.40; 95%CI 0.21, 0.75; $p < 0.005$). This finding was robust in a proportional hazards model, also containing FVC, age and gender as covariates (Table 6).

Safety
In the UHH cohort, 30 patients (33,3%) reported gastrointestinal discomfort and 17 patients (18,8%) have experienced photosensitivity. Finally, 3 patients (3.3%) discontinued treatment due to gastrointestinal adverse events, 9 (10%) patients discontinued due to photosensitivity and 10 (11.1%) due to non-compliance to treatment. The long-term safety results from this study are consistent with the known safety profile of pirfenidone, with no new safety signals observed.

Discussion
This is a single-center observational, intention to treat study of efficacy and safety of Pirfenidone in IPF. We observed that treatment adherent patients had an increased 3 years survival rate of 73% despite the inclusion of patients who would normally be excluded from pharmaceutical trials. The approval of the antifibrotic agents has marked the end of the placebo-controlled studies in IPF. Nowadays, it is not ethical to withhold Pirfenidone therapy to establish a true control group and therefore we chose to use a historical cohort as a control group. Importantly, the use of Pirfenidone was associated with a significantly higher survival compared to a historical cohort studied in the pre-pirfenidone era after adjustment for demographic characteristics and baseline disease severity as judged by FVC. When we examined age and follow-up time between the two cohorts as confounding factors, the

Table 3 Demographic characteristics of the patients from the UHH and RBH cohort included in the survival analysis. Seven patients with DLco< 30 were excluded from the initial UHH cohort

Patients data	UHH (n = 75)	RBH (n = 136)	P value
Age	72.5 ± 7.6^a	62.5 ± 9.9^a	$P < 0.0001$
Gender (male/female)	64/11	96/40	$P < 0.01$
Smoking status			
Never smokers	26	27	$P = 0.08$
Smokers	49	109	$P = 0.34$
Radiological pattern (Definite UIP/Possible UIP)	41/34	56/55	$P = 0.7$
Biopsy proven UIP	9	25	
FEV$_1$	87.4 ± 21.5^a	78.9 ± 15.6^a	$P < 0.0006$
FVC	81.8 ± 17.8^a	79.3 ± 18.0^a	$P = 0.16$
DLco	56.7 ± 16.0^a	46 ± 12.4^a	$P < 0.0001$

UIP usual interstitial pneumonia, *FEV$_1$* forced expiratory volume in 1 s, *FVC* forced vital capacity, *DLco* diffusing capacity of the lung for carbon monoxide
[a]The values are expressed as mean ± SD

Table 4 Survival analysis. Proportional hazards model containing FVC, age and gender as covariates

	HR	95% CI	P value
Centre	0.28	0.16, 0.48	$P<0.0001$
Gender	1.96	1.19, 3.22	$P<0.008$
Age	1.03	1.01, 1.05	$P<0.002$
FVC	0.97	0.96, 0.98	$P<0.0001$

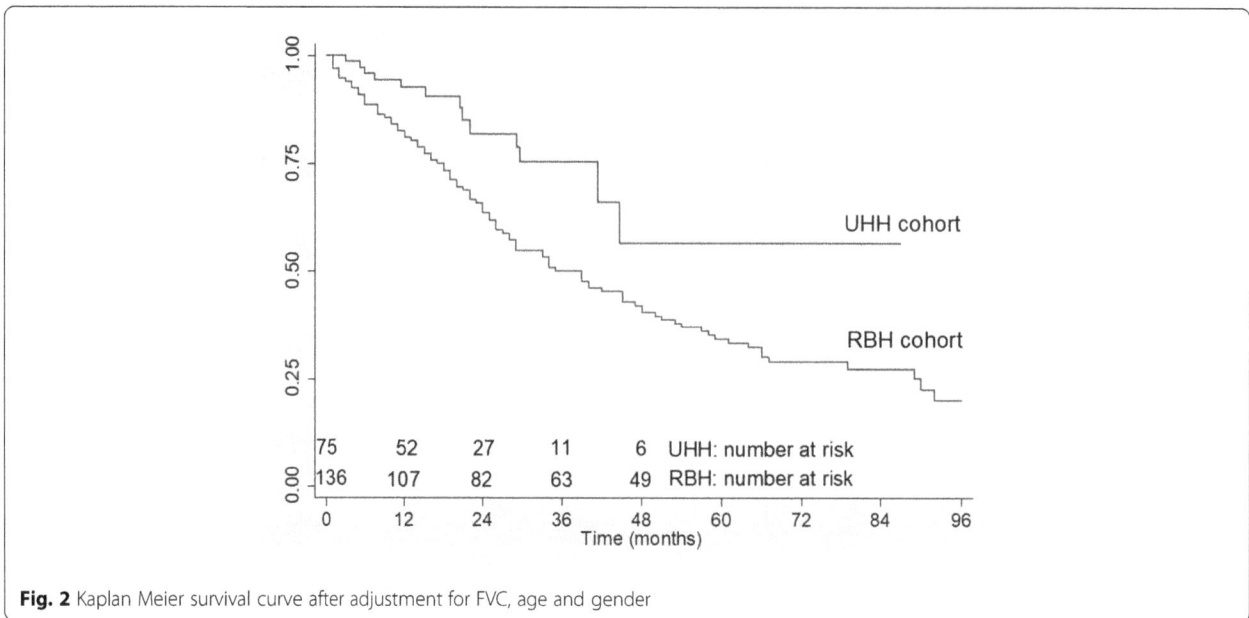

Fig. 2 Kaplan Meier survival curve after adjustment for FVC, age and gender

effect of Pirfenidone on survival remained robust. We chose to use survival as a "response measure" instead of long-term pulmonary function trends which are seriously biased by the fact that they can only be evaluated in survivors. This is a major problem in open-label studies and has been explored in a recent commentary in Lancet Respiratory Medicine [16]. The safety profile was comparable to that reported in phase III and extension trial analysis [6, 9].

It is well known that phase III IPF trials have not been designed to estimate long-term survival. Designing and conducting an adequately powered survival study in IPF is challenging due to the rare nature of the disease and the need for extended follow-up. Open-label extension studies in patients with IPF who completed the phase III trials are expected to provide answers on the survival benefit. However, patients participating in randomized controlled trials (RCTs) represent a highly selected group of patients fulfilling strict inclusion and exclusion criteria as shown by the high screen failure of 70% in the ASCEND study [6]. Real world observational studies could provide evidence regarding the efficacy of the antifibrotic compounds although patients are often different than

those enrolled in clinical trials for the presence of co-morbidities and for advanced disease at presentation as judged by pre-treatment FVC and DLco values. In the UHH cohort, seven patients with advanced disease (DLCO< 30%) and a significant number of patients with more than one comorbidities such as emphysema, is-chemic heart disease and diabetes were included. Therefore, a significant number of our real-world patients would not fulfil the inclusion criteria for clinical trials.

Despite the inclusion of these patients, we still observed a relatively high 3-years survival rate. When we excluded from the analysis the patients who discontinued the treatment due to side effects or lack of adherence, the survival benefit remained unchanged. To strengthen our results, we compared the survival in our intention to treat cohort to a non-intention to treat historical cohort. We found that, in unadjusted analysis, the UHH cohort had a 30% increased survival and the survival benefit remained significant after adjustment for age, gender and baseline severity. In order to exclude the likelihood that the observed survival benefit was due to the inclusion of less cases with advanced disease in the UHH cohort, we repeated the analysis after excluding patients with a DLco< 30%.

Table 5 Age-matched model comparing survival between cohorts in 64 age-matched patient couples

	HR	95% CI	P value
Centre	0.27	0.14, 0.55	$P < 0.0001$
Gender	1.96	0.99, 3.88	$P < 0.053$
Age	1.00	0.96, 1.04	$P < 0.838$
FVC	0.98	0.97, 1.00	$P < 0.204$

Table 6 Survival sub-analysis at 40 months

	HR	95% CI	P value
Centre	0.28	0.14,0.54	$P < 0.0001$
Gender	1.72	0.94,3.16	$P < 0.077$
Age	1.02	1.00,1.05	$P < 0.033$
FVC	0.97	0.96,0.98	$P < 0.0001$

The results did not change. Plainly, we cannot exclude whether the observed benefit was due to the adverse effect of the immunosuppressive treatment used as standard IPF therapy in the pre-antifibrotic era. It is now well known that the combination of low dose of prednisolone with azathioprine and N-acetyl-cysteine has been proved not efficacious and deleterious in IPF [17]. However, it is also acknowledged that the increased number of deaths and hospitalizations due to infections was observed when the patients were receiving significantly higher doses of prednisolone [17]. According to the therapeutic algorithm of the RBH hospital, doses of prednisolone higher than 10 mg were not used when the RBH cohort was studied. Keeping this in mind, we can conclude that not using immunosuppression and using pirfenidone instead, provides a 30% survival benefit in IPF. A recent study confirmed that the use of pirfenidone is associated with a survival benefit. The authors observed that pirfenidone treated patients have a 2.47 years longer life expectancy than IPF patients receiving best supportive care [18]. Best supportive care includes interventions such as pulmonary rehabilitation, supplemental oxygen therapy, and/or other symptomatic treatments, which do not have any effect on IPF survival.

Our finding is important because the 3 years survival rate did not change regardless the exclusion of the cases, which discontinued Pirfenidone. In our survival analysis, we included all patients who received Pirfenidone at baseline, even those who interrupted the treatment for different reasons. In the open-label extension RECAP study the median on-treatment survival from the first dose of 2403 mg/day pirfenidone was 77.2 months [9]. However, patients who interrupted the treatment were not included in this analysis and as observed in trials outside IPF, withdrawals from drug trials have worse outcome [19–21]. Therefore, the open-label data do not actually show true mortality outcome on intention to treat with Pirfenidone.

In the UHH cohort, 30 patients reported gastrointestinal discomfort and 17 patients have experienced photosensitivity. Three patients discontinued treatment due to gastrointestinal adverse events, 9 due to photosensitivity and 10 due to non-compliance. The rate of discontinuation due to adverse effects is 13.3% which is similar to the rate observed in the ASCEND and CAPACITY trials (14.4% and 15 respectively in the treatment arms) [6, 22]. One of the most frequent adverse events was a photosensitivity reaction, which is totally expected keeping in mind the weather condition in south Greece. The rate of discontinuation due to a photosensitivity reaction is lower than in phase III tri-

als and recently published real-life studies [6, 22–25]. This is mainly due to a very detailed discussion between the treating physicians and the patient prior to the introduction of treatment. A leaflet with helpful recommendations was given to every patient as a skin protection guide. The use of wide-brimmed hats, sunglasses, long-sleeved shirts, trousers, gloves if possible, and sunscreens with high sun protection factor (ie, > 50) with UV-A/UV-B protection is recommended [4]. Real-life studies have highlighted the importance of a frequent review of the patients by a specialist nurse as well as the importance of a contact number given to the patients so that they can communicate whenever they have questions about the drug or when they experience side effects. In UHH, a dedicated research fellow provides regular specialist input to provide support and education in order to improve concordance to treatment.

Conclusion

To the best of our knowledge, this is the first intention to treat real-life study showing an increased 3 years survival rate in patients treated with Pirfenidone and a survival benefit of 30% compared to patients treated with no antifibrotic agents. The effect of Pirfenidone on survival is remarkable if ones takes into account that patients with comorbidities and severe disease have been included in the UHH cohort unlike what happens in pharmaceutical trials. We confirmed the safety profile of Pirfenidone and observed a lower rate of discontinuation due to photosensitivity reactions and stressed the importance of patient's counselling before the initiation of treatment. More real life studies with a higher number of patients who are unlikely to be eligible for inclusion in pharmaceutical trials are needed to evaluate the effect of Pirfenidone on disease progression.

Abbreviations

DL$_{CO}$: Diffusing capacity for carbon monoxide; FEV$_1$: Forced expiratory volume in 1 s; FVC: Forced vital capacity; HR: Hazard ratio; HRCT: High resolution computed tomography; IPF: Idiopathic pulmonary fibrosis; MDT: Multidisciplinary team; NPP: Named Patient Program; PFTs: Pulmonary function tests; RBH: Royal Brompton Hospital; RCTs: Randomized controlled trials; UHH: University Hospital of Herakleion; UIP: Usual interstitial pneumonia

Acknowledgements

The authors would like to thank Dr. Konstantinos Karagiannis, Dr. Evangelia Stamataki and Mrs. Despoina Moraitaki (Respiratory Medicine Department, University Hospital of Heraklion, Crete, Greece) for their participation in the collection of the data and for the performance of the lung function tests.

Funding

Not applicable

Authors' contribution

GAM, AT, AUW, EB, EV, GP, SD, NT and KMA made substantial contributions to conception, design, data analysis and manuscript preparation. AT, EV, EB and GP were involved in acquisition of data. SD, GAM, KMA, AUW were responsible for the assessment of HRCT. All authors have read and approved the manuscript. All authors read and approved the final manuscript and have given their consent to publish.

Competing interests

The authors declare that they have no competing interests.

Author details

¹Respiratory Medicine Department, University Hospital of Heraklion, Crete, Greece. ²Interstitial Lung Disease Unit, Royal Brompton Hospital, London, UK. ³Radiology Department, University Hospital of Heraklion, Crete, Greece.

References

1. Margaritopoulos GA, Romagnoli M, Poletti V, Siafakas NM, Wells AU, Antoniou KM. Recent advances in the pathogenesis and clinical evaluation of pulmonary fibrosis. Eur Respir Rev. 2012;21:48-56.

2. Siegel RL, Miller KD, Jemal A. Cancer statistics, 2016. CA Cancer J Clin. 2016; 66(1):7–30.

3. Hutchinson J, Fogarty A, Hubbard R, McKeever T. Global incidence and mortality of idiopathic pulmonary fibrosis: a systematic review. Eur Respir J. 2015;46(3):795–806.

4. Margaritopoulos GA, Vasarmidi E, Antoniou KM. Pirfenidone in the treatment of idiopathic pulmonary fibrosis: an evidence-based review of its place in therapy. Core Evidence. 2016;11:11–22.

5. Raghu G, Rochwerg B, Zhang Y, Garcia CA, Azuma A, Behr J, Brozek JL, Collard HR, Cunningham W, Homma S, et al. An official ATS/ERS/JRS/ALAT clinical practice guideline: treatment of idiopathic pulmonary fibrosis. An update of the 2011 clinical practice guideline. Am J Respir Crit Care Med. 2015;192(2):e3–19.

6. King TE Jr, Bradford WZ, Castro-Bernardini S, Fagan EA, Glaspole I, Glassberg MK, Gorina E, Hopkins PM, Kardatzke D, Lancaster L, et al. A phase 3 trial of pirfenidone in patients with idiopathic pulmonary fibrosis. N Engl J Med. 2014;370(22):2083–92.

7. Nathan SD, Albera C, Bradford WZ, Costabel U, Glaspole I, Glassberg MK, Kardatzke DR, Daigl M, Kirchgaessler KU, Lancaster LH, et al. Effect of pirfenidone on mortality: pooled analyses and meta-analyses of clinical trials in idiopathic pulmonary fibrosis. Lancet Respir Med. 2017;5(1):33–41.

8. Wells AU, Behr J, Costabel U, Cottin V, Poletti V, Richeldi L. Hot of the breath: mortality as a primary end-point in IPF treatment trials: the best is the enemy of the good. Thorax. 2012;67(11):938–40.

9. Costabel U, Albera C, Lancaster LH, Lin CY, Hormel P, Hulter HN, Noble PW. An open-label study of the long-term safety of pirfenidone in patients with idiopathic pulmonary fibrosis (RECAP). Respiration. 2017;94(5):408–15.

10. Raghu G, Collard HR, Egan JJ, Martinez FJ, Behr J, Brown KK, Colby TV, Cordier JF, Flaherty KR, Lasky JA, et al. An official ATS/ERS/JRS/ALAT statement: idiopathic pulmonary fibrosis: evidence-based guidelines for diagnosis and management. Am J Respir Crit Care Med. 2011;183(6):788–824.

11. Margaritopoulos GA, Antoniou KM, Wells AU. Comorbidities in interstitial lung diseases. Eur Respir Rev. 2017;26(143):160027.

12. Mura M, Porretta MA, Bargagli E, Sergiacomi G, Zompatori M, Sverzellati N, Taglieri A, Mezzasalma F, Rottoli P, Saltini C, et al. Predicting survival in newly diagnosed idiopathic pulmonary fibrosis: a 3-year prospective study. Eur Respir J. 2012;40(1):101–9.

13. Wells AU, Desai SR, Rubens MB, Goh NS, Cramer D, Nicholson AG, Colby TV, du Bois RM, Hansell DM. Idiopathic pulmonary fibrosis: a composite physiologic index derived from disease extent observed by computed tomography. Am J Respir Crit Care Med. 2003;167(7):962–9.

14. Richeldi L, du Bois RM, Raghu G, Azuma A, Brown KK, Costabel U, Cottin V, Flaherty KR, Hansell DM, Inoue Y, et al. Efficacy and safety of nintedanib in idiopathic pulmonary fibrosis. N Engl J Med. 2014;370(22):2071–82.

15. Raghu G, Wells AU, Nicholson AG, Richeldi L, Flaherty KR, Le Maulf F, Stowasser S, Schlenker-Herceg R, Hansell DM. Effect of nintedanib in

16. Wells AU. Efficacy data in treatment extension studies of idiopathic pulmonary fibrosis: interpret with caution. Lancet Respir Med. 2018; [Epub ahead of print].

17. Raghu G, Anstrom KJ, King TE Jr, Lasky JA, Martinez FJ. Prednisone, azathioprine, and N-acetylcysteine for pulmonary fibrosis. N Engl J Med. 2012;366(21):1968–77.

18. Fisher M, Nathan SD, Hill C, Marshall J, Dejonckheere F, Thuresson PO, Maher TM. Predicting life expectancy for pirfenidone in idiopathic pulmonary fibrosis. J Manag Care Spec Pharm. 2017;23(3-b Suppl):S17–s24.

19. Collet JP, Montalescot G, Steg PG, Steinhubl SR, Fox KA, Hu TF, Johnston SC, Hamm CW, Bhatt DL, Topol EJ. Clinical outcomes according to permanent discontinuation of clopidogrel or placebo in the CHARISMA trial. Arch Cardiovasc Dis. 2009;102(6–7):485–96.

20. Calverley PM, Spencer S, Willits L, Burge PS, Jones PW. Withdrawal from treatment as an outcome in the ISOLDE study of COPD. Chest. 2003;124(4):1350–6.

21. Vestbo J, Anderson Julie A, Calverley Peter Mark A, Celli B, Ferguson Gary T, Jenkins C, Yates Julie C, Jones Paul W. Bias due to withdrawal in long-term randomised trials in COPD: evidence from the TORCH study. Clin Respir J. 2010;5(1):44–9.

22. Noble PW, Albera C, Bradford WZ, Costabel U, Glassberg MK, Kardatzke D, King TE Jr, Lancaster L, Sahn SA, Szwarcberg J, et al. Pirfenidone in patients with idiopathic pulmonary fibrosis (CAPACITY): two randomised trials. Lancet (London, England). 2011;377(9779):1760–9.

23. Salih GN, Shaker SB, Madsen HD, Bendstrup E. Pirfenidone treatment in idiopathic pulmonary fibrosis: nationwide Danish results. Eur Clin Respir J. 2016;3. https://doi.org/10.3402/ecrj.v3403.32608.

24. Hughes G, Toellner H, Morris H, Leonard C, Chaudhuri N. Real world experiences: pirfenidone and nintedanib are effective and well tolerated treatments for idiopathic pulmonary fibrosis. J Clin Med. 2016;5(9):78.

25. Tzouvelekis A, Karampitsakos T, Ntolios P, Tzilas V, Bouros E, Markozannes E, Malliou I, Anagnostopoulos A, Granitsas A, Steiropoulos P, et al. Longitudinal "real-world" outcomes of pirfenidone in idiopathic pulmonary fibrosis in Greece. Front Med. 2017;4:213.

17

Metallic small y stent placement at primary right carina for bronchial disease

Yonghua Bi[1†], Jindong Li[2†], Zepeng Yu[1], Jianzhuang Ren[1], Gang Wu[1*] and Xinwei Han[1*] (iD)

Abstract

Background: Metallic large Y stent placement has been used mainly for airway disease around the main carina. However, few studies have reported this treatment for bronchial disease around the primary right carina.

Methods: Twenty-eight patients were treated by small y stent. All stents were custom-designed and placed under fluoroscopic guidance. Clinical and imaging data were analyzed retrospectively.

Results: Thirty-one stents were successfully inserted in 28 patients. Twenty-five patients succeed at the first attempt (89.3%), and 3 patients needed a second attempt. Twelve complications occurred in 10 patients (35. 7%). Stent restenosis and sputum retention were the most common complications. Five patients underwent successful stent removal due to complications or cure efficacy. During follow up, 17 patients died of tumors and one died of myocardial infarction. The 1-, 3-, and 5-year survival rates were 49.3, 19.6 and 19.6%, respectively.

Conclusions: Metallic small y stent placement is technically feasible, effective and safe for bronchial disease around the primary right carina.

Keywords: Bronchial fistula, Bronchial stenosis, Sten, Primary right carina, Fluoroscopy

Background

Metallic stent placement has been known as an effective treatment for patients with airway disease [1–10]. Metallic large Y stent placement has been used mainly for airway disease around the main carina [11, 12]. Clinically, bronchial disease is also common shown around the primary right carina. For example, silicone small y stents have been used to treat airway disease around the left carina [13]. Placement of metallic small y stents can be less traumatizing with the help of guide wires [14], and may well be an alternative to the silicone y stent [14]. Unfortunately, few studies have reported the use of metallic small y stents for the treatment of bronchial disease around primary right carina. In this study, we used the metallic y stent to treat bronchial disease that involved primary right carina, and aimed to determine the safety, feasibility and efficacy of this stenting technique.

* Correspondence: wuganghenan2004@126.com; dreamweaver08@126.com
†Yonghua Bi and Jindong Li contributed equally to this work.
[1]Department of Interventional Radiology, the First Affiliated Hospital of Zhengzhou University, Zhengzhou, China
Full list of author information is available at the end of the article

Materials and methods

Patients

From January 2011 to May 2017, 28 patients were treated for bronchial disease by metallic small y stent in our department. Bronchoscopy and chest spiral computed tomography (SCT) was used for the diagnosis of bronchial disease. The medical records of these patients were retrospectively reviewed. Bronchoscopy and chest SCT were used to confirm the diagnosis and determine the location of fistula or stenosis. Metallic airway stents were manufactured by Nanjing Micro-Tech Medical Company (Nanjing, China), and were woven with a nickel–titanium alloy wires (Fig. 1). The airway stents were designed according to the diameter and length of the bronchus (Fig. 2, a; Fig. 3, a, b). All the Y shape stent was custom manufactured by Micro-Tech Co. Ltd. (Nanjing, China). [12]

Stenting procedure

The stenting procedure was performed under fluoroscopic guidance [12]. A vertebral artery catheter (Cook Corporation, Bloomington, Ind, USA) was introduced

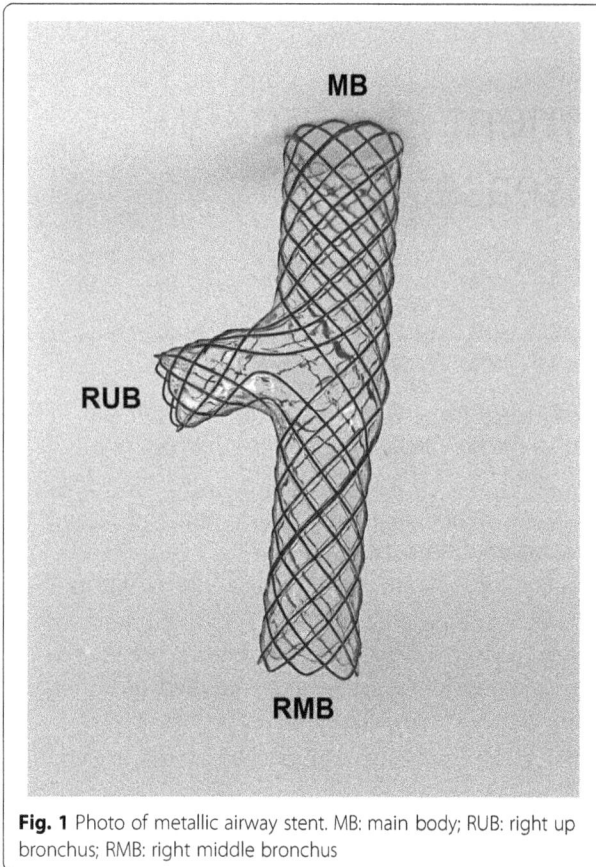

Fig. 1 Photo of metallic airway stent. MB: main body; RUB: right up bronchus; RMB: right middle bronchus

into the distal end of the right lobar bronchi. The location and size of the fistula or stenosis was confirmed by radiography. Then two stiff guide wires (Cook Corporation) were inserted into the distal end of the lobar bronchus. The small y stent was introduced into the primary right carina. The branches of the small y stent were deployed first, and the main body of the stent was deployed at the right main bronchus (Fig. 2, b). For stent removal, a long sheath and retrieval hook was inserted (Fig. 2, e; Fig. 4, c). The tip of the hook was placed next to the end of the stent and withdrawn from the airway wall (Fig. 2, f; Fig. 4, d). Radiography was performed again to show sealing of the fistula or patency of the stent immediately after stenting (Fig. 4, e).

Follow up
During follow up, bronchoscopy and chest SCT were used to show sealing of the bronchial fistula and stent patency, and radiography was performed if necessary (Fig. 2, c, d; Fig. 3, c, D; Fig. 4, f). Stent removal was conducted once a severe complication was found or patients were cured.

Statistical analysis
Data were expressed as mean ± standard deviation, and analyzed by ANOVA. Qualitative data were expressed in percentage. Survival rate was compared by Log-rank (Mantel-Cox) Test (GraphPad Software, Inc., USA). Statistical significance was considered when $p < 0.05$.

Results
Patient characteristics
Twenty-two patients were diagnosed with esophageal cancer; 4 patients, with lung cancer; and 2 patients, with tuberculosis or pulmonitis. Twenty-two patients underwent lobectomy due to lung cancer ($n = 1$) or resection of esophageal carcinoma ($n = 21$). After a median interval of 1.5 month, patients exhibited airway symptoms, with a median symptom duration of 1.0 month. Thoracogastric airway fistula (71.4%) was the main indication for stent placement in this study. Other indications included airway stenosis and bronchopleural fistula (Table 1).

Stenting procedure
Stents were successfully inserted in 25 patients at the first attempt (89.3%). Three patients underwent a successful second attempt, including 2 migrations during withdrawal of the guide wires and one partial obstruction of the left main bronchus due to stent retraction. A total of 31 small y stents were inserted. The median diameter of the stent is 14 mm for main body (Interquartile range, IQR 12, 16), 10 mm for the limb in the right upper bronchus (IQR 10, 12) and 10 mm for another limb in the right middle bronchus (IQR 8, 13). The median length of stent is 15 mm for the main body (IQR 10, 18), 12 mm for the limb in right upper bronchus (IQR 10, 15) and 20 mm for another limb in the right middle bronchus (IQR 15, 25). Five patients underwent successful stent removal due to stent migration ($n = 1$), restenosis (n = 1) or cure efficacy ($n = 3$), with a median time of 76 days (IQR 25.5, 497.5). All of these stents were removed successfully at the first attempt with no complications.

Complications
No perioperative deaths or severe complications (massive hemorrhage or airway rupture) occurred during stent placement or removal. A total of 12 major complications occurred in 10 patients (35.7%). Four patients showed stent restenosis after a median time of 65 days. Six patients showed sputum retention after a median time of 10.5 days, and endoscopic sputum aspiration was performed for these patients. Migration of two stents was found during withdrawal of the delivery system. One patient showed stent migration 11 days later due

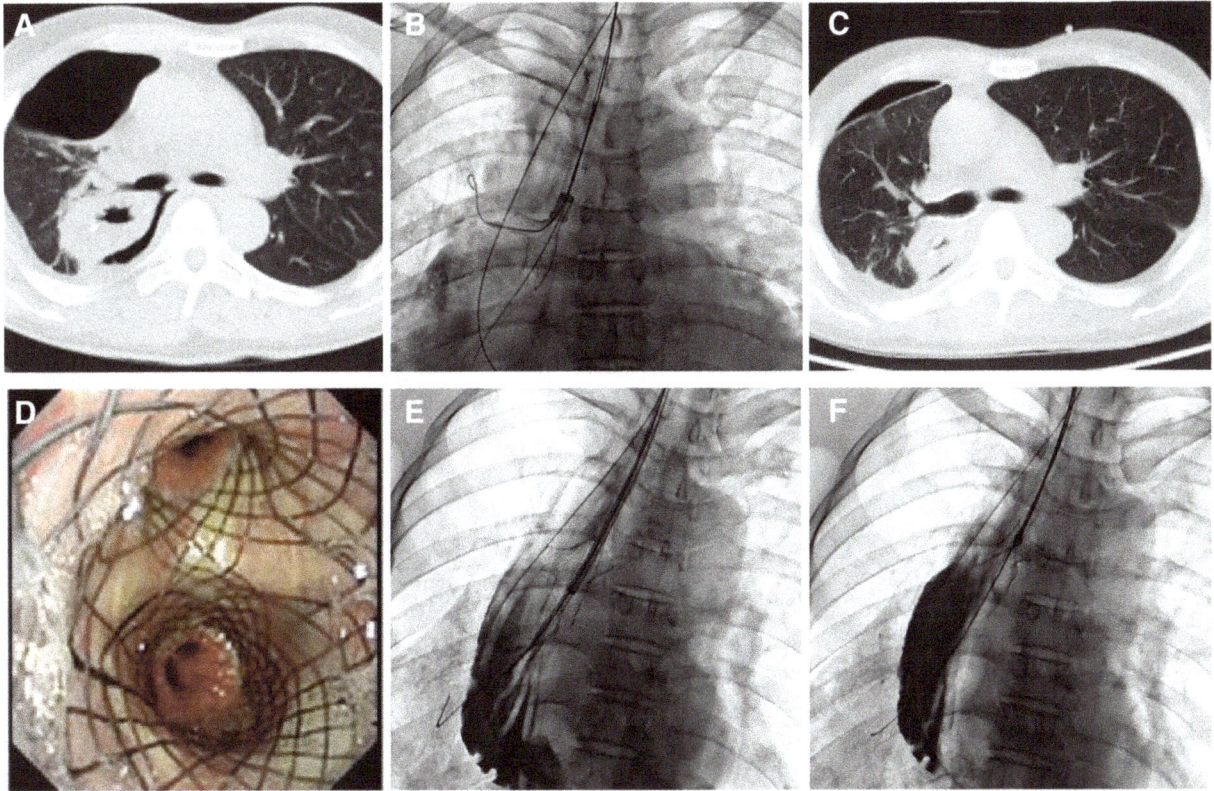

Fig. 2 Treatment of a 59-year-old man with fistula in right main bronchus. a, Chest SCT showed fistula in right main bronchus with right pneumothorax. b, Small y covered stent inserted in primary right carina. c, Chest SCT shows sealing of bronchial fistula with decreased right pneumothorax. d, Bronchoscopy confirmed complete seal of the fistula. E, A long sheath was introduced for stent removal after 167 days due to patient cure. F, Tip of hook was placed next to end of stent and stent was withdrawn from the airway wall

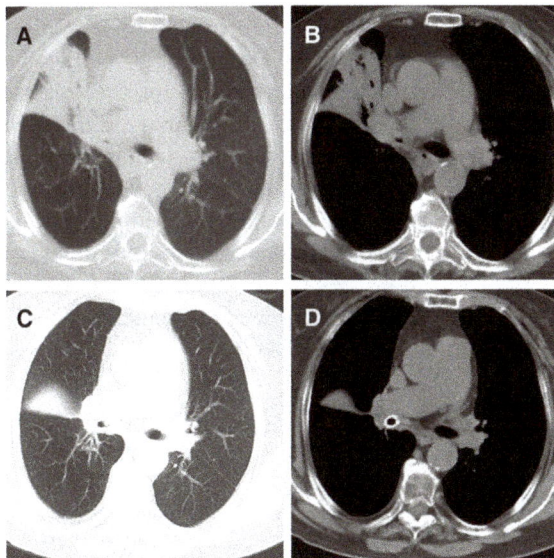

Fig. 3 Treatment of a 77-year-old woman with severe stenosis in right main bronchus. a, b, Chest SCT showed severe stenosis in right main bronchus and atelectasis. c, d After small y stent placement, chest SCT confirmed patency of right main bronchus and disappearance of atelectasis

to frequent cough and a second small y stent was inserted after removal of the migrated one. All patients tolerated the stent well and had good palliation of airway symptoms (Table 2).

Follow up
Two patients were lost to follow up. The remaining 26 patients were followed up for a median time of 9.2 months (IQR 3.5–23.8 months). Seventeen patients died of tumors and one died of myocardial infarction during follow up. The 1-, 3-, and 5-year survival rates were 49.3, 19.6 and 19.6%, respectively. The median survival was 12 months.

Discussion
Airway stents of various types and materials have been used for the treatment of airway disease, such as silicone stents [15–17] and metallic stents [1–9, 11, 12]. Small y stent placement may be applicable for patients with bronchial disease around the primary right carina. For example, the silicone y stent

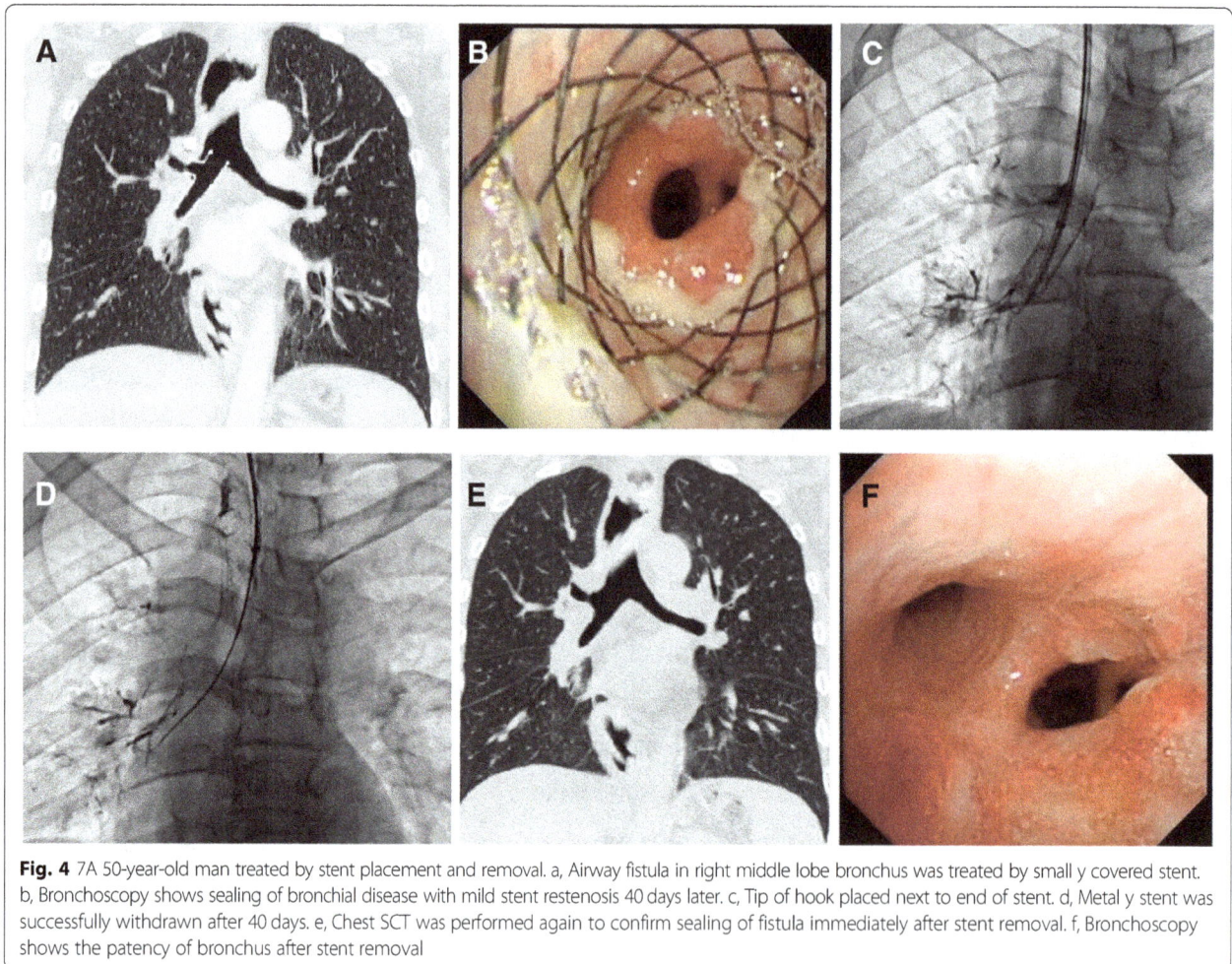

Fig. 4 7A 50-year-old man treated by stent placement and removal. a, Airway fistula in right middle lobe bronchus was treated by small y covered stent. b, Bronchoscopy shows sealing of bronchial disease with mild stent restenosis 40 days later. c, Tip of hook placed next to end of stent. d, Metal y stent was successfully withdrawn after 40 days. e, Chest SCT was performed again to confirm sealing of fistula immediately after stent removal. f, Bronchoscopy shows the patency of bronchus after stent removal

Table 1 The patients' characteristics

Characteristics	Median (IQR) or No. (%)
Patients, No.	28
Age, years	59 (51–64.5)
Male gender	22 (78.6%)
Duration of symptom, Months	1.0 (0.4–4.8)
Interval between surgery and symptom, Months	1.5 (0.5–13.8)
Duration of stenting procedure, Minutes	31.5 (19.5–44.3)
Previous disease	
Esophageal cancer	22 (78.6%)
Lung cancer	4 (14.3%)
Tuberculosis/pulmonitis	2 (7.1%)
Indications for stent placement	
Airway stenosis	5 (17.9%)
Thoracogastric airway fistula	20 (71.4%)
Bronchopleural fistula	3 (10.7%)
Location of fistula/stenosis	
Right bronchus	22 (78.6%)
Right middle lobe bronchus	6 (21.4%)

has been used for the treatment of airway disease around the left carina [13]. However, few studies have reported the use of metallic y stents for the treatment of bronchial disease around the primary right carina. Our study demonstrated that this technique is safe and feasible for these patients with good efficacy. In our study, stents were successfully inserted in all patients with no perioperative death or severe complications, such

Table 2 Clinic effect and complications of stenting

	N (%)	Days after stenting
Clinic efficacy		
Cure or improved	8 (28.6%)	31.8 (25.6, 34.4)
Death	18 (64.3%)	9 (3.9, 53.4)
Loss of follow	2 (7.1%)	–
Complications		
Stent restenosis	4 (14.3%)	65 (43.5, 186.3)
Bronchus obstruction	1 (3.6%)	0
Stent migration	3 (10.7%)	0 (0,11)
Retention of sputum	6 (21.4%)	1.5 (5.3, 169.3)

as massive hemorrhage or airway rupture. Twelve complications occurred in 10 patients. Stent restenosis and sputum retention were the most common complications, occurring in 4 and 6 patients, respectively. All of these complications were successfully treated by endoscopy or re-intervention.

Owing to easy removal, durability and low cost, the silicone stent is widely used clinically [13, 18–20]. However, metallic stents show good support and flexibility, can be placed with the help of guide wires, may be less traumatizing and minimize the procedures in cases with a fistula [14]. Currently, individualized metallic stents are available and can be produce upon request [1, 7, 21]. Metallic large Y stents were designed to be inserted for airway disease at the main carina. Owing to a low rate of stent migration, the metallic large Y stent placement on the primary carina may be an alternative to conventional straight stent placement. In this study, metallic small y stents were customized and used for airway disease around the primary right carina. According to our experience, metallic small y stent placement can be an alternative to silicone y stenting for airway disease around the primary right carina. In addition, implanted Y stents show excellent stability, with a low migration rate [22].

Oki et al. reported 3 cases of malignant disease treated with silicone y stent placement around the primary right carina [17]. The sample size of our study is significantly larger than that of his study, which helps to provide more reliable clinical experience. Metallic stent placement under fluoroscopic guidance dose not require the complex skills needed for rigid bronchoscopy, and this will contribute to the popularization and application of this technology. It needs to be pointed out that silicone stents have to be placed under rigid bronchoscopy only. In addition, rigid bronchoscopy is not only a way to access the airway but also a tool to achieve tumor debulking and dilation of stenosis.

The limitation of this study is its small retrospective nature. A larger prospective study is necessary to further investigate outcomes. In addition, good results of this study might not be reproduced at a less treatment experienced center. In conclusion, metallic small y stent placement is technically feasible, effective and safe for bronchial disease around primary right carina.

Conclusions

Metallic small y stent placement is technically feasible, effective and safe for bronchial disease around the primary right carina.

Abbreviations
IQR: interquartile range; SCT: spiral computed tomography

Acknowledgements
Not applicable.

Funding
This work was supported by National Natural Science Foundation of China (Grant No. 81501569). No funding body participated in the design of the study and collection, analysis, and interpretation of data and in writing the manuscript.

Authors' contributions
BYH, LJD, WG and HXW designed study. BYH, LJD, YZP performed study. YZP, RJZ collected and analyzed data. WG revised the manuscript. All authors wrote the paper and finally approved of the version to be published.

Competing interests
The authors declare that they have no competing interests.

Author details
[1]Department of Interventional Radiology, the First Affiliated Hospital of Zhengzhou University, Zhengzhou, China. [2]Department of Thoracic Surgery, the First Affiliated Hospital of Zhengzhou University, Zhengzhou, China.

References
1. Han X, Li L, Zhao Y, Liu C, Jiao D, Ren K, Wu G. Individualized airway-covered stent implantation therapy for thoracogastric airway fistula after esophagectomy. Surg Endosc. 2017;31:1713–8.
2. Han X, Wu G, Li Y, Li M. A novel approach: treatment of bronchial stump fistula with a plugged, bullet-shaped, angled stent. Ann Thorac Surg. 2006; 81:1867–71.
3. Wu G, Li ZM, Han XW, Wang ZG, Lu HB, Zhu M, Ren KW. Right bronchopleural fistula treated with a novel, Y-shaped, single-plugged, covered, metallic airway stent. Acta Radiol. 2013;54:656–60.
4. Li TF, Duan XH, Han XW, Wu G, Ren JZ, Ren KW, Lu HB. Application of combined-type Y-shaped covered metallic stents for the treatment of gastrotracheal fistulas and gastrobronchial fistulas. J Thorac Cardiovasc Surg. 2016;152:557–63.
5. Stockton PA, Ledson MJ, Hind CR, Walshaw MJ. Bronchoscopic insertion of Gianturco stents for the palliation of malignant lung disease: 10 year experience. Lung Cancer. 2003;42:113–7.
6. Prasad M, Bent JP, Ward RF, April MM. Endoscopically placed nitinol stents for pediatric tracheal obstruction. Int J Pediatr Otorhinolaryngol. 2002;66: 155–60.
7. Han X, Al-Tariq Q, Zhao Y, Li L, Cheng Z, Wang H, Liu C, Jiao D, Wu G. Customized hinged covered metallic stents for the treatment of benign Main bronchial stenosis. Ann Thorac Surg. 2017;104:420–5.
8. Thornton RH, Gordon RL, Kerlan RK, LaBerge JM, Wilson MW, Wolanske KA, Gotway MB, Hastings GS, Golden JA. Outcomes of tracheobronchial stent placement for benign disease. Radiology. 2006;240:273–82.
9. Park JH, Kim PH, Shin JH, Tsauo J, Kim MT, Cho YC, Kim JH, Song HY. Removal of retrievable self-expandable metallic tracheobronchial stents: an 18-year experience in a single center. Cardiovasc Intervent Radiol. 2016;39: 1611–9.
10. Ma J, Han X, Wu G, Jiao D, Ren K, Bi Y. Outcomes of temporary partially covered stent placement for benign tracheobronchial stenosis. Cardiovasc Intervent Radiol. 2016;39:1144–51.
11. Buskens CJ, Hulscher JB, Fockens P, Obertop H, van Lanschot JJ. Benign tracheo-neo-esophageal fistulas after subtotal esophagectomy. Ann Thorac Surg. 2001;72:221–4.
12. Han XW, Wu G, Li YD, Zhang QX, Guan S, Ma N, Ma J. Overcoming the delivery limitation: results of an approach to implanting an integrated self-

expanding Y-shaped metallic stent in the carina. J Vasc Interv Radiol. 2008; 19:742–7.

13. Oki M, Saka H. New dedicated bifurcated silicone stent placement for stenosis around the primary right carina. Chest. 2013;144:450–5.

14. Oki M, Saka H. Silicone Y-stent placement on the secondary left Carina. Respiration. 2015;90:493–8.

15. Machuzak MS, Santacruz JF, Jaber W, Gildea TR. Malignant tracheal-mediastinal-parenchymal-pleural fistula after chemoradiation plus bevacizumab: management with a Y-silicone stent inside a metallic covered stent. J Bronchology Interv Pulmonol. 2015;22:85–9.

16. Murgu SD, Colt HG. Silicone Y stent placement at secondary left carina for malignant central airway obstruction. J Thorac Cardiovasc Surg. 2010;139: 494–5.

17. Oki M, Saka H, Kitagawa C, Kogure Y. Silicone y-stent placement on the carina between bronchus to the right upper lobe and bronchus intermedius. Ann Thorac Surg. 2009;87:971–4.

18. Bolliger CT, Sutedja TG, Strausz J, Freitag L. Therapeutic bronchoscopy with immediate effect: laser, electrocautery, argon plasma coagulation and stents. Eur Respir J. 2006;27:1258–71.

19. Dahlqvist C, Ocak S, d'Odemont JP. New bifurcated silicone stent for the treatment of posttransplant bronchus intermedius stenosis: new silicone stent in posttransplant stenosis. Chest. 2014;145:429.

20. Lopez-Padilla D, Garcia-Lujan R, de Pablo A, de Miguel Poch E. Oki stenting for anastomotic bronchomalacia in lung transplantation. Eur J Cardiothorac Surg. 2015;48:e53–4.

21. Gompelmann D, Eberhardt R, Schuhmann M, Heussel CP, Herth FJ. Self-expanding Y stents in the treatment of central airway stenosis: a retrospective analysis. Ther Adv Respir Dis. 2013;7:255–63.

22. Dutau H, Toutblanc B, Lamb C, Seijo L. Use of the Dumon Y-stent in the management of malignant disease involving the carina: a retrospective review of 86 patients. Chest. 2004;126:951–8.

18

Predictors of positive airway pressure therapy termination in the first year: analysis of big data from a German homecare provider

Holger Woehrle[1*], Michael Arzt[2], Andrea Graml[3], Ingo Fietze[4], Peter Young[5], Helmut Teschler[6] and Joachim H. Ficker[7,8*]

Abstract

Background: There is a lack of robust data about factors predicting continuation (or termination) of positive airway pressure therapy (PAP) for sleep apnea. This analysis of big data from a German homecare provider describes patients treated with PAP, analyzes the therapy termination rate over the first year, and investigates predictive factors for therapy termination.

Methods: Data from a German homecare service provider were analyzed retrospectively. Patients who had started their first PAP therapy between September 2009 and April 2014 were eligible. Patient demographics, therapy start date, and the date of and reason for therapy termination were obtained. At 1 year, patients were classified as having compliance-related therapy termination or remaining on therapy. These groups were compared, and significant predictors of therapy termination determined.

Results: Of 98,329 patients included in the analysis, 11,702 (12%) terminated PAP therapy within the first year (after mean 171 ± 91 days). There was a U-shaped relationship between therapy termination and age; therapy termination was higher in the youngest (< 30 years, 15.5%) and oldest (≥ 80 years, 19.8%) patients, and lower in those aged 50–59 years (9.9%). Therapy termination was significantly more likely in females versus males (hazard ratio 1. 48, 95% confidence interval 1.42–1.54), in those with public versus private insurance (1.75, 1.64–1.86) and in patients whose first device was automatically adjusting or fixed-level continuous positive airway pressure versus bilevel or adaptive servo-ventilation (1.28, 1.2–1.38).

Conclusions: This analysis of the largest dataset investigating PAP therapy termination identified a number of predictive factors. These can help health care providers chose the most appropriate PAP modality, identify specific patient phenotypes at higher risk of stopping PAP and target interventions to support ongoing therapy to these groups, as well as allow them to develop a risk stratification tool.

Keywords: Positive airway pressure, Compliance, Patient phenotype, Therapy termination

* Correspondence: hwoehrle@lungenzentrum-ulm.de; ficker@klinikum-nuernberg.de
[1]Sleep and Ventilation Center Blaubeuren, Respiratory Center Ulm, Ulm, Germany
[7]Department of Respiratory Medicine, Allergology and Sleep Medicine, General Hospital Nuremberg, Nuremberg, Germany
Full list of author information is available at the end of the article

Background

Poor compliance with long-term therapies compromises the effectiveness of treatment and, on average, half of patients with a chronic illness don't adhere to their prescribed therapy [1]. Continuous positive airway pressure (CPAP) is the gold standard treatment for obstructive sleep apnea (OSA). However, long-term compliance with CPAP therapy is important for the achievement of therapeutic goals, including improvements in daytime sleepiness [2–6] and memory [7], reductions in blood pressure and the incidence of hypertension [8–13], and decreased cardiovascular risk [9, 14, 15]. The Sleep Apnea cardio-Vascular Endpoints (SAVE) study (NCT00738179) was the first large randomized controlled trial to investigate the effects of CPAP therapy on morbidity and mortality in patients with sleep apnea at risk for cardiovascular events [16]. The trial included nonsleepy patients with OSA who were randomized to CPAP or usual care. The results showed no significant difference in the rates of hospitalization or mortality between the CPAP and usual care groups. However, mean CPAP usage was only 3.3 h/night during the trial, and this low compliance might have contributed to the negative result of this study.

Rates of noncompliance with CPAP (defined as device use for < 4 h/night) have been reported to range from 29 to 83% in OSA patients receiving long-term therapy [17]. Although a number of studies have investigated compliance with positive airway pressure (PAP) therapy, the results have not always been consistent [18–24]. In addition, while the pattern of compliance within first weeks of CPAP therapy appears to be predictive of longer term compliance [25] – highlighting the importance of achieving good compliance early to ensure adequate long-term device use – there is a general lack of robust data from big data analyses [26] on specific predictors of PAP therapy persistence or termination. Identifying patients who are at risk of stopping CPAP therapy and the time course of when this might occur could help to optimize and target the provision of support strategies designed to increasing compliance [17, 19, 27, 28].

Therapy termination, with return of the PAP device to the service provider, represents a definitive form of non-compliance. Even though noncompliant, a patient who retains the device still has the potential to re-start therapy. This is much less likely once the device has been returned. However, very little data exist on the rates of therapy termination in patients using PAP therapy.

This big data analysis uses information from the database of a German homecare provider to describe the patient population treated with PAP therapy, analyze termination rates over the first year of therapy, and investigate factors predictive of therapy termination.

Methods

Patient population/sample

Observational study data were obtained from the database of a Germany homecare service provider (ResMed Healthcare Germany). Patients who had a physician diagnosis of sleep apnea and were prescribed PAP therapy, started PAP therapy for the first time between 1 September 2009 and 30 April 2014, and were being treated with fixed-pressure CPAP, automatically adjusting continuous positive airway pressure (APAP), bilevel PAP or adaptive servo-ventilation (ASV) devices, using a nasal mask, nasal pillows or a full face mask interface, were eligible for inclusion in this analysis. The presence of sleep apnea was based on diagnosis by each patient's treating physician.

Data extraction and definitions

The commercial homecare provider database contains information relevant to the provision of PAP therapy rather than individual clinical data. Therefore, it stores less information than a full electronic medical record, and did not record the severity of sleep apnea, mode of diagnosis, and comorbidities. The following variables were extracted from the database for each patient: therapy start date, and the date of and reason for therapy termination. A de-identified copy of all information available (to protect patient privacy) was provided to the scientific committee analyzing the data. German data protection law allows for the use of such data, if strictly anonymized, for scientific purposes. Therefore, patient informed consent and ethical approval were not required.

Therapy termination was then described as compliance related if it occurred as the result of patient decision or behavior due to patient-reported problems with the PAP interface or device (i.e. not accepting or tolerating PAP therapy). Terminations that occurred when a patient was lost to follow-up, transferred to a ventilation device or died, or were related to insurance coverage issues or patient transfer to another homecare provider were classified as not compliance related.

Patients were assigned to one of two groups based on their PAP usage status at 1 year: on therapy or therapy terminated. Data were censored whereby all patients who had not terminated therapy by 1 year were assigned to the "on therapy" group. All included patients had data available on the status at last observation (event occurrence or censoring) and time to event (or censoring). A flow diagram showing the patient selection pathway is presented in Fig. 1.

Data analysis

Age was regarded as plausible if the value was between 0 and 100 years, and termination date was regarded as

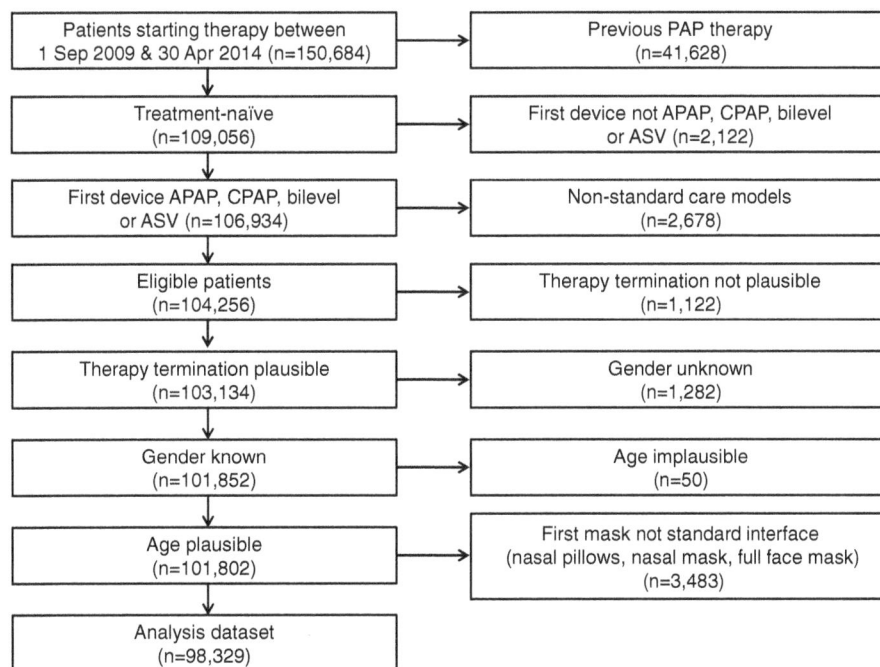

Fig. 1 Flow diagram of patient selection

plausible if it took place between therapy start date and the date that data were extracted. Several variables were used as covariates in the model (i.e. gender, age, insurance, and device), and complete observations were required for these data.

Numerical data are presented as mean ± standard deviation (SD). Differences between groups were analyzed using a t-test because the patient numbers allow for normal approximation. Ordinal and nominal data was presented as absolute and relative frequency. Differences in proportion were assessed with Z-tests. The time-to-event data were analyzed using Kaplan-Meier-plots and Cox proportional hazards regression. An event was defined as the compliance-related termination of PAP therapy, whereas compliance not related to therapy termination was defined as right censoring. Time was defined as time on therapy in the first year (i.e. time between therapy start registered in the ResMed database system and time of therapy termination, or 365 days for patients who did not terminate therapy). For compliance-related therapy termination, this is time to termination and for compliance not related to termination, this is time to censoring.

In general, p values of < 0.05 were considered statistically significant. All statistical analyses were performed using IBM SPSS Statistics 22 and R version 2.15.

Results

A total of 98,329 patients were included in the analysis dataset (Fig. 1). Of these, 12% ($n = 11,702$) terminated PAP therapy within the first year. Mean time to therapy

termination was 171 ± 91 days. Available demographic and clinical data for patients who continued PAP therapy or had compliance-related termination within the first year are shown in Table 1. Patients who terminated therapy were significantly older, significantly more likely to be female and to have APAP or CPAP as their first PAP device, and significantly less likely to have private insurance compared with those who remained on therapy (Table 1).

Reasons for therapy termination in the first year of PAP therapy were patient-related in 70% of subjects, administration- or insurance-related in 24%, based on medical decision in 1% and due to death in 5%. Cox proportional hazards regression analysis shows that the risk of therapy termination was significantly increased in female patients (hazard ratio [HR] 1.48, 95% confidence interval [CI] 1.42–1.54; $p < 0.001$; Fig. 2), when the first device was APAP or CPAP (HR 1.28, 95% CI 1.2–1.38; $p < 0.001$; Fig. 3), and when patients had public insurance (HR 1.75, 95% CI 1.64–1.86; Fig. 4). There was a U-shaped relationship between age and therapy termination rate. Compared with patients aged 50–59 years, the rate of therapy termination was significantly higher in younger patients (age < 30 years: HR 1.58, 95% CI 1.34–1.87; age 30–39 years: HR 1.15, 95% CI 1.05–1.27; $p = 0.003$) and in older patients (age 60–69 years: HR 1.15, 95% CI 1.10–1.22; p < 0.001; age 70–79 years: HR 1.56, 95% CI 1.48–1.64; p < 0.001; age ≥ 80 years: HR 2.19, 95% CI 2.04–2.37; p < 0.001); the rate of therapy termination in those aged 40–49 years did not differ

Table 1 Baseline demographic and clinical characteristics of patients who continued or terminated positive airway pressure therapy in the first year

	On Therapy (n = 86,627)	Terminating therapy (n = 11,702)	Total (n = 98,329)
Age, years	61 ± 12	63 ± 13*	61 ± 13
Gender, n (%)			
Male	66,755 (77)	8063 (69)*	74,818 (76)
Female	19,872 (23)	3639 (31)*	23,511 (24)
Insurance, n (%)			
Public	73,949 (85)	10,694 (91)*	84,643 (86)
Private	12,678 (15)	1008 (9)*	13,686 (14)
First PAP device, n (%)			
APAP/CPAP	78,357 (90)	10,827 (93)*	89,184 (91)
Bilevel/ASV	8270 (10)	875 (7)*	9145 (9)

Values are mean ± standard deviation, or number of patients (%)
*$p < 0.05$ vs patients who remained on therapy
APAP automatic continuous positive airway pressure, *ASV* adaptive servo-ventilation, *Bilevel* bilevel positive airway pressure, *CPAP* continuous positive airway pressure, *PAP* positive airway pressure

significantly from that in those aged 50–59 years (HR 1.05, 95% CI 0.98–1.11; $p = 0.167$). Time to therapy termination in the different age groups is shown in Fig. 5. Presentation of the Cox model data in a Forest plot confirmed the above significant predictors of therapy termination, and highlights the U-shaped relationship between age and therapy termination (Fig. 6).

Discussion

To the best of our knowledge, this big data analysis includes the largest dataset investigating predictors of current PAP therapy termination in practice to date. We identified a U-shaped relationship between age and

therapy termination, with significantly higher therapy termination rates in younger and older age groups compared with patients aged 50–59 years. In geriatric patients aged 80 years or older, the therapy termination rate was double that in patients aged 50–59 years. Female patients were 1.4 times more likely to terminate therapy than males, while the risk of therapy termination was increased by 41% in patients who had public versus private insurance and there was a 26% higher rate of therapy termination in the first year when the first device was APAP or CPAP versus bilevel or ASV.

The overall PAP termination rate in the first year of therapy was 12% in our study, substantially lower than the 26% of patients who stopped PAP therapy in the first year of another large European analysis conducted in Switzerland ($n = 2187$) [29]. There are a number of factors that could have contributed to this difference, including the slightly newer technology used in our study, differences in diagnostic and treatment algorithms, and different patient population characteristics. In contrast to our findings and those of other studies [19, 30], age and gender were not significant independent predictors of PAP compliance in the Swiss study [29]. Instead, a low oxygen desaturation index (ODI) and Epworth Sleepiness Scale score, and high body mass index and apnea-hypopnea index were significantly associated with better compliance with PAP therapy [29]. Baseline sleep apnea severity has also been identified as a significant predictor of PAP compliance in a number of other studies [4, 19–23, 30], although the relationship has been described as relatively weak, especially when other factors are taken into account [28].

Existing data on the influence of age on compliance with CPAP therapy are conflicting. Increasing age has

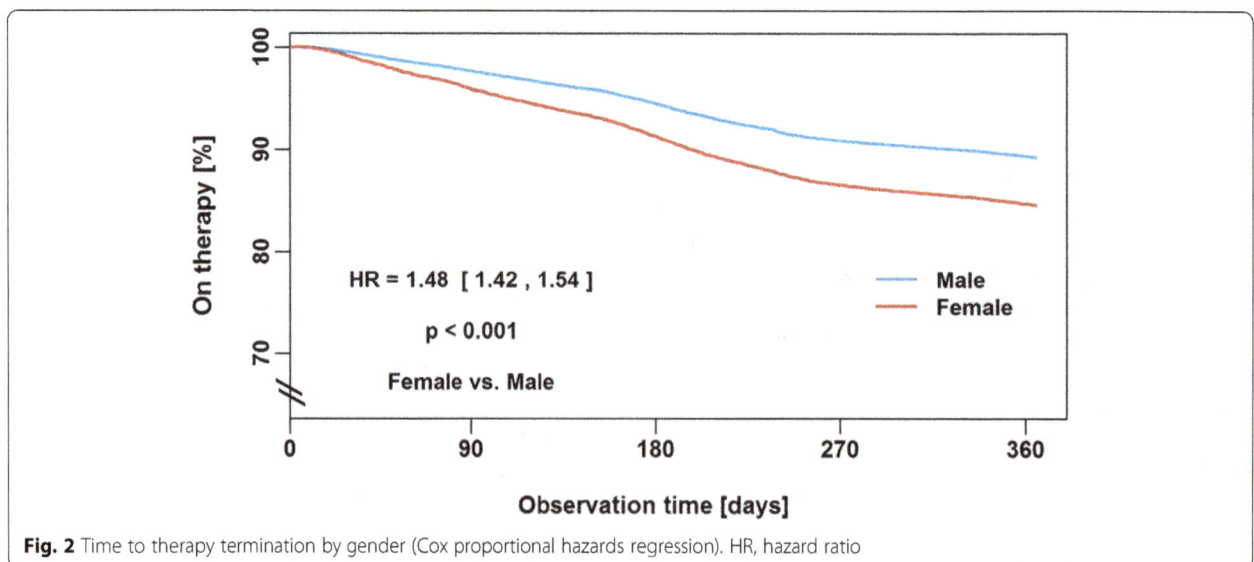

Fig. 2 Time to therapy termination by gender (Cox proportional hazards regression). HR, hazard ratio

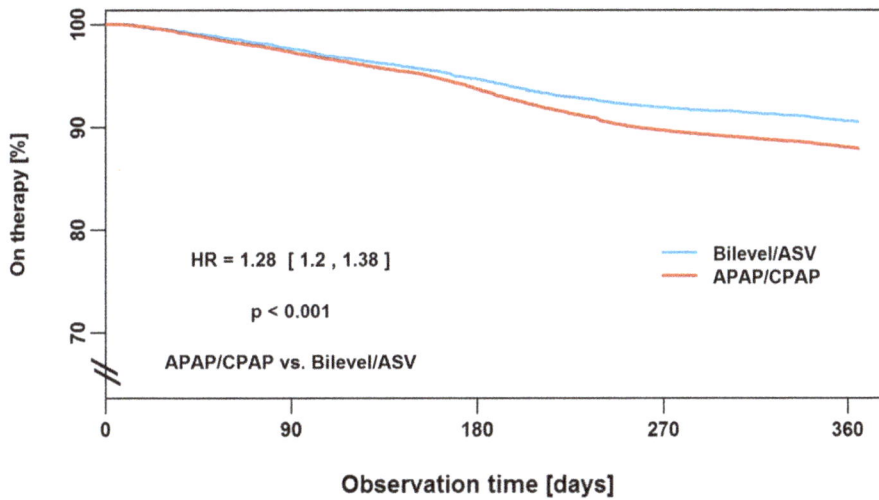

Fig. 3 Time to therapy termination by first device used (Cox proportional hazards regression). APAP, automatic continuous positive airway pressure; ASV, adaptive servo-ventilation; Bilevel, bilevel positive airway pressure; CPAP, continuous positive airway pressure; HR, hazard ratio

been shown to be associated with decreased CPAP usage [31]. However, this is far from a consistent observation, with several studies having failed to identify such an association [32–34], and older or increasing age has also been associated with better nightly CPAP usage [23, 35]. It has been suggested that other factors might attenuate the effects of advancing age on PAP compliance [22, 28]. The U-shaped relationship identified for the first time in our analysis could be one possible contributor to the inconsistent results reported to date. Only large data sets like ours allow five different age groups to be analyzed separately, which resulted in the identification of a

U-shaped relationship between age and therapy termination. It would not be possible to identify such a relationship in studies comparing only very old and very young patients.

The results of the present analysis indicated a higher therapy termination rate in women compared with men. Evidence from existing literature in this area is again inconsistent. Although many studies have failed to find an association between gender and PAP usage [19, 25, 30, 36], others have shown female gender to be significantly associated with both better [23, 32] and worse [22, 37] CPAP compliance. The results of the current larger

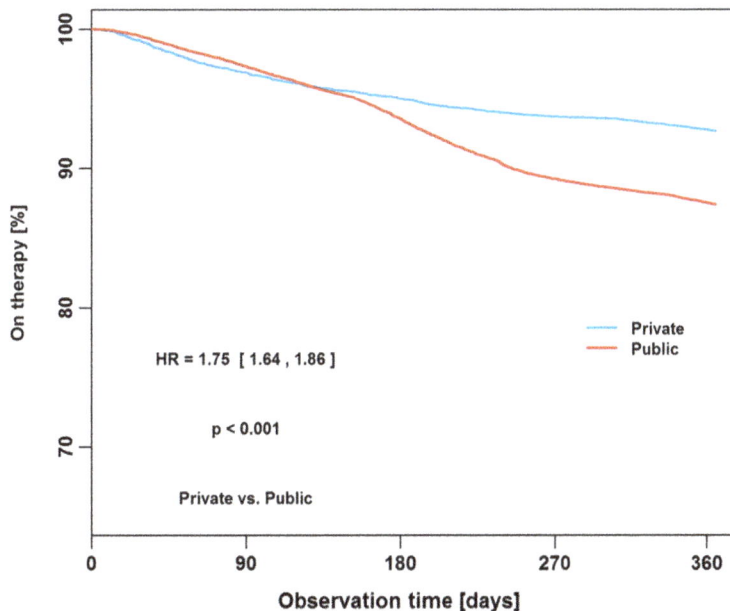

Fig. 4 Time to therapy termination by insurance type (Cox proportional hazards regression). HR, hazard ratio

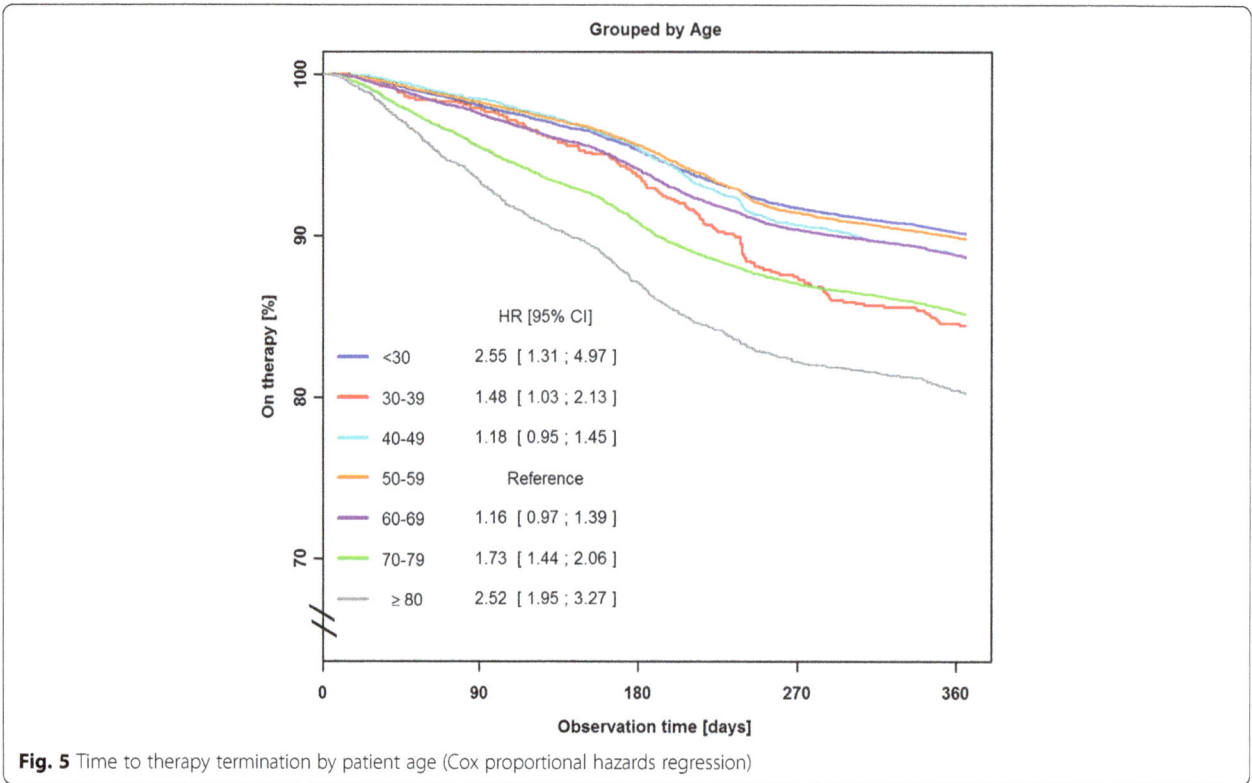

Fig. 5 Time to therapy termination by patient age (Cox proportional hazards regression)

analysis identified female gender as a significant predictor of PAP therapy termination (i.e. poor compliance with therapy). Clearly the role of gender in compliance with PAP therapy is a topic that needs to be investigated further. Reasons underlying the higher therapy termination rate we observed in women versus men are also not clearly defined. It is possible that women dislike the aesthetics of PAP treatment more than men or have less tolerant partners. A dislike of the PAP therapy equipment could also be one potential explanation for

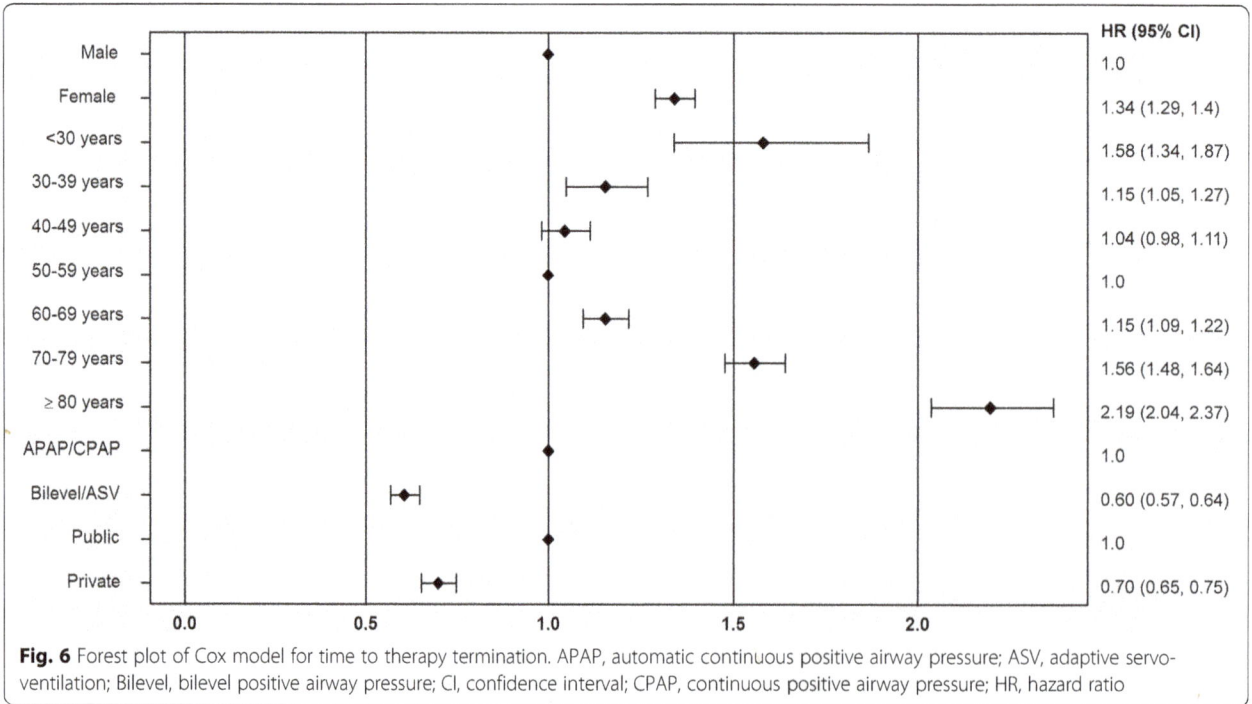

Fig. 6 Forest plot of Cox model for time to therapy termination. APAP, automatic continuous positive airway pressure; ASV, adaptive servo-ventilation; Bilevel, bilevel positive airway pressure; CI, confidence interval; CPAP, continuous positive airway pressure; HR, hazard ratio

higher therapy termination in the youngest group of patients. Furthermore, privately insured patients may have a better awareness of the cost of PAP therapy, increasing the likelihood of persevering with therapy. However, these suggestions are speculative and hypothesis generating only, and need to be investigated in future studies.

Interestingly, compliance rates in the long-term Swiss analysis that collected data over the period 2001 to 2011 were significantly higher in patients who started PAP therapy in the final 2 years of data analysis compared with those whose therapy was initiated earlier [29]. One possible explanation for this is that improvements in technology over time contributed to better compliance, highlighting the importance of data obtained in patients being treated with the latest devices and technologies.

This appears to be the first study to use big data to investigate predictors of PAP therapy termination. Analysis of big data allows inclusion of a very large population of patients and means that subgroup analyses include adequate numbers of patients to allow statistically meaningful comparisons. However, there are also some limitations associated with conducting scientific research using databases that were created for administrative, rather than scientific, purposes [26]. Such databases, including the one used in this analysis, include limited baseline clinical and demographic data, and no information about the severity of sleep-disordered breathing, method of diagnosis and comorbidities. The retrospective nature of the analysis is another limitation. In addition, compared with previous studies, we examined the rate of therapy termination rather than compliance. Therapy termination represents the most extreme form of non-compliance. There are other usage and behavior patterns that might fulfill criteria for non-compliance but not therapy termination, such as keeping the PAP device but never using it. The impact of telemonitoring on compliance with any type of PAP therapy was not evaluated in the current analysis (patients undergoing telemonitoring were excluded), but the impact of different telemedicine strategies on therapy termination rates have been reported separately [38, 39]. It is also important to note that the type of PAP device used depends on the type of sleep-disordered breathing being treated, with fixed pressure or automatically-titrating CPAP used to manage OSA, while bilevel PAP and ASV are better options when central sleep apnea is persistent or emerges during CPAP. Use of different devices in different settings could contribute to differences in compliance and therapy termination rates. Strengths of this analysis include the very large data set and the inclusion of a significant number of elderly and younger patients, and a large number of females. These groups are often under-represented in clinical

trials, but were included in large numbers in this analysis, making the sample highly representative of clinical practice and improving the generalizability of the results. Nevertheless, caution needs to be exercised in extrapolating the results to other healthcare settings where differences in clinical practice might influence therapy termination rates [40]. Another important point to note is that our study analyzed different PAP devices together. The majority of previous studies investigating predictors of compliance have focused on CPAP, and variations in predictors of therapy termination between the different types of therapy (i.e. CPAP, ASV, etc.) cannot be ruled out. Nevertheless, the exploratory results are based on a very broad range of patients and provide useful information about which patient groups could be targeted to improve continuous use of PAP therapy, and serve as a guide for generating hypotheses and designing studies for future research.

Conclusions

In this big database analysis of a large, unselected group of anonymized patients receiving PAP therapy in a real-world setting, gender, age, type of insurance, and device type were associated with therapy termination. These exploratory data highlight the importance of individualized approaches to PAP therapy management, and could help health care providers identify specific patient phenotypes that are at higher risk of stopping PAP therapy in the first year after treatment initiation. This would facilitate the choice of most appropriate PAP modality, targeting of interventions to support ongoing therapy to these groups, maximizing both the efficiency of resource use, service provision, and patient outcomes.

Abbreviations
APAP: automatically adjusting continuous positive airway pressure; ASV: adaptive servo-ventilation; CI: confidence interval; CPAP: continuous positive airway pressure; HR: hazard ratio; OSA: obstructive sleep apnea; PAP: positive airway pressure; SD: standard deviation

Acknowledgements
Medical writing assistance was provided by Nicola Ryan, independent medical writer, funded by ResMed.

Funding
This study was funded by ResMed Germany Healthcare. Study design, data collection, analysis, interpretation and manuscript preparation were undertaken by the listed authors, without influence from the funder.

Authors' contributions
HW was involved in the conception and design of the study. Data collection and analysis was performed by HW, AG and JF, with critical review by MA, IF,

PY and HT. All authors were involved in preparation of the manuscript, revising it for important intellectual content, and approved the final version.

Competing interests

HW is a paid consultant to ResMed and has received research grants. MW reports grants and personal fees from ResMed and Philips Respironics, outside the submitted work. AG is an employee of ResMed Germany; IF reports grants from ResMed, Philips, Fisher & Paykel, Hoffrichter, Heinen & Löwenstein and Weinmann, and personal fees from ResMed, outside the submitted work; PY reports personal fees from Sanofi Genzyme, Biomarin, UCB Pharma, Medice, ResMed, Heinen & Loewenstein and Vanda, and grants from Lowensteinstiftung and the German Ministry of Education and Science (BMBF), outside the submitted work; HT reports grants, personal fees and non-financial support from ResMed both during the conduct of the study and outside the submitted work; JHF reports personal fees and non-financial support from ResMed and Weinmann, outside the submitted work.

Author details

[1]Sleep and Ventilation Center Blaubeuren, Respiratory Center Ulm, Ulm, Germany. [2]Department of Internal Medicine II, University Hospital Regensburg, Regensburg, Germany. [3]ResMed Science Center, ResMed Germany, Martinsried, Germany. [4]Charité – University Medical Center Berlin, Center for Cardiovascular and Vascular Medicine, Interdisciplinary Sleep Medicine Center, Berlin, Germany. [5]Clinic for Sleep Medicine and Neuromuscular Diseases, University Hospital Münster, Münster, Germany. [6]Department of Pneumology, Ruhrlandklinik, West German Lung Center, University Hospital Essen, University Duisburg-Essen, Essen, Germany. [7]Department of Respiratory Medicine, Allergology and Sleep Medicine, General Hospital Nuremberg, Nuremberg, Germany. [8]Paracelsus Medical University, Nuremberg, Germany.

References

1. Sabate E. Adherence to long-term therapies: evidence for action: World Health Organization; 2003. http://apps.who.int/iris/bitstream/handle/10665/42682/9241545992.pdf;jsessionid=23CC7EEFE0CADC14992C86EA65954C35?sequence=1.
2. Antic NA, Catcheside P, Buchan C, Hensley M, Naughton MT, Rowland S, et al. The effect of CPAP in normalizing daytime sleepiness, quality of life, and neurocognitive function in patients with moderate to severe OSA. Sleep. 2011;34:111–9.
3. Barnes M, Houston D, Worsnop CJ, Neill AM, Mykytyn IJ, Kay A, et al. A randomized controlled trial of continuous positive airway pressure in mild obstructive sleep apnea. Am J Respir Crit Care Med. 2002;165:773–80.
4. Engleman HM, Kingshott RN, Wraith PK, Mackay TW, Deary IJ, Douglas NJ. Randomized placebo-controlled crossover trial of continuous positive airway pressure for mild sleep apnea/hypopnea syndrome. Am J Respir Crit Care Med. 1999;159:461–7.
5. Stradling JR. Davies RJ. Is more NCPAP better? Sleep. 2000;23(Suppl 4):S150–3.
6. Weaver TE, Maislin G, Dinges DF, Bloxham T, George CF, Greenberg H, et al. Relationship between hours of CPAP use and achieving normal levels of sleepiness and daily functioning. Sleep. 2007;30:711–9.
7. Zimmerman ME, Arnedt JT, Stanchina M, Millman RP, Aloia MS. Normalization of memory performance and positive airway pressure adherence in memory-impaired patients with obstructive sleep apnea. Chest. 2006;130:1772–8.
8. Barbe F, Duran-Cantolla J, Capote F, de la Pena M, Chiner E, Masa JF, et al. Long-term effect of continuous positive airway pressure in hypertensive patients with sleep apnea. Am J Respir Crit Care Med. 2010;181:718–26.
9. Barbe F, Duran-Cantolla J, Sanchez-de-la-Torre M, Martinez-Alonso M, Carmona C, Barcelo A, et al. Effect of continuous positive airway pressure on the incidence of hypertension and cardiovascular events in nonsleepy patients with obstructive sleep apnea: a randomized controlled trial. JAMA. 2012;307:2161–8.
10. Duran-Cantolla J, Aizpuru F, Montserrat JM, Ballester E, Teran-Santos J, Aguirregomoscorta JI, et al. Continuous positive airway pressure as treatment for systemic hypertension in people with obstructive sleep apnoea: randomised controlled trial. BMJ. 2010;341:c5991.
11. Lozano L, Tovar JL, Sampol G, Romero O, Jurado MJ, Segarra A, et al. Continuous positive airway pressure treatment in sleep apnea patients with resistant hypertension: a randomized, controlled trial. J Hypertens. 2010;28:2161–8.
12. Marin JM, Agusti A, Villar I, Forner M, Nieto D, Carrizo SJ, et al. Association between treated and untreated obstructive sleep apnea and risk of hypertension. JAMA. 2012;307:2169–76.
13. Montesi SB, Edwards BA, Malhotra A, Bakker JP. The effect of continuous positive airway pressure treatment on blood pressure: a systematic review and meta-analysis of randomized controlled trials. J Clin Sleep Med. 2012;8:587–96.
14. Campos-Rodriguez F, Martinez-Garcia MA, Reyes-Nunez N, Caballero-Martinez I, Catalan-Serra P, Almeida-Gonzalez CV. Role of sleep apnea and continuous positive airway pressure therapy in the incidence of stroke or coronary heart disease in women. Am J Respir Crit Care Med. 2014;189:1544–50.
15. Martinez-Garcia MA, Campos-Rodriguez F, Catalan-Serra P, Soler-Cataluna JJ, Almeida-Gonzalez C, De la Cruz Moron I, et al. Cardiovascular mortality in obstructive sleep apnea in the elderly: role of long-term continuous positive airway pressure treatment: a prospective observational study. Am J Respir Crit Care Med. 2012;186:909–16.
16. McEvoy RD, Antic NA, Heeley E, Luo Y, Ou Q, Zhang X, et al. CPAP for prevention of cardiovascular events in obstructive sleep apnea. N Engl J Med. 2016;375:919–31.
17. Weaver TE, Grunstein RR. Adherence to continuous positive airway pressure therapy: the challenge to effective treatment. Proc Am Thorac Soc. 2008;5:173–8.
18. Collen J, Lettieri C, Kelly W, Roop S. Clinical and polysomnographic predictors of short-term continuous positive airway pressure compliance. Chest. 2009;135:704–9.
19. Kohler M, Smith D, Tippett V, Stradling JR. Predictors of long-term compliance with continuous positive airway pressure. Thorax. 2010;65:829–32.
20. Krieger J, Kurtz D, Petiau C, Sforza E, Trautmann D. Long-term compliance with CPAP therapy in obstructive sleep apnea patients and in snorers. Sleep. 1996;19:S136–43.
21. McArdle N, Devereux G, Heidarnejad H, Engleman HM, Mackay TW, Douglas NJ. Long-term use of CPAP therapy for sleep apnea/hypopnea syndrome. Am J Respir Crit Care Med. 1999;159:1108–14.
22. Pelletier-Fleury N, Rakotonanahary D, Fleury B. The age and other factors in the evaluation of compliance with nasal continuous positive airway pressure for obstructive sleep apnea syndrome. A Cox's proportional hazard analysis. Sleep Med. 2001;2:225–32.
23. Sin DD, Mayers I, Man GC, Pawluk L. Long-term compliance rates to continuous positive airway pressure in obstructive sleep apnea: a population-based study. Chest. 2002;121:430–5.
24. Sucena M, Liistro G, Aubert G, Rodenstein DO, Pieters T. Continuous positive airway pressure treatment for sleep apnoea: compliance increases with time in continuing users. Eur Respir J. 2006;27:761–6.
25. Budhiraja R, Parthasarathy S, Drake CL, Roth T, Sharief I, Budhiraja P, et al. Early CPAP use identifies subsequent adherence to CPAP therapy. Sleep. 2007;30:320–4.
26. Martinez-Garcia MA, Dinh-Xuan AT. Deriving information from external big databases and big data analytics: all that glitters is not gold. Eur Respir J. 2016;47:1047–9.
27. Rose MW. Positive airway pressure adherence: problems and interventions. Sleep Med Clin. 2006;1:533–9.
28. Sawyer AM, Gooneratne NS, Marcus CL, Ofer D, Richards KC, Weaver TE. A systematic review of CPAP adherence across age groups: clinical and empiric insights for developing CPAP adherence interventions. Sleep Med Rev. 2011;15:343–56.
29. Schoch OD, Baty F, Niedermann J, Rudiger JJ, Brutsche MH. Baseline predictors of adherence to positive airway pressure therapy for sleep apnea: a 10-year single-center observational cohort study. Respiration. 2014;87:121–8.
30. Gagnadoux F, Le Vaillant M, Goupil F, Pigeanne T, Chollet S, Masson P, et al. Influence of marital status and employment status on long-term adherence with continuous positive airway pressure in sleep apnea patients. PLoS One. 2011;6:e22503.
31. Janson C, Noges E, Svedberg-Randt S, Lindberg E. What characterizes patients who are unable to tolerate continuous positive airway pressure (CPAP) treatment? Respir Med. 2000;94:145–9.
32. Amfilochiou A, Tsara V, Kolilekas L, Gizopoulou E, Maniou C, Bouros D, et al. Determinants of continuous positive airway pressure compliance in a group of Greek patients with obstructive sleep apnea. Eur J Intern Med. 2009;20:645–50.
33. Galetke W, Anduleit N, Richter K, Stieglitz S, Randerath WJ. Comparison of

automatic and continuous positive airway pressure in a night-by-night analysis: a randomized, crossover study. Respiration. 2008;75:163–9.

34. Poulet C, Veale D, Arnol N, Levy P, Pepin JL, Tyrrell J. Psychological variables as predictors of adherence to treatment by continuous positive airway pressure. Sleep Med. 2009;10:993–9.

35. Budhiraja R, Kushida CA, Nichols DA, Walsh JK, Simon RD, Gottlieb DJ, et al. Impact of randomization, clinic visits, and medical and psychiatric Cormorbidities on continuous positive airway pressure adherence in obstructive sleep apnea. J Clin Sleep Med. 2016;12:333–41.

36. Campos-Rodriguez F, Martinez-Alonso M, Sanchez-de-la-Torre M, Barbe F, Spanish Sleep N. Long-term adherence to continuous positive airway pressure therapy in non-sleepy sleep apnea patients. Sleep Med. 2016;17:1–6.

37. Woehrle H, Graml A, Weinreich G. Age- and gender-dependent adherence with continuous positive airway pressure therapy. Sleep Med. 2011;12:1034–6.

38. Woehrle H, Arzt M, Graml A, Fietze I, Young P, Teschler H, et al. Effect of a patient engagement tool on positive airway pressure adherence: analysis of a German healthcare provider database. Sleep Med. 2018;41:20–6.

39. Woehrle H, Ficker JH, Graml A, Fietze I, Young P, Teschler H, et al. Telemedicine-based proactive patient management during positive airway pressure therapy: impact on therapy termination rate. Somnologie (Berl). 2017;21:121–7.

40. Mayer G, Apelt S, Hessmann P, Rees J-P, Dodel R, Heitmann J. Versorgung von Schlafapnoe-Patienten in Hessen. Somnologie. 2015;19:145–53.

19

Atrial septostomy and disease targeting therapy in pulmonary hypertension secondary to neurofibromatosis

George Giannakoulas[1*], Panagiotis Savvoulidis[1] (iD), Vasilios Grosomanidis[2], Sophia-Anastasia Mouratoglou[1], Haralambos Karvounis[1] and Stavros Hadjimiltiades[1]

Abstract

Background: Neurofibromatosis type 1 (NF1) is a rare multisystem genetic disorder. During the course of the disease it can be rarely complicated with pulmonary hypertension (PH) which confers a dismal prognosis.

Case presentation: We describe the case of a 57-year-old female patient with NF1 complicated by severe precapillary PH despite dual disease-specific oral combination therapy. The patient was treated with initial atrial septostomy followed by administration of high-dose subcutaneous treprostinil with a favorable medium-term clinical and hemodynamic response.

Conclusions: PH secondary to NF1 may be successfully treated with the combination of atrial septostomy and PH targeted therapy in selected patients.

Keywords: Neurofibromatosis, Pulmonary hypertension, Septostomy, Case report

Background

Neurofibromatosis type 1 (NF1) is a genetic disease with a prevalence of 1:3500 in the general population, transmitted with the autosomal dominant inheritance pattern and with full penetrance characterized by prominent skin features (hyperpigmented macules, termed café-au-lait spots and nerve tumors), optical tumors and other central nervous system tumors, certain bony abnormalities, some learning deficits and an increased risk of certain non-nervous system cancers [1]. Mutations of the NF1 gene, which encodes neurofibromin and is located at chromosome 17q11.2, a negative regulator of the ras signal transduction pathway that has a role in both tumor suppression and regulation of cell growth and proliferation, are responsible for the NF1 [2].

A rare still morbid complication of NF1 is pulmonary hypertension (PH) which confers a dismal prognosis overall. To the best of our knowledge this is the first documented report of successful treatment of PH secondary to NF1 with atrial septostomy followed by escalation of PH targeted treatment.

Case presentation

A 57-year-old female patient with a history of NF1 and PH initially diagnosed 3 years ago, already on conventional treatment with supplemental oxygen and anticoagulation, as well as disease-specific double oral combination therapy (ambrisentan 10 mg od and tadalafil 40 mg od) was admitted to the hospital because of worsening dyspnea on mild exertion and a presyncopal episode.

Her past medical history was notable for surgically repaired pyloric stenosis and 2 abortions during the third trimester of gestation due to intrauterine fetal death, followed by a successful pregnancy. The patient had already undergone an extensive workup which excluded known causes of PH. Lung ventilation/perfusion scan was not suggestive for chronic thromboembolic disease and high-resolution CT of the lungs was negative for interstitial lung disease. Blood tests excluded other causes of pulmonary hypertension.

* Correspondence: giannak@med.auth.gr
[1]Department of Cardiology, AHEPA University Hospital, Aristotle University of Thessaloniki, Stilp. Kiriakidi 1, Thessaloniki 54637, Greece

Considering the patient's clinical deterioration, the decision was made to proceed immediately with atrial septostomy, due to inherent difficulties in the reimbursement of prostanoids in our hospital at that time. The patient had an uneventful procedure with graded balloon dilation of the interatrial septum with gradually increasing inflated balloons diameter of 6, 8 and 10 mm. A moderate decrease in right atrial pressure (Fig. 1), a mild increase in cardiac index and, as expected, a decrease in SaO2 was noted (Table 1) due to the right-to-left shunting through the atrial septum. The patient remained clinically and hemodynamically stable and was discharged a few days later.

After an initial modest improvement in symptoms, six-minute walk test (6MWT) and NT-proBNP at 2 months, access to prostanoids was eventually gained and the patient was started on subcutaneous treprostinil with gradual increase in the administered dose up to 100 ng/kg/min in a time period of 7 months.

The patient during a follow-up period of 2 years demonstrated gradual improvement and at present remains in World Health Organization class 2 with significant hemodynamic improvement (Table 1). A recent transthoracic echocardiogram demonstrated the positive remodeling of the right ventricle (Fig. 2a, b) and the persistence of the atrial septostomy (Fig. 2c). The shunt flow was small and at rest was from the left atrium to the right atrium but after 2 min of isometric exercise (hand grip and feet in cycling position) the shunt became right-to-left (Fig. 2d).

Discussion

A few cases suggesting an association of NF1 gene mutation and precapillary PH have been published [3, 4]. Plexiform lesions similar to those observed in human idiopathic PAH have been described, implying that vasculopathy of neurofibromatosis might underlie the pathophysiology of PH, a severe complication, which seems to show a predilection for women with severe clinical and hemodynamic impairment and a poor outcome [5].

Herein, we report a case of a patient with NF1 and severe precapillary PH, without parenchymal lung disease, yet with prominent pulmonary vascular involvement, treated with atrial septostomy, followed by the administration of subcutaneous treprostinil. The medium-term clinical response after 2 years was impressive with improvement in her functional class, 6MWT distance, hemodynamic parameters and NT-proBNP. To the best of our knowledge this is the first published case of PH secondary to neurofibromatosis treated successfully with the combination of atrial septostomy and aggressive PH targeted therapy.

The favorable clinical response of our patient to the atrial septostomy and the further gradual, but more pronounced, improvement with the chronic administration of subcutaneous treprostinil suggests that pulmonary vasculopathy is the underlying mechanism of PH in these patients. The creation of a shunt that decreases the preload of the right ventricle and increases that of the left ventricle with concomitant increase in the cardiac output makes it easier to initiate and uptitrate the prostanoid infusion. The long-term effect of the persistence of the

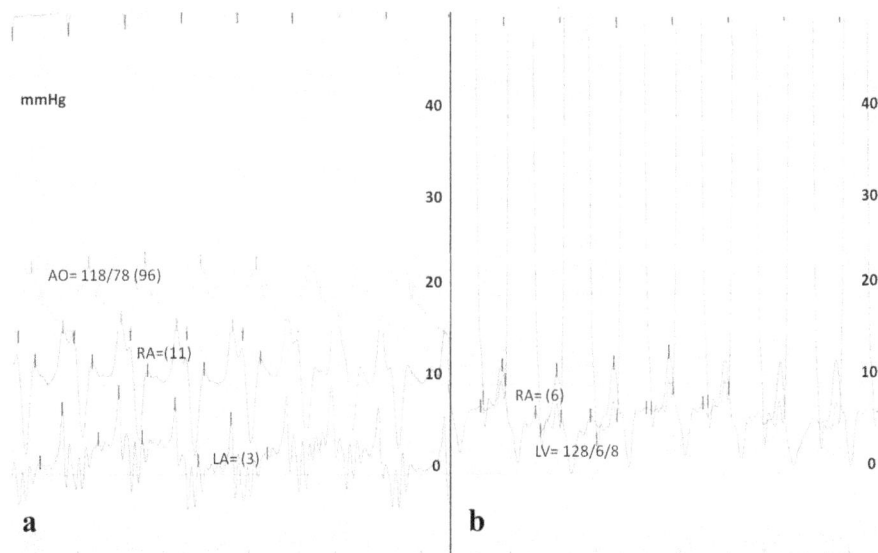

Fig. 1 a Simultaneous recording of *right atrial* (RA) and *left atrial* (LA) pressures, before the creation of the balloon atrial septostomy. b Simultaneous recording of *right atrial* (RA) and *left ventricular* (LV) pressures, demonstrating the fall in the mean RA and the increase in the LV diastolic pressures as compared to the LA pressure in A. The aortic pressure (AO) is recorded on a pressure scale of 0–200 mmHg. Mean pressures are in parentheses

Table 1 Serial hemodynamic, functional and neurohormonal measurements

Parameter	Jan 2011	PreBAS Mar 2014	PostBAS	Trepostinil Mar 2015	Trepostinil Feb 2016
HR (beats/min)	76	91	90	71	70
RAP (mmHg)	(3)	(11)	(7)	(4)	(6)
PAP (mmHg)	68/26 (43)	130/57 (84)	135/56 (84)	106/36 (63)	77/30 (49)
PAWP/LAP* (mmHg)	(6)	(2)*	(7)*	(7)	(9)*
Ao (mmHg)	130/68 (93)	122/65 (84)	124/65 (84)	119/71 (87)	128/65 (85)
PVR (WU)	8.3	27.1	26.3	11.6	6.8
CI (l/min/m^2)	2.9	1.9	2.0	3.1	3.7
SaO2 (%)	97 at rest 90 (during exercise)	98	93	95 at rest (70 during exercise)	98 at rest (75 during exercise)
6MWT (m)	489	230[a]	335[b]	345	399
NT-proBNP (pg/ml)	125	3402[a]	1507[b]	NA	161

Mean pressures are shown in parentheses

BAS: balloon atrial septostomy, HR: heart rate, RAP: Right atrial pressure, PAP: Pulmonary artery pressure, LAP: Left atrial pressure, PCWP: Pulmonary capillary wedge pressure, Ao: Aortic pressure, PVR: Pulmonary vascular resistance, CI: Cardiac index, WU: Wood Units, 6MWT: 6-min walking test, NT-proBNP: N-terminal pro-brain natriuretic peptide, NA: not available

*Asterisk indicates that the pressure was measured in the left atrium

[a]2 weeks prior to the procedure

[b]1 month after the procedure

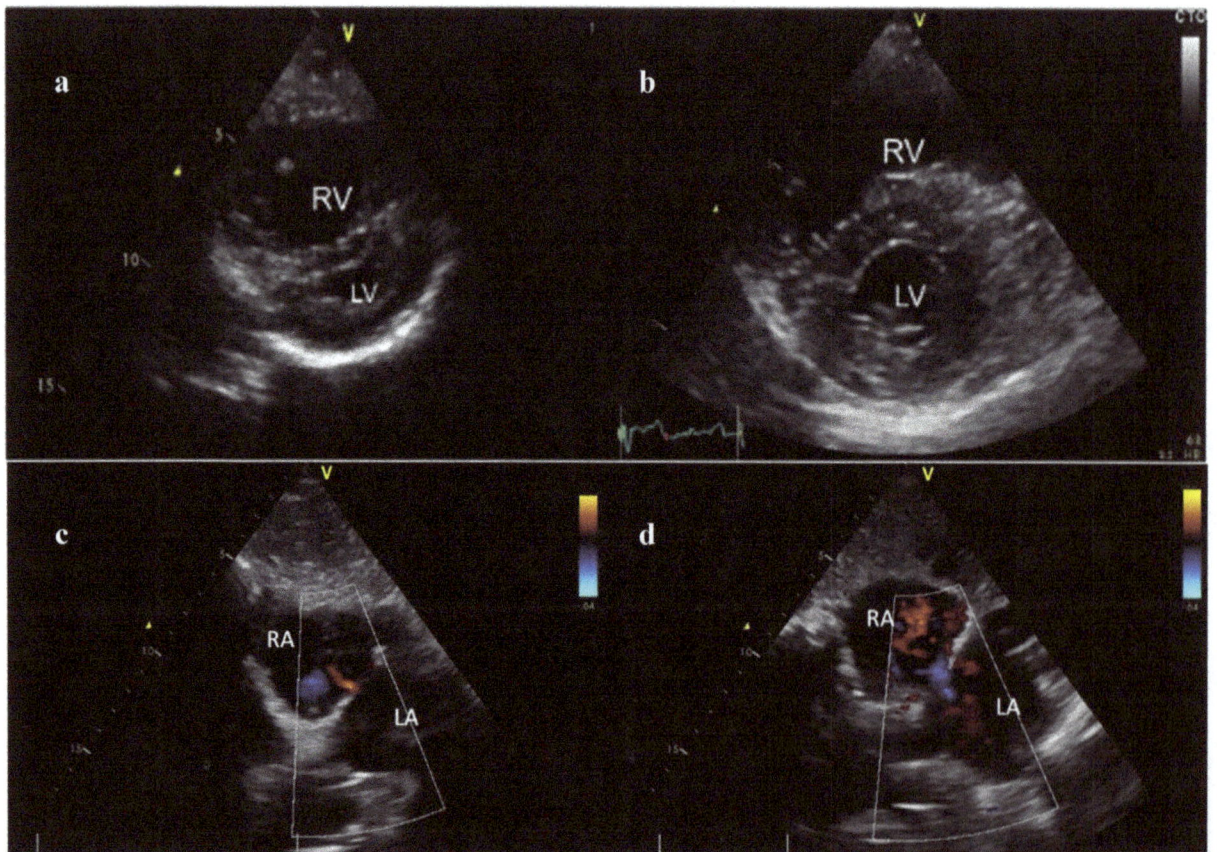

Fig. 2 a, **b** Short-axis transthoracic echocardiographic view demonstrating the positive remodelling of the *right ventricle* (RV) 2 years after the atrial septostomy and the initiation of subcutaneous treprostinil. LV = *left ventricle* **c** Subxiphoid echocardiographic view of the persistent flow from the *left atrium* (LA) to the *right atrium* (RA) at rest **d** Reversal of flow from RA to LA after isometric exercise

shunt in our case, following the decrease in the right sided pressures on chronic treprostinil therapy, is not known; whether the reversal of the shunt during exercise by decreasing the load on the right ventricle will continue to be beneficial, despite the arterial oxygen desaturation, is not clear [6].

There are very few cases in the literature with the utilization of PAH-targeted therapies in these patients [7–9]. Our patient improved significantly after the initiation of treprostinil, while double oral therapy had initially failed. The development of PH in patients with NF1 confers a dismal prognosis and therefore, the earlier and aggressive treatment with prostanoids should be considered. Finally, listing these patients for lung transplantation is a matter of debate, since a higher than the general population incidence of malignancies has been described [10].

Conclusions

This report demonstrates the successful management of a patient with PH secondary to NF1 with atrial septostomy in conjunction with PAH targeted therapy. Looking ahead, national and international prospective registries will shed light on the pathophysiology, and especially optimal therapy and prognosis of neurofibromatosis-associated PH especially in the modern era of targeted PAH treatment.

Abbreviations
6MWT: Six minute walk test; NF1: Neurofibromatosis type I; NT-proBNP: N-terminal pro-brain natriuretic peptide; PH: Pulmonary hypertension; PAH: Pulmonary arterial hypertension

Acknowledgements
Not applicable.

Funding
This work was not funded by any grant.

Authors' contributions
All authors actively participated in the conception, case interpretation and writing of this article. All authors read and approved the final manuscript.

Competing interests
The authors declare that they have no competing interests.

Author details
[1]Department of Cardiology, AHEPA University Hospital, Aristotle University of Thessaloniki, Stilp. Kiriakidi 1, Thessaloniki 54637, Greece. [2]Department of Anesthesiology and Intensive Care Medicine, AHEPA University Hospital, Aristotle University of Thessaloniki, Stilp. Kiriakidi 1, Thessaloniki 54637, Greece.

References
1. Korf BR. Malignancy in neurofibromatosis type 1. Oncologist. 2000;5:477–85.
2. Gutmann DH, Collins FS. The neurofibromatosis type 1 gene and its protein product, neurofibromin. Neuron. 1993;10:335–43.
3. Stewart DR, Cogan JD, Kramer MR, et al. Is pulmonary arterial hypertension in neurofibromatosis type 1 secondary to a plexogenic arteriopathy? Chest. 2007;132:798–808.
4. Montani D, Coulet F, Girerd B, et al. Pulmonary hypertension in patients with Neurofibromatosis type 1. Med. 2011;90:201–10.
5. Hamilton SJ, Friedman JM. Insights into the pathogenesis of neurofibromatosis 1 vasculopathy. Clin Genet. 2000;58:341–4.
6. Koeken Y, Kuijpers NH, Lumens J, Arts T, Delhaas T. Atrial septostomy benefits severe pulmonary hypertension patients by increase of left ventricular preload reserve. Am J Physiol Heart Circ Physiol. 2012;302:2654–62.
7. Kamdar F, Thenappan T, Missov E. Pulmonary arterial hypertension in von Recklinghausen's disease. Am J Med. 2015;128:39–40.
8. Engel PJ, Baughman RP, Menon SG, Kereiakes DJ, Taylor L, Scott M. Pulmonary hypertension in neurofibromatosis. Am J Cardiol. 2007;99:1177–8.
9. Tamura Y, Ono T, Sano M, Fukuda K, Kataoka M, Satoh T. Favorable effect of sorafenib in a patient with neurofibromatosis-associated pulmonary hypertension. Am J Respir Crit Care Med. 2012;186:291–2.
10. Uusitalo E, Rantanen M, Kallionpää RA, et al. Distinctive cancer associations in patients with neurofibromatosis type I. J Clin Oncol. 2016;34:1978–86.

20

Safety and efficacy of bridging to lung transplantation with antifibrotic drugs in idiopathic pulmonary fibrosis

Isabelle Delanote[1], Wim A. Wuyts[1,2], Jonas Yserbyt[1], Eric K. Verbeken[3], Geert M. Verleden[1,2] and Robin Vos[1,2*] (iD)

Abstract

Background: Following recent approval of pirfenidone and nintedanib for idiopathic pulmonary fibrosis (IPF), questions arise about the use of these antifibrotics in patients awaiting lung transplantation (LTx).

Methods: Safety and efficacy of antifibrotic drugs in IPF patients undergoing LTx were investigated in a single-centre retrospective cohort analysis.

Results: A total of nine patients, receiving antifibrotic therapy for 419 ± 315 days until subsequent LTx, were included. No major side effects were noted. Significant weight loss occurred during antifibrotic treatment ($p = 0.0062$). FVC tended to stabilize after 12 weeks of treatment in most patients. A moderate decline in FVC, TLC and DLCO was noted during the whole pretransplant time period of antifibrotic therapy. Functional exercise capacity and lung allocation score remained unchanged. No post-operative thoracic wound healing problems, nor severe early anastomotic airway complications were attributable to prior antifibrotic treatment. None of the patients developed chronic lung allograft dysfunction after a median follow-up of 19.8 (11.2–26.5) months; and post-transplant survival was 100% after 1 year and 80% after 2 years.

Conclusions: Antifibrotic drugs can probably be safely administered in IPF patients, possibly attenuating disease progression over time, while awaiting LTx.

Keywords: Antifibrotics, IPF, Lung transplantation, Nintedanib, Pirfenidone, Safety

Background

Idiopathic pulmonary fibrosis (IPF) is a progressive and lethal disease characterized by chronic, fibrosing interstitial pneumonitis of unknown cause, associated with a histopathologic and/or radiologic pattern of usual interstitial pneumonia (UIP) [1]. The course of the disease is unpredictable. Most patients demonstrate a slow, gradual progression; some patients remain stable; while others have an accelerated decline, sometimes due to repeated exacerbations. Consequently, respiratory failure is the most common cause of death in IPF. Once diagnosed, timely referral to an expert centre is therefore essential to assess eligibility for pharmacological therapy and/or lung transplantation (LTx) [2].

In October 2014, the US Food and Drug Administration (FDA) approved two anti-fibrotic drugs for IPF - pirfenidone and nintedanib - based on the results of large randomized clinical trials (CAPACITY-1, CAPACITY-2 and ASCEND with pirfenidone; TOMORROW, INPULSIS-1 and INPULSIS-2 with nintedanib) demonstrating a reduction in the rate of decline in forced vital capacity (FVC) in mild to moderate IPF [3–5]. Post-hoc analysis also demonstrated a risk reduction for IPF-related mortality with pirfenidone compared to placebo (HR 0.32, 95% CI 0.14–0.76, $p = 0.006$) [6], a same trend which was also observed with nintedanib (HR 0.70; 95% CI 0.46–1.08; $p = 0.0954$) [7].

Despite these positive findings, it should be emphasized that both antifibrotic drugs do not represent a 'cure' for IPF, but only aim to attenuate the decline in FVC, at best resulting in temporary disease stabilization. Moreover, side

* Correspondence: robin.vos@uzleuven.be

[1]Department of Respiratory Diseases, Interstitial Lung Disease and Lung Transplant Unit, University Hospitals Leuven, Leuven, Belgium

[2]KULeuven, Department of Clinical and Experimental Medicine, Division of Respiratory Diseases, Laboratory of Respiratory Diseases, Lung Transplantation Unit, KU Leuven, Herestraat 49, B-3000 Leuven, Belgium

effects (typically nausea, anorexia, malaise, or rash for pirfenidone; and diarrhea for nintedanib) or adverse events (mainly toxic hepatitis) may force some patients to reduce or even stop treatment, which may again accelerate disease progression. Hence, early evaluation and referral for LTx, which presently remains the only definitive treatment option for well-selected IPF patients, is highly recommendable, particularly since IPF patients have the highest waiting list mortality, due to disease progression. The recent introduction of the lung allocation score (LAS) in some countries may nevertheless decrease future waiting list mortality in IPF. Implementation of the LAS indeed has already led to a substantial increase in the proportion of LTx performed for IPF, making it the most common indication for LTx and reducing waiting list time for IPF in these countries [8].

With increasing use of antifibrotics following recent FDA approval, questions arise about their safety in IPF patients undergoing LTx, yet safety data in this specific setting are currently lacking. The antifibrotic properties of pirfenidone result from inhibition of transforming growth factor (TGF)-β expression, thus attenuating myofibroblast differentiation and fibroblast activity [9]. Nintedanib is a tyrosine kinase inhibitor, which blocks receptors for platelet-derived growth factor (PDGF), fibroblast growth factor (FGF), and vascular endothelial growth factor (VEGF), thus inhibiting downstream signaling in (myo-)fibroblasts [10]. Both antifibrotics may hence theoretically impair post-operative wound healing and/or cause bronchial anastomotic complications following LTx. Nintedanib, by inhibition of VEGF and PDGF, may in theory also result in an increased peri-operative bleeding risk. Moreover, it is unclear whether antifibrotic treatment, when effectively achieving disease stabilization for several months, would influence LAS or may even interfere with referral for LTx, given an upper age limit for LTx used in most centres.

In the current study we therefore report on safety and efficacy of pretransplant antifibrotics in IPF patients undergoing LTx. Pretransplant pulmonary function, functional exercise capacity; and immediate and long-term post-operative outcomes, including the early post-operative course, presence of bronchial anastomotic complications, chronic lung allograft dysfunction (CLAD) and survival, were retrospectively assessed.

Methods
Study design and population
This is a single-centre, retrospective analysis of IPF patients undergoing LTx in a large volume transplant centre at a tertiary care hospital. The current study was approved by the Leuven University Hospital Ethical Review Board (S51577) and patients gave informed consent. IPF diagnosis was confirmed in by a multidisciplinary board discussion, including

an expert chest physician specialized in interstitial lung disease (ILD) (WW), an experienced chest imaging radiologist and a specialized lung-pathologist (EKV). For the current study, we included all IPF patients up to December 2015 who had undergone LTx in our centre whilst being treated with either pirfenidone or nintedanib. There were no IPF patients receiving antifibrotic drugs who died on the waiting list before LTx.

Pirfenidone was initiated between September 2008 and September 2013; and patients were subsequently transplanted between November 2008 and April 2015. Nintedanib was started between August 2010 and January 2012; and patients were transplanted between March 2011 and October 2014. In Belgium, pirfenidone was approved for mild to moderate IPF (FVC >50%predicted (%pred) and Diffusion Capacity (DL_{CO}) >35%pred) in December 2012 and nintedanib has been approved for mild to severe IPF (FVC ≥50%pred and DL_{CO} ≥30%pred) since December 2015. Patients in whom antifibrotic therapy was initiated before these respective dates thus received the drugs in the context of clinical trials, thereafter patients received open-label treatment according to reimbursement rules. All IPF patients were evaluated on regular intervals (every 3 to 4 months) at a specialized outpatient ILD consultation by a specialized physician (WW) and nurse, who checked compliance and tolerance of their antifibrotic therapy.

Data collection
Data were retrospectively collected from the patients' electronical medical files, including clinical and demographical variables, duration of antifibrotic treatment, laboratory results, anastomotic problems (scored according to MDS classification as previously reported, [11]), evolution of pulmonary function and functional exercise capacity. The estimated annual decline in pulmonary function parameters (FVC, Total Lung Capacity (TLC) and DL_{CO}) was calculated based on the difference in pulmonary function parameters between the start of antifibrotic therapy ('baseline') and at the time of LTx, adjusted for the number of months therapy was taken (monthly decline) and extrapolated to 1 year (monthly decline x12). The same approach was used regarding the decrease in six minute walking test (6MWT) between start of therapy and LTx. LAS was retrospectively assessed at start of antifibrotic therapy, at LTx listing (data summarized in Table 1) and at LTx. However, we used LAS at start of antifibrotic therapy for further statistical analyses regarding pre-LTx evolution of LAS, because most patients were initiated on antifibrotics before LTx listing.

Historical controls
We additionally identified a comparable group of historical controls ($n = 6$), which consisted of IPF patients who

Table 1 Recipient and donor demographics of the IPF treatment group and historical control group

ID	Recipient Gender (M/F)	Recipient Age (Years)	Anti-fibrotic Drug	Cardio-Pulmonary Rehabilitation	Time on Therapy (Days)	FVC at start (%pred)	TLC at start (%pred)	DLco at start (%pred)	6MWT at start (m)	Time on WL (Days)	LAS at listing	Type of LTx (S/SS)	Donor Gender (M/F)	Donor Age (Years)	Type of Donor	CMV Donor/Recipient
1	F	62	PFD	no	735	91	72	46	529	762	32	SS	F	17	DBD	D+/R+
2	M	61	PFD	CPR	545	71	61	37	379	179	31	SS	F	67	DCD cat III	D-/R-
3	M	51	PFD	CPR	387	88	80	47	552	29	35	SS	M	37	DBD	D+/R-
4	M	63	PFD	CPR	539	52	45	32	384	51	30	SS	M	55	DBD	D-/R+
5	M	55	PFD	CPR	188	56	52	35	631	25	29	SS	M	23	DBD	D+/R-
6	M	64	PFD	no	115	62	48	39	503	163	33	SS	M	35	DCD cat V	D+/R+
7	M	64	PFD	no	65	79	56	28	267	419	37	S	F	42	DBD	D+/R-
8	M	65	NIN	no	1003	80	69	58	598	155	31	SS	M	62	DBD	D+/R-
9	M	56	NIN	no	194	58	56	29	275	74	32	SS	M	39	DCD cat III	D-/R-
Mean or Median		60.1 ± 4.9			419 ± 315	70.8 ± 14.5	59.9 ± 11.7	39.0 ± 9.8	457.6 ± 135.6	155 (40–299)	32.2 ± 2.5			43.6 ± 17.1		
1	M	57	/	no	/	/	/	/	/	279	33	SS	F	48	DCD cat III	D-/R+
2	M	62	/	no	/	/	/	/	/	153	35	SS	F	66	DBD	D+/R+
3	M	55	/	no	/	/	/	/	/	17	34	SS	M	74	DBD	D+/R+
4	M	59	/	CPR	/	/	/	/	/	274	32	SS	M	22	DCD cat III	D-/R+
5	M	59	/	CPR	/	/	/	/	/	253	29	SS	M	57	DBD	D-/R-
6	M	65	/	CPR	/	/	/	/	/	112	26	S	M	37	DBD	D+/R+
Mean or Median		59.5 ± 3.6[a]								203 (88–275)[a]	31.5 ± 3.4[a]			50.7 ± 19.[a]		

ID	Ischemic Time 1st/2nd Lung (min)	Immunosuppressive Regimen	Time to Extubation (Hours)	PGD at 72 h	Time on ICU (Days)	Time in Hospital (Days)	AR or LB Episodes (Number)	Most Severe AR or LB (Grade)	Respiratory infection before Discharge (Presence = 1)	Respiratory Pathogen before Discharge	Anastomotic Complications (Details in Text)
1	187/320	rATG/FK/MMF/CS	34	0	6	16	0	0	0	/	0
2	432/580	rATG/FK/MMF/CS	20	3	7	20	1	1	1	E. coli, S. viridans	M2aD0aS0 (POD 30)
3	498/694	No ATG, FK/MMF/CS	37	0	4	16	2	2	1	A. baumanii, E. coli, S. aureus	M3bD2cS2f (POD 204)
4	417/631		65	1	13	26	1	1	0	/	

Table 1 Recipient and donor demographics of the IPF treatment group and historical control group (Continued)

		rATG/FK/ MMF/CS									M2aD0aS0 (POD 30)
5	366/515	rATG/FK/ MMF/CS	41	2	6	17	0	0	1	C. freundii	0
6	385/582	rATG/FK/ MMF/CS	37	1	4	16	3	2	0	/	0
7	341	rATG/FK/ MMF/CS	33	2	3	21	0	0	1	H. influenza, MRSA	0
8	180/356	rATG/FK/ MMF/CS	178	3	10	28	1	3	1	H. influenza, S. pneumoniae	M1aD0aS0 (POD 90)
9	239/356	rATG/FK/ MMF/CS	38	2	5	23	1	2	0	/	0
	338 ± 113/504 ± 142		37 (33.5–53)	2 (0.5–2.5)	6.4 ± 3.2	20.3 ± 4.6	1 (0–1.5)	1 (0–2)			
1	404/626	rATG/FK/ MMF/CS	72	0	7	19	1	2	0	/	0
2	220/412	rATG/FK/ MMF/CS	16	1	7	25	2	3	1	S. aureus	M3bD0aS0 (POD 30)
3	288/431	rATG/FK/ MMF/CS	432	3	60	253	1	1	1	P. aeruginosa, K. pneumoniae,	M3bD2bS0 (POD 40)
4	276/423	rATG/FK/ MMF/CS	48	2	15	32	1	1	1	E. faecalis	M2aD0aS0 (POD 14)
5	209/439	rATG/CsA/ AZA/CS	48	2	23	32	0	0	1	K. oxytoca	M3aD0S0 (POD 17)
6	186	rATG/CsA/ AZA/CS	24	1	8	20	2	1	0	/	0
	264 ± 79[a]/466 ± 90[a]		48 (22–162)[a]	1.5 (0.8–2.3)[a]	20.0 ± 20.6[b]	63.5 ± 93[a]	1 (0.75–2.0)[a]	1 (0.75–2.25)[a]			

ID	Time of Follow-up (Months)	Status (Dead = 1)		Last FVC Post-LTx (%pred)	Last FEV$_1$ Post-LTx (%pred)	Last FEV$_1$/FVC Post-LTx (%pred)
1	7.7	0		145	147	86
2	8.6	0		106	90	66
3	16.9	0		70	68	77
4	21.9	0		90	67	58
5	25.8	0		93	93	80
6	27.1	0		123	126	79

Table 1 Recipient and donor demographics of the IPF treatment group and historical control group (Continued)

7	19.8	1	110	107	76
8	13.8	0	119	115	75
9	56.3	0	132	141	84
	19.8 (11.2–26.5)		109 ± 23.1	106 ± 29.1	75.7 ± 8.8
1	14.9	0	117	76	66
2	23.5	0	104	99	76
3	37.0	0	67	61	73
4	38.6	0	107	92	67
5	52.4	0	104	58	43
6	12.2	1	79	82	81
	30.3 (14.2–42.1)		96.3 ± 19.1	78.0 ± 16.4	67.7 ± 13.3

Data are expressed as mean ± SD, median (interquartile range) or as total values where appropriate

Abbreviations: *6MWT* 6 min walking test, *AR* Acute (cellular) Rejection, *AZA* azathioprine, *cat* category, *CMV* Cytomegalovirus, *CPR* Cardio-Pulmonary Rehabilitation, *CS* corticosteroids, *CsA* cyclosporine A, *D* donor, *DBD* donation after brain death, *DCD* donation after cardiac death, *DLCO* diffusion capacity, *F* Female, *FK* tacrolimus, *FVC* Forced Vital Capacity, *ICU* Intensive Care Unit, *ID* identification, *LAS* lung allocation score, *LB* lymphocytic bronchiolitis, *LTx* lung transplantation, *M* male, *MDS* severity of anastomotic complication according to MDS classification, *MMF* mycophenolate mofetil, *NIN* nintedanib, *PFD* pirfenidone, *PGD* primary graft dysfunction, *R* recipient, *rATG* rabbit Anti-Thymocyte Globulin, *S* single, *SS* sequential single, *TLC* Total Lung Capacity, *WL* waiting list

[a]*p* > 0.05 (not statistically significant compared to treated group). [b]*p* = 0.021 compared to treated group

did not receive antifibrotic therapy before LTx, but were transplanted in the same era (7/2010 to 9/2014), had comparable age and lung function at the time of LTx compared to the treatment group: FVC 57.0 (43.0–69.8) %pred ($p = 0.69$ vs. treatment), TLC 53.0 (42.5–71.0) %pred ($p = 1.0$ vs. treatment) and DL_{CO} 21.5 (17.0–29.2) %pred ($p = 0.11$ vs. treatment). Given the small number of available patients, it was impossible to match both groups any further regarding concurrent emphysema (but TLC and DL_{CO} were comparable between both groups, thus excluding major differences due to emphysema), pulmonary hypertension (was not routinely assessed in non-treated IPF patients, no comparison possible with treated group who were all screened at start of antifibrotic therapy) or cardiovascular disease (but major cardiovascular disease is generally an exclusion-criterion to proceed to LTx in any patient). Reasons for not starting antifibrotic therapy in these matched historical controls were: absence of consent ($n = 3$), DL_{CO} too low for study-inclusion ($n = 2$) and pending approval by the health care authorities whilst awaiting LTx ($n = 1$). These historical controls were only used as comparator for the IPF group treated with antifibrotics regarding the annual pre-transplant decline in pulmonary function; and some mportant early post-transplant outcome parameters, including rates of PGD, infection, rejection and anastomotic complications. These historical patients were not the main aim of this study, which focusses on reporting safety and efficacy of antifibrotics in IPF patients undergoing LTx.

Statistical analysis

All analyses were performed using Graphpad Prism 5a software (San Diego, USA). Results are expressed as mean (± standard deviation) or median (interquartile range) where appropriate. Group means were compared using paired or unpaired t-test; Mann-Whitney test or Wilcoxon signed rank test for normally or not-normally distributed variables, respectively. All reported p-values are two-tailed and $p < 0.05$ was considered significant.

Results

Patients' characteristics

A total of 9 IPF patients were treated with antifibrotics and subsequently underwent LTx: pirfenidone $n = 7$ ($n = 2$ study vs. $n = 5$ open-label treatment), nintedanib $n = 2$ (both in study). All patients, but one, underwent bilateral LTx and all, but one, were male. Age at LTx was 60.1 ± 4.9 years. Five patients were on continuous oxygen therapy (4 (3.5–4.0) Liters/min) before LTx, while 4 were not (Table 1). Antifibrotic therapy had been initiated 362 (152–578) days before listing for LTx in 6/9 patients, whereas in 3/9 patients antifibrotics were started 48 (27–354) days after transplant listing. In all 9 cases

antifibrotic therapy was continued until the day of transplant procedure. Total duration of antifibrotic therapy until LTx was 419 ± 315 days, or 13.8 ± 10.3 months. All patients received the full, recommended dose (i.e. 801 mg tid for pirfenidone and 150 mg bid for nintedanib).

Nausea was reported as main side-effect of antifibrotic therapy in 9/9 patients; and 7/9 patients lost weight during treatment ($n = 6$ pirfenidone, $n = 1$ nintedanib), in one patient (on pirfenidone) weight remained stable and one patient (on nintedanib) gained 1 kg. Overall, body mass index (BMI) decreased from 27.3 ± 3.2 kg/m^2 to 25.8 ± 3.3 kg/m^2 ($p = 0.0063$) during antifibrotic treatment, with an absolute weight loss of 329 ± 360 g per month of treatment ($p = 0.0062$). None of the patients developed toxic hepatitis, nor discontinued their therapy due to other severe side-effects or adverse events. No acute IPF exacerbations occurred in any of the patients during antifibrotic treatment.

Evolution of pretransplant pulmonary function, functional exercise capacity, pulmonary hypertension, renal function and LAS

Spirometry was performed at the start of antifibrotic treatment ('baseline') and during subsequent follow-up. Consecutive spirometry after six months of antifibrotic therapy was only available in 6/9 patients, as 3 patients ($n = 2$ pirfenidone, $n = 1$ nintedanib) underwent LTx within 6 months after initiating therapy (Fig. 1). In these 6/9 patients ($n = 5$ pirfenidone, $n = 1$ nintedanib), the absolute decline in FVC *after 12 weeks* of treatment compared to baseline was −7.0%pred (−1.8 to −11.5), with 4/6 (66.6%) patients having <10% decline in FVC %pred; and only 2/6 (33.3%) patients demonstrating a ≥10% decline in FVC %pred ($p = 0.063$ vs. start). Nevertheless, an overall absolute decrease in FVC, TLC and DL_{CO} during the *whole* pretransplant antifibrotic treatment period (i.e. 419 ± 315 days or 59 ± 44 weeks) was observed in these 6/9 patients (Fig. 2).

The calculated *annual* decline during treatment for all included patients was: FVC 322.0 (148.3–1074.0) mL or 6.6 (0–23.8) %pred, TLC 360.0 (157.5–1818.0) mL or 6.0 (2.0–25.7) %pred; and DL_{CO} 0.77 (0.40–1.96) mmol/min/Kpa or 7.5 (4.7–18.6) %pred. Interestingly, the measured annual rate of decline in the matched historical controls (without antifibrotic therapy) during the year preceding LTx appeared to be somewhat more severe compared to the group with antifibrotics, although no significant differences were seen: FVC 460.0 (215.0–732.5) mL or 13.0 (4.8–18.0) %pred ($p = 0.69$); TLC 945.0 mL (362.5–1490) or 10.0%pred (2.0–20.0) ($p = 1.0$); and DL_{CO} 1.26 (0.38–2.09) mmol/min/Kpa or 14.0 (4.0–24.8) %pred ($p = 0.94$).

6MWT was performed before the start of antifibrotic therapy and consecutive 6MWT was available in 5/9

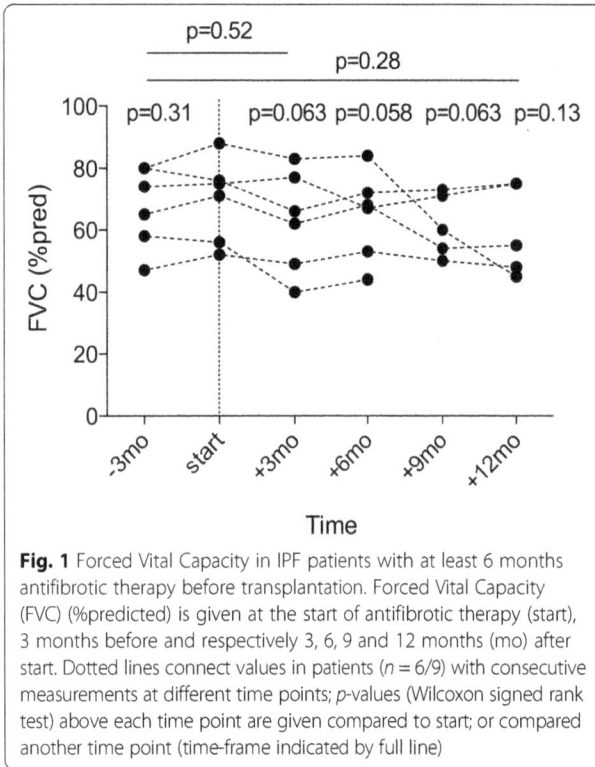

Fig. 1 Forced Vital Capacity in IPF patients with at least 6 months antifibrotic therapy before transplantation. Forced Vital Capacity (FVC) (%predicted) is given at the start of antifibrotic therapy (start), 3 months before and respectively 3, 6, 9 and 12 months (mo) after start. Dotted lines connect values in patients ($n = 6/9$) with consecutive measurements at different time points; p-values (Wilcoxon signed rank test) above each time point are given compared to start; or compared another time point (time-frame indicated by full line)

patients (all on pirfenidone), of whom 3/5 were enrolled in a pretransplant cardio-pulmonary rehabilitation (CPR) program upon transplant listing and 2/5 were not. 6MWT overall increased with 54 (−260.0–95.5) m *after 12 weeks* of treatment compared to baseline ($p = 0.62$), with an improved in 4/5 patients of 74.5 (21.8–95.8) m, while one patient demonstrated a decline of 531 m (patient n°5 in Table 1, no CPR, concomitant decline in FVC of 12%pred during these 12 weeks of treatment). During the *whole* pretransplant time period of antifibrotic treatment (59 ± 44 weeks), 6MWT did not significantly change compared to baseline ($p = 0.89$): 6MWT improved compared to baseline in 2/5 patients (+63 m (no CPR) and +142 m (with CPR), respectively), while 6MWT deteriorated in 3/5 patients (one no CPR, two with CPR), in whom there was an absolute decline of −172 (34–531) meters or a *monthly* decline of −5.2 (2.7–85.7) meters during treatment (Fig. 2). In the historical controls, unfortunately, 6MWD was only available upon listing for LTx, thus no consecutive 6MWT were available for further comparison.

Transthoracic echocardiography performed before start of antifibrotic therapy (pulmonary arterial pressure (PAP) 31.1 ± 7.4 mmHg) and consecutive echocardiography was available in 4/9 patients, in whom PAP tended to increase during antifibrotic treatment (PAP +9.5 (2.0–15.5) mmHg: $p = 0.090$). Renal function remained stable during antifibrotic treatment: serum creatinine was 0.96 ± 0.14 mg/dL at start versus $0.95 \pm$ 0.17 mg/dL at LTx ($p = 0.97$), estimated glomerular filtration rate was 83 ± 13 mL/min/1.73 m^2 at start versus 82 ± 14 mL/min/1.73 m^2 at LTx ($p = 0.83$). No hepatic dysfunction was observed in any patient during treatment. LAS did not significantly change during antifibrotic treatment: 32.2 ± 2.5 at start of therapy versus 32.3 ± 1.0 at LTx ($p = 0.13$).

Post-transplant outcomes

Patients receiving antifibrotics were listed for 155 (40–299) days before subsequent LTx. Transplant procedures were overall uneventful and only one patient (who had received pirfenidone, had the highest pretransplant PAP of 48 mmHg and underwent single sided LTx) required peri-operative support with veno-arterial extracorporeal membrane oxygenation. There were no bleeding problems (i.e. no need for re-thoracotomy for hemothorax, no additional transfusion of blood products for blood loss) in any patient, including those on nintedanib. Overall, patients were extubated after 37.0 (33.5–53.0) hours of ventilation, discharged from the intensive care unit after 6.4 ± 3.2 days and discharged home after a hospital stay of 20.3 ± 4.6 days. There were no problems with postoperative thoracic wound healing or dehiscence in any patient. All patients, but one, received post-operative induction therapy with anti-thymocyte globulin for 3 days; and post-operative immunosuppressive regimen consisted of tacrolimus, mycophenolate mofetil and steroids in all patients, except one (transplanted in 2008) who received cyclosporine, azathioprine and steroids (our standard regimen before 2010). No major side effects due to possible drug-interactions with prior antifibrotics were seen in the first days post-LTx.

A total of 4/9 patients were included in a clinical trial immediately following LTx: 2 in a therapeutic trial with azithromycin (AZI003, NCT01915082), 1 in an ex-vivo normothermic machine perfusion trial (EXPANDLung, NCT01963780) and 1 in a Diaphragm Pacing trial (NCT02411383), which may obviously influence early and/or late outcomes (including post-transplant evolution of pulmonary function, anastomotic airway complications, primary graft dysfunction (PGD), rejection, infection, CLAD) in these transplant recipients compared to those not included in a trial or historical controls. Overall, incidence of PGD (PGD ≥ 2 in 5/9 patients), early post-operative infection (5/9 patients) and acute cellular rejection (4/9 patients) or lymphocytic bronchiolitis (4/9) during the first 6 months were comparable to findings in the historical controls (all $p > 0.5$) (Table 1).

Anastomotic airway complications were present in 4/9 patients: in two patients (prior pirfenidone) mild anastomotic necrosis without dehiscence or airway narrowing was noted upon discharge after LTx (post-operative day

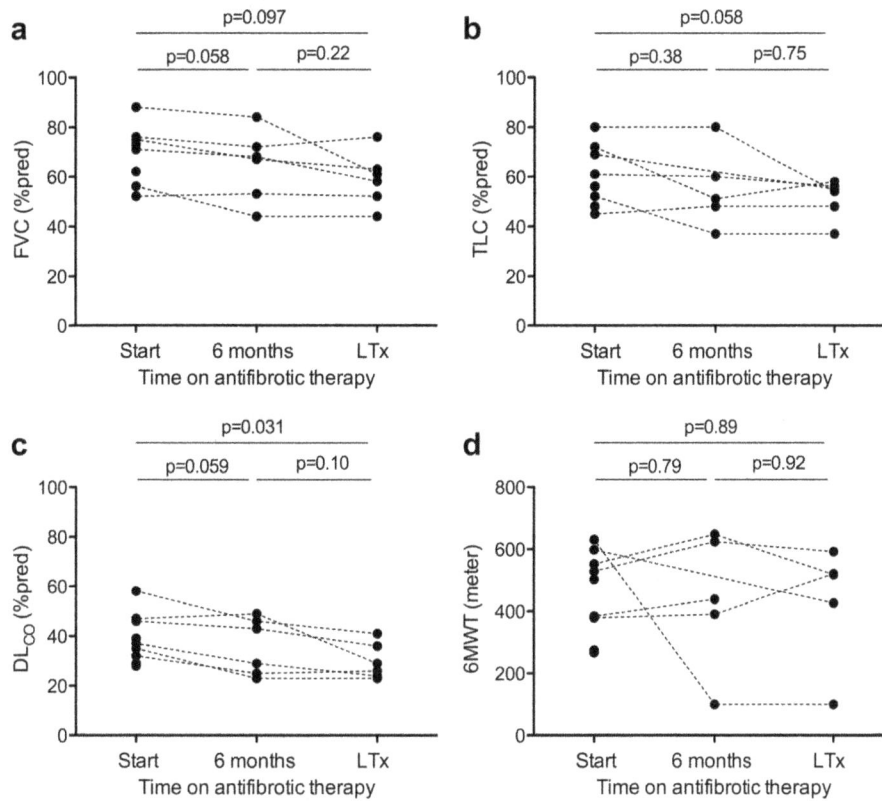

Fig. 2 Pretransplant evolution of pulmonary function and functional exercise capacity following treatment with antifibrotic drugs. Forced Vital Capacity (FVC) (**a**), Total Lung Capacity (TLC) (**b**), Diffusion capacity (DL$_{CO}$) (**c**) (all in (%predicted) and 6 min walk test (6MWT, meter) (**d**) at start of antifibrotic therapy (start) and at the moment of lung transplantation (LTx) in the included IPF patients. Dotted lines connect values in patients (n = 6/9) with a consecutive measurement at six months and just before transplantation; p-values (Wilcoxon signed rank test) are given for patients that had consecutive measurements

(POD) 30; MDS classification M2aD0aS0 for right-sided anastomosis and M0aD0aS0 for left-sided anastomosis in both patients), with spontaneous and uncomplicated resolution thereafter. In a third patient (initially no anastomotic complications, prior nintedanib), there was mild protrusion of cartilage on POD 90 (M0aD0aS0 for right-sided anastomosis and M1aD0aS0 for left-sided anastomosis), with spontaneous and uncomplicated resolution thereafter. In the fourth patient (initially no anastomotic complications, prior pirfenidone), following infection with *Aspergillus fumigatus* at POD 186, late-onset (POD 204) anastomotic necrosis occurred with bronchial narrowing and extensive dehiscence (M0aD0aS0 for right-sided anastomosis and M3bD2cS2f for left-sided anastomosis). Despite antifungal treatment, he developed severe symptomatic anastomotic stenosis, which finally required surgical sleeve-resection and reconstruction of the left main bronchus on POD 410. Thereafter, no other problems occurred and the patient currently has a stable pulmonary function at POD 525. The observed anastomotic airway complications, however, did not appear to be more severe or prevalent compared to previously reported data from our centre [11] or to the historical controls, of whom

4/6 controls had early anastomotic airway complications (ranging from M2aD0aS0 to M3bD2bS0; Table 1).

Overall, long-term outcome in our cohort was good: after a median follow-up of 19.8 (11.2–26.5) months, currently all patients have a stable pulmonary function (Table 1) and none of the patients has developed CLAD. One patient (who underwent single sided LTx), unfortunately, has died because of non-squamous large cell lung carcinoma of his native IPF lung on POD 615, all other patients are alive and ambulatory at present. Overall survival was 100% after 1 year and 80% after 2 years, respectively.

Discussion

Little is known about safety of antifibrotic therapy with pirfenidone or nintedanib in patients undergoing LTx. Actually only 11 IPF patients receiving pirfenidone; and none receiving nintedanib, included in the large randomized trials with these drugs (comprising a total of 2832 study-subjects) were reported as having been transplanted during antifibrotic treatment, yet detailed outcome data for these patients are lacking [3–7]. Only 1 case report has currently been published on pretransplant pharmacological bridging with pirfeni-done, allowing stabilization of respiratory function and subsequent single sided LTx in IPF. Anastomic airway complications, however, were not reported in this case [12]. Next to this, there have been two abstracts report-ing on this topic, which did not yet result in peer-reviewed papers, but in which, apparently, pirfenidone therapy was not linked to adverse post-transplant events, however follow-up was limited and detailed outcome data missing [13, 14]. In the current case series, we therefore report on pre-operative evolution and post-transplant outcomes of 9 IPF patients, treated with either pirfenidone or nintedanib for a mean of 13.4 months until subsequent LTx and with a median post-transplant follow-up of 19.8 months.

According to the same definitions used in larger IPF trials [6, 15], we noted relative stabilization (i.e. < 10% change) of FVC during the first 12 weeks of antifibrotic treatment. Importantly, this early stabilization, or per-haps better attenuated rate of decline, in FVC may by no means be a reason to deny subsequent LTx to eligible patients, because further decline in FVC, lung volumina and DL_{CO} is to be expected despite antifibrotic treat-ment, as was obvious from our results. The estimated annual decline in FVC during treatment in our cohort, however, would be around 6.6%pred, which corroborates recent findings that both pirfenidone and nintedanib re-duce the proportion of patients with a ≥10% decline in FVC %pred after 1 year of treatment [5, 6]. As they may attenuate disease progression, these antifibrotics may thus allow for valuable added time on the LTx waiting list. Next to FVC, 6MWT has also been shown to be a valid outcome measure, both in IPF, in whom the clinic-ally important difference in 6MWT distance is reported to be 24–45 m [3–5] and in whom 6MWT is associated with changes in pulmonary function and quality-of-life [16]; and in patients awaiting LTx, in whom it is associ-ated with post-transplant survival [17]. A reduction of the decline in 6MWT was also observed in treated pa-tients compared to placebo in pooled analyses of IPF tri-als [3–5], which may partly explain why 6MWT overall remained relatively stable during treatment in our co-hort, next to the obvious beneficial effects of cardio-pulmonary rehabilitation is some patients. Although the LAS is actually not used in Belgium for prioritizing organ allocation, the calculated LAS (which includes FVC and 6MWT among other parameters) did not sig-nificantly change during pretransplant antifibrotic treat-ment in our cohort. An average LAS of 32 at the time of LTx in our study may seem fairly low for IPF patients, yet LAS was quite comparable between our treated patients and historical controls; and was in the same range (median of ±35) as previously described for IPF patients at LTx listing [18]. We therefore believe that

our cohort indeed reflects the general population of IPF patients transplanted during the past 5–10 years. How-ever, in the last few years, as seen in the US, an increase in LAS is also noted in our centre, with more sicker pa-tients (LAS > 40) being listed for LTx [19].

No serious side effects were noted during antifibrotic therapy. However, significant weight loss occurred, which is most likely due to drug-induced anorexia or possibly due to respiratory cachexia in end-stage lung disease. Post-operatively, no problems with bleeding or thoracic wound healing were observed. One patient, treated with nintedanib; and three patients who had received pirfeni-done developed, mostly mild and uneventful, anastomic airway complications. Intervention for anastomotic sten-osis was needed for one case, which only occurred late-onset after prior fungal infection. Overall, it is unlikely that any of these anastomotic problems were directly related to prior antifibrotic treatment given the time of onset/clinical context of anastomotic complications, comparable anasto-motic problems in the historical controls; and rather short half-life of both drugs (for pirfenidone 3 h, for nintedanib 9.5 h) [20, 21]. The short half-life of both antifibrotic drugs is important, as drug-interactions with calcine-urin inhibitors, by altered hepatic (CYP3A4) metaboli-sation leading to changes in tacrolimus/cyclosporine trough levels, are a feared iatrogenic adverse event in LTx. However, hepatic metabolism of pirfenidone primarily oc-curs through the CYP1A2 enzyme; whereas nintedanib is mainly a substrate of P-glycoprotein (P-gp) and only weakly interferes with CYP3A4. This probably also ex-plains why no major side effects due to drug-interactions with peri-operatively used drugs were noted in our cohort. Finally, long-term outcomes regarding pulmonary func-tion and overall survival were overall good in our current case series, suggesting that antifibrotic agents can prob-ably be safely given without deleterious effects on peri-operative or medium-term outcomes.

Possible limitations of the current study, of course, are its retrospective design, the small number of included patients; and historical controls as comparator for some outcomes, which of course limits interpretations regarding antifibrotic drug efficacy and safety. Also, disease severity ranged from mild to severe IPF, which may bias the observed effects of pretransplant antifibrotic therapy; and post-transplant evo-lution, including pulmonary function, may be biased by in-clusion of some patients in various randomized clinical trials. Larger, preferably prospective, case-series are there-fore undeniably needed to confirm our findings, especially for nintedanib additional safety data are needed before fir-mer conclusions can be made regarding its safety.

Conclusion

In summary, we conclude that antifibrotic drugs are prob-ably safe in IPF patients undergoing LTx. By attenuating disease progression while awaiting LTx, these antifibrotics may perhaps further help to reduce the number of IPF patients dying on the waiting list.

Abbreviations

6MWT: Six minute walking test; BMI: Body mass index; CLAD: Chronic lung allograft dysfunction; CPR: Cardio-pulmonary rehabilitation; DLCO: Diffusion capacity; FDA: Food and Drug Administration; FGF: Fibroblast growth factor; FVC: Forced vital capacity; ILD: Interstitial lung disease; IPF: Idiopathic pulmonary fibrosis; LAS: Lung allocation score; LTx: Lung transplantation; MDS: Macroscopic Diameter Sutures (MDS Classification); PDGF: Platelet-derived growth factor; PGD: Primary graft dysfunction; POD: Post-operative day; TGF- β: Transforming growth factor –beta; TLC: Total lung capacity; UIP: Usual interstitial pneumonia; VEGF: Vascular endothelial growth factor

Acknowledgments

Not applicable.

Funding

RV is supported by the Starting Grant (STG/15/023) and JY is supported by the Clinical Research Fund (KOF), UZLeuven, Belgium. WW and RV are senior research fellows of the Research Foundation Flanders (FWO), Belgium (12G8715N). GMV is supported by the FWO (G.0723.10, G.0679.12 and G.0679.12).

Competing interests

The authors declare that they have no competing interests.
The authors confirm that that the work described has not been published previously, that it is not under consideration for publication elsewhere, that its publication is approved by all authors and tacitly or explicitly by the responsible authorities where the work was carried out, and that, if accepted, it will not be published elsewhere in the same form in English or in any other language, without the written consent of the copyright holder.

Authors' contributions

ID: performed data collection, wrote the paper and helped with its critical appraisal. WW: is responsible ILD physician during pretransplant period and helped with critical appraisal of the manuscript. JY: is responsible ILD physician during pretransplant period and helped with critical appraisal of the manuscript. EV: is responsible ILD pathologist during pretransplant period and helped with critical appraisal of the manuscript. GV: is responsible ILD physician during pretransplant period and responsible LTx physician during post-LTx period, helped with critical appraisal of the manuscript. RV: is responsible LTx physician during post-LTx period, performed design of the study, data collection, statistical analyses, and helped with critical appraisal of the manuscript. All authors read and approved the final manuscript.

Author details

[1]Department of Respiratory Diseases, Interstitial Lung Disease and Lung Transplant Unit, University Hospitals Leuven, Leuven, Belgium. [2]KULeuven, Department of Clinical and Experimental Medicine, Division of Respiratory Diseases, Laboratory of Respiratory Diseases, Lung Transplantation Unit, KU Leuven, Herestraat 49, B-3000 Leuven, Belgium. [3]KULeuven, Department of Histopathology, Leuven, Belgium.

References

1. Raghu G, Collard HR, Egan JJ, Martinez FJ, Behr J, Brown KK, et al. ATS/ERS/JRS/ALAT Committee on Idiopathic Pulmonary Fibrosis. An official ATS/ERS/JRS/ALAT statement: idiopathic pulmonary fibrosis: evidence-based guidelines for diagnosis and management. Am J Respir Crit Care Med. 2011;183(6):788–824.
2. National Clinical Guideline Centre (UK). Diagnosis and management of suspected idiopathic pulmonary fibrosis: idiopathic pulmonary fibrosis, National Institute for Health and Care Excellence: clinical guidelines. London: Royal College of Physicians (UK); 2013.
3. Noble PW, Albera C, Bradford WZ, Costabel U, Glassberg MK, Kardatzke D, CAPACITY Study Group, et al. Pirfenidone in patients with idiopathic pulmonary fibrosis (CAPACITY): two randomised trials. Lancet. 2011; 377(9779):1760–9.
4. King Jr TE, Bradford WZ, Castro-Bernardini S, Fagan EA, Glaspole I, Glassberg MK, ASCEND Study Group, et al. A phase 3 trial of pirfenidone in patients with idiopathic pulmonary fibrosis. N Engl J Med. 2014;370(22):2083–92.
5. Richeldi L, du Bois RM, Raghu G, Azuma A, Brown KK, Costabel U, INPULSIS Trial Investigators, et al. Efficacy and safety of nintedanib in idiopathic pulmonary fibrosis. N Engl J Med. 2014;370(22):2071–82.
6. Noble PW, Albera C, Bradford WZ, Costabel U, du Bois RM, Fagan EA, et al. Pirfenidone for idiopathic pulmonary fibrosis: analysis of pooled data from three multinational phase 3 trials. Eur Respir J. 2016;47(1):243–53.
7. Mazzei ME, Richeldi L, Collard HR. Nintedanib in the treatment of idiopathic pulmonary fibrosis. Ther Adv Respir Dis. 2015;9(3):121–9.
8. Kistler KD, Nalysnyk L, Rotella P, Esser D. Lung transplantation in idiopathic pulmonary fibrosis: a systematic review of the literature. BMC Pulm Med. 2014;14:139.
9. Conte E, Gili E, Fagone E, Fruciano M, Iemmolo M, Vancheri C. Effect of pirfenidone on proliferation, TGF-β-induced myofibroblast differentiation and fibrogenic activity of primary human lung fibroblasts. Eur J Pharm Sci. 2014;58:13–9.
10. Wollin L, Wex E, Pautsch A, Schnapp G, Hostettler KE, Stowasser S, et al. Mode of action of nintedanib in the treatment of idiopathic pulmonary fibrosis. Eur Respir J. 2015;45(5):1434–45.
11. Yserbyt J, Dooms C, Vos R, Dupont LJ, Van Raemdonck DE, Verleden GM. Anastomotic airway complications after lung transplantation: risk factors, treatment modalities and outcome-a single-centre experience. Eur J Cardiothorac Surg. 2016;49(1):e1–8.
12. Paone G, Sebastiani A, Ialleni E, Diso D, Rose D, Quagliarini F, et al. A combined therapeutic approach in progressive idiopathic pulmonary fibrosis-pirfenidone as bridge therapy for ex vivo lung transplantation: a case report. Transplant Proc. 2015;47(3):855–7.
13. Riddell P, Minnis P, Ging P, Egan JJ. Pirfenidone as a bridge to lung transplantation in patients with progressive IPF. Thorax. 2014;69:A183.
14. Mortensen A, Cherrier L, Walia R. Lung transplantation on pirfenidone: a single center experience. J Heart Lung Transplant. 2016;35(4S):883.
15. Taniguchi H, Kondoh Y, Ebina M, Azuma A, Ogura T, Taguchi Y, Pirfenidone Clinical Study Group in Japan, et al. The clinical significance of 5% change in vital capacity in patients with idiopathic pulmonary fibrosis: extended analysis of the pirfenidone trial. Respir Res. 2011;12:93.
16. Nathan SD, du Bois RM, Albera C, Bradford WZ, Costabel U, Kartashov A, et al. Validation of test performance characteristics and minimal clinically important difference of the 6-min walk test in patients with idiopathic pulmonary fibrosis. Respir Med. 2015;109(7):914–22.
17. Castleberry AW, Englum BR, Snyder LD, Worni M, Osho AA, Gulack BC, et al. The utility of preoperative six-minute-walk distance in lung transplantation. Am J Respir Crit Care Med. 2015;192(7):843–52.
18. Egan TM, Murray S, Bustami RT, Shearon TH, McCullough KP, Edwards LB, et al. Development of the new lung allocation system in the United States. Am J Transplant. 2006;6(5 Pt 2):1212–27.
19. Egan TM, Edwards LB. Effect of the lung allocation score on lung transplantation in the United States. J Heart Lung Transplant. 2016;35(4): 433–9.
20. ESBRIET® (pirfenidone) hard capsules, for oral use. electronic Medicines Compendium. Genentech. Accessed 12 Dec 2015.
21. OFEV® (nintedanib) capsules, for oral use. electronic Medicines Compendium. Boehringer Ingelheim. Accessed 12 Dec 2015.

21

Corticosteroids in treatment of aspiration-related acute respiratory distress syndrome

Jiang-nan Zhao[1], Yao Liu[2] and Huai-chen Li[2*]

Abstract

Background: Acute stroke patients suffering from aspiration may present with acute respiratory distress syndrome (ARDS). There is still a lack of convincing data about the efficacy of corticosteroids in the treatment of aspiration-related ARDS. Therefore, we evaluated the clinical impact of corticosteroids on aspiration-related ARDS.

Methods: Between 2012 and 2014, we conducted a retrospective study among acute stroke patients diagnosed with aspiration-related ARDS. The data analyzed included demographic characteristics, clinical manifestations, laboratory examinations, chest imaging, and hospital discharge status.

Results: Seventy-three acute stroke patients were diagnosed with aspiration-related ARDS. The hospital mortality rate was 39.7 %. Corticosteroids were administered in 47 patients (64.4 %). The mean dosage was 1.14 (standard deviation [SD] 0.47) mg/kg daily of methylprednisolone (or an equivalent) by intravenous infusion for a period of 7.3 (SD 3.8) days. Ground glass opacities in chest computed tomography images were resolved when corticosteroids were administered. The admission National Institute of Health Stroke Scale score (odds ratio [OR] 5.17, 95 % confidence interval [CI] 1.27–10.64) and Acute Physiology and Chronic Health Evaluation II score (OR 2.00, 95 % CI 1.12–3.56) were associated with an increased risk of hospital mortality, while albumin (OR 0.81, 95 % CI 0.64–0.92) and corticosteroids therapy (OR 0.50, 95 % CI 0.35–0.70) were associated with a decreased risk.

Conclusions: Low-dose and short-term corticosteroid therapy may have an impact on survival in aspiration-related ARDS. The presence of ground glass opacities on the chest computed tomography, performed to rule out aspiration-related ARDS, could be translated into an increased possibility of positive response to corticosteroid therapy.

Background

Aspiration of oropharyngeal or gastric contents flowing into the lower respiratory tract may result in several pulmonary diseases [1–3], such as airway obstruction, aspiration lung abscess, aspiration pneumonia, aspiration pneumonitis, and even acute respiratory distress syndrome (ARDS) [3, 4]. Among stroke patients, ARDS caused by aspiration is a major cause of death. The early diagnosis of aspiration-related ARDS is crucial to improve patient outcomes, as well as to choose the optimal treatment, including mechanical ventilation

settings [5, 6]. Little is known about the clinical features and outcomes of aspiration-related ARDS.

Because dysregulated inflammation is the cardinal feature of ARDS [7, 8], it seems to be a rational choice to use corticosteroids as part of the treatment. In the early 1980s, clinical investigators found that the inflammatory exudation in patients with ARDS could be decreased with systemic corticosteroid therapy [9]. Meduri and colleagues found that peripheral blood leukocytes, which are exposed to plasma from patients with ARDS, can produce inflammatory cytokines. If methylprednisolone was given to these patients, the inflammation reaction could be reduced [10]. Conversely, Sukumaran and colleagues found that patients who were given corticosteroids experienced longer stay in the intensive care unit. However, there were no significant differences in the outcome [11]. Moreover,

* Correspondence: zjn911016@126.com
[2]Department of Respiratory Medicine, Shandong Provincial Hospital Affiliated to Shandong University, Jinan, Shandong 250021, China
Full list of author information is available at the end of the article

in a case–control study, patients treated with corticosteroids were more easily infected by gram-negative bacteria and developed pneumonia more frequently [12].

In current clinical practice, systemic corticosteroids are often used as part of the treatment of aspiration-related ARDS, depending on the discretion of individual pulmonologist. However, the effect of systemic corticosteroids on the prognosis of the disease has not yet been revealed. Therefore, we conducted a retrospective study of acute stroke patients with aspiration-related ARDS aiming to evaluate the efficacy of corticosteroids and to identify predictors of hospital mortality.

Methods

The study was approved by the Ethics Committee of Shandong Provincial Hospital, Shandong Province, China. Patient records were anonymized and de-identified prior to analysis.

Our study was a retrospective single-center study that included about 2986 consecutive acute stroke patients admitted to the adult medical neurology department between 1 January 2012 and 31 July 2014. All patients were selected at the Shandong Provincial Hospital, a tertiary-care, university-affiliated hospital. To be eligible, all acute stroke patients had to meet all of the following criteria [13, 14]: (1) aged 18 years or older; (2) diagnosed with rapidly developed clinical signs of cerebral function disturbance of vascular origin, and classified based on results from the first brain scan into cerebral infarct, intracerebral hemorrhage, and subarachnoid hemorrhage, according to the World Health Organization definition; (3) presented within 24 h of the onset of acute stroke; (4) confirmed by head computerized tomography (CT) or brain magnetic resonance imaging (MRI).

Inclusion criteria

For inclusion, the following clinical signs and symptoms after the episode of aspiration had to be present: (1) a subjective worsening of dyspnea, development of hypoxia with pulse oxygen saturation (SPO2) < 90 mmHg, radiographic pulmonary abnormalities presented by chest radiography or CT that were reviewed by two radiologists; (2) or abnormal breath sounds, fever ($\geq$37.5 °C) or leukocytosis; (3) or requirement for intensive care (defined as the use of mechanical ventilation or the need for treatment with vasopressors against shock). To be included, all patients had to conform to the first item. Either the aspiration (following an episode of dysphagia, choking, vomiting or regurgitation) had been observed, or gastric contents had been suctioned from the endotracheal tube following intubation. Although, it is difficult to monitor the occurrence of aspiration, if one person with healthy lungs showed the above mentioned clinical symptoms, we considered aspiration as the root cause. After the diagnosis of aspiration-related lung injury, all patients were managed by both neurologists and pulmonologists.

The diagnosis of ARDS was established by the treating physician, and it was based on the Berlin definition [8]. Aspiration-related ARDS was defined as ARDS developed after aspiration. Other etiologies of ARDS such as sepsis, major trauma, multiple transfusions, pulmonary contusion, and acute pancreatitis were excluded. Conditions in which patients frequently have hypoxia and diffuse pulmonary infiltration, such as pulmonary edema, congestive heart failure, interstitial lung disease, active tuberculosis, radiation pneumonitis, pulmonary infiltration with eosinophilia, widespread infection, pulmonary alveolar hemorrhage alveolar proteinosis, bronchioloalveolar cell carcinoma were also ruled out.

Exclusion criteria

Patients with the following conditions were excluded: nosocomial pneumonia; severe immunosuppression (Acquired Immune Deficiency Syndrome (AIDS), use of immuno-suppressant such as cytotoxic drugs, cyclosporine, monoclonal antibodies, among others); preexisting medical condition with life expectancy lower than 3 months (i.e., malignancy); pregnancy; major gastrointestinal bleeding (GIB) within 3 months of the current hospitalization; acute asthma, chronic obstructive pulmonary disease or autoimmune disorders (i.e., any condition requiring more than 0.5 mg/kg/day of prednisone equivalent); and hepatic cirrhosis.

Data collection

For the present study, the following data were analyzed: age, sex, National Institutes of Health Stroke Scale (NIHSS) score on admission, Glasgow Coma Scale (GCS) score on admission, smoking history, excess alcohol consumption ($\geq$2 standard alcohol beverages per day), preexisting comorbidities (hypertension, diabetes, coronary heart disease, liver disease, kidney disease, among others), clinical symptoms on admission and new symptoms and signs after admission, PaO_2/FiO_2, mechanical devices (invasive/non-invasive mechanical ventilation used after admission for unsolved hypoxia despite of high-flow oxygen), time from diagnosis to corticosteroid therapy, chest radiological findings, and Acute Physiology and Chronic Health Evaluation II (APACHE II) score for patients with ARDS, laboratory indices (routine blood counts, liver function indicators, routing chemistry tests laboratory, blood gas analysis, and others), hospital length-of-stay (LOS) (days), hospital discharge status (survivor, dead). All data were extracted from the electronic medical record (EMR) system by trained research coordinators.

Corticosteroid therapy

The dose and administration intervals of corticosteroid therapy were collected from EMR records. Patient response to treatment and outcome were evaluated by the following criteria: decrease in respiratory rate (≤ 20/min), increase in oxygenation at rest and sleep ($SPO_2 \geq$ 90 mmHg), and improvement in chest CT images.

The commonly expected adverse events included new infection, hyperglycemia with additional glucose-lowering therapy, GIB, and neuromyopathic complications. A new infection was defined as an infection, not present or incubating before the administration of corticosteroids. Infections sites included pulmonary, blood, urinary, skin wound and other organs/tissues. Pulmonary infection was indicated by newly emerging increase in temperature, leukocytosis, radiological abnormalities, and decline in PaO_2 compared with the initial observations (before the administration of corticosteroid therapy).

Statistical analysis

Continuous variables were summarized with mean and standard deviation (SD); categorical variables were summarized as proportions. In univariate analysis, a X^2 test was used to compare categorical variables, and a t test with equal variance was used to compare continuous variables. To identify independent factors that were associated with hospital mortality, multivariate logistic regression analysis was used. The adjusted odds ratios (OR) and the 95 % confidence interval (CI) and P values for individual variables were obtained using a logistic regression model. $P < 0.05$ was considered statistically significant. All analyses were performed with SPSS version 17.0 for Windows (SPSS Inc., Chicago, IL, USA).

Results

Patient population

Of the 2286 acute stroke patients enrolled in the study, 551 patients were diagnosed with aspiration pneumonia. According to the inclusion and exclusion criteria, 73 patients were diagnosed with aspiration-related ARDS. Patients' clinical characteristics are shown in Table 1. Of these, 52 patients were men, and the mean age was 67 (SD 14.1) years. The mean NIHSS and GCS scores were 9.3 (SD 3.2) and 5.6 (SD 2.0), respectively. The mean hospital LOS was 23 (SD 7.0) days.

Of the 73 patients with aspiration-related ARDS, mechanical ventilation (MV) was required in 63 patients, including invasive MV (IMV) ($n = 49$, 77.8 %) and non-invasive MV ($n = 14$, 22.2 %). According to the EMR records, the surrogates of 10 patients with aspiration-related ARDS refused to use MV care and signed the informed consent for refusing treatment. The mean duration of IMV was 8.5 (SD, 5.5) days. In total, 29 patients died with a mortality rate of 39.7 %.

Table 1 Baseline characteristics of enrolled patients

Characteristics	Total (n, %)
Number	73
Age (years)	67.0 (SD 14.1)
Sex male	52 (71.2)
Admission NIHSS score	9.3 (SD 3.2)
Admission GCS score	5.6 (SD 2.0)
Smoking	30 (41.1)
Excess alcohol consumption	22 (30.1)
Pre-existing illnesses	
Hypertension	53 (72.6)
Diabetes	36 (49.3)
Coronary heart disease	14 (19.2)
Liver disease (except for hepatic cirrhosis)	0 (0)
Kidney disease	2 (2.7)
Chest X ray	73 (100)
Chest CT	58 (79.5)
GGOs	40/58 (69.0)
Consolidation opacities	31/58 (53.4)
Pleural effusions	14/58 (24.1)
Air bronchogram	11/58 (19.0)
Tachypnea (RR $\geq$ 25 breaths/min)	67 (91.8)
Fever (T $\geq$ 37.5 °C)	43 (58.9)
PaO_2/FiO_2 (mmHg)	143.5 (SD 59.0)
APACHE II score	28.2 (SD 10.4)
pH value	7.38 (SD 0.57)
Acidosis (pH < 7.35)	11 (15.1)
Albumin (g/L)	26.1 (SD 9.2)
Treatment	
Corticosteroids	47 (64.4)
No respiratory response	16/47 (34.0)
Respiratory response	31/47 (66.0)
Ventilatory support	63 (86.3)
Non-invasive ventilation alone	14/63 (22.2)
Non-invasive ventilation followed by intubation	16/63 (25.4)
First line invasive ventilation	33/63 (52.4)
Time from diagnosis to corticosteroids (days)	6.5 (SD 3.5)
Outcomes	
Duration of IMV (days)	8.5 (SD 5.5)
Hospital LOS (days)	23.0 (SD 7.0)
Hospital mortality	29 (39.7)

Abbreviation: *SD* standard deviation, *NIHSS* National Institutes of Health Stroke Scale, *GCS* Glasgow Coma Scale, *GGOs* ground glass opacities, *RR* respiratory rate, *APACHE* Acute Physiology and Chronic Health Evaluation, *PaO₂* partial pressure of oxygen in arterial blood, *FiO₂* fraction of inspired oxygen, *IMV* invasive mechanical ventilation, *LOS* length-of-stay

Corticosteroid therapy

Corticosteroid therapy was used in 47 (64.4 %) patients after the onset of aspiration-related ARDS. On average, it took 6.5 (SD 3.5) days from ARDS diagnosis to corticosteroid therapy initiation. Of the 47 patients, 31 (66 %) met the criteria for responsiveness (Figs. 1 and 2). Among the 21 patients who underwent IMV who responded to corticosteroid therapy, 17 patients were successfully extubated within 15 days. The remaining four patients experienced fatal complications. The corticosteroid dose ranged from 20 mg/day to 160 mg/day of methylprednisolone (or its equivalent), and the duration ranged from 2 to 17 days. The mean daily dose of methylprednisolone (or its equivalent) was 1.14 (SD 0.47) mg/kg, and the mean duration was 7.3 (SD 3.8) days.

By univariate analysis, the proportion of patients with GGOs in chest images differed significantly ($P < 0.05$) in the responsive and nonresponsive groups (Table 2). There was no significant difference in any adverse event between two groups. The adverse events of patients treated with and without systemic corticosteroids are shown in Table 3.

Risk factors of hospital mortality

The 10 patients, whose surrogates refused MV, were excluded from the analysis. By univariate analysis, age, male sex, admission NIHSS score, excess alcohol consumption, hypertension, GGOs in chest CT images, PaO_2/FiO_2, APACHE II score, albumin, corticosteroid therapy with response, and IMV support were significantly (p values < 0.05) associated with hospital mortality.

The significant risk factors for hospital mortality according to multiple logistic regression analysis are shown in Table 4. The analysis showed that the protective roles of hospital mortality were albumin (OR 0.81, 95 % CI

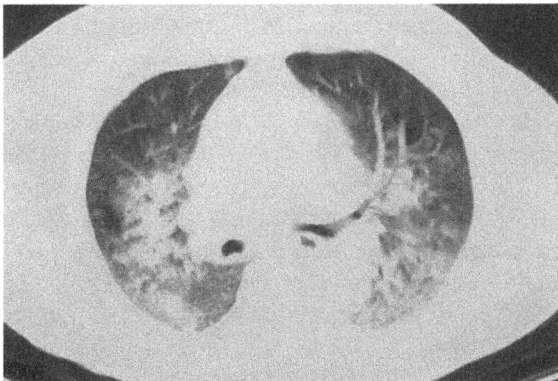

Fig. 1 Radiologic finding in a 78-year-old cerebral infarct man with aspiration-related ARDS. Chest CT showed ground-glass opacities, inhomogenous patchy consolidations and pleural effusion in bilateral lobes

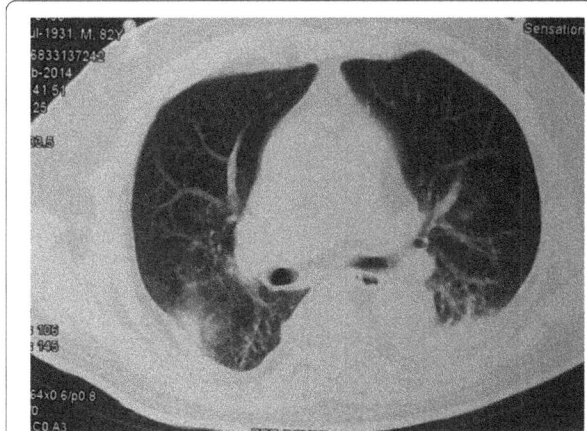

Fig. 2 The patient (weight = 73 kg) was treated with intravenous methylprednisolone (80 mg/day for 8 consecutive days). Chest CT scan demonstrated decreased density and extent of pulmonary opacification involving both lungs

0.64–0.92) and corticosteroid therapy (OR 0.50, 95 % CI 0.35–0.70). The two factors that were independently associated with hospital mortality were admission NIHSS score (OR 5.17, 95 % CI 1.27–10.64) and APACHE II score (OR 2.00, 95 % CI 1.12–3.56).

Discussion

Acute respiratory distress syndrome causes severe acute respiratory failure with dynamic impairment in oxygen and carbon dioxide transfer, and it is associated with the need for mechanical ventilation to provide high levels of supplementary oxygen [7, 8]. Given the impaired consciousness and swallowing difficulty, acute stroke patients are at great risk for aspiration [14, 15]. Patients who have aspirated gastric material may present with dramatic signs and symptoms, such as gastric material in the oropharynx as well as wheezing, coughing, dyspnea, cyanosis, pulmonary edema, and hypoxia. Any of these signs or symptoms could rapidly progress to ARDS [3]. Until now, no study has comprehensively described the clinical characteristics and outcomes of aspiration-related ARDS. After the first few victims were encountered at our institution, we became alert to patients with similar clinical courses because of their bad prognosis and high mortality rate.

In the present study, we found a high hospital mortality rate of 39.7 % for stroke patients with aspiration-related ARDS, among whom 86.3 % underwent MV, including IMV and non-invasive MV. As dysregulated inflammation is the cardinal feature of ARDS, corticosteroids are often added to the treatment based on the discretion of the treating pulmonologist. In our retrospective study, we found that corticosteroids therapy was administered in about two-thirds of patients, among which 66 % responded to the treatment. Patients with

Table 2 Univariate analyses of factors associated with corticosteroids responsiveness

	Response (n = 31,%)	Non-response (n = 16,%)	P value
Age (years)	65.8 (SD 9.5)	67.1 (SD 14.2)	0.21
Sex male	21 (67.4)	13 (68.4)	0.49
NIHSS score	9.0 (SD 3.2)	9.3 (SD 2.8)	0.50
GCS score	6.0 (SD 2.1)	5.8 (SD 2.1)	0.72
Smoking	12 (38.7)	7 (43.6)	0.76
Excess alcohol consumption	9 (29.0)	5 (31.3)	1.00
Pre-existing illnesses			
Hypertension	22 (71.0)	11 (68.9)	0.90
Diabetes	16 (51.6)	8 (50.0)	0.17
Coronary heart disease	6 (19.4)	3 (18.9)	1.00
Chest CT			
GGOs	23 (74.2)	7 (43.8)	0.04
Consolidation opacities	16 (51.6)	9 (56.3)	1.00
Pleural effusions	10 (32.3)	4 (25.0)	0.74
Air bronchogram	6 (19.4)	4 (25.0)	0.72
PaO_2/FiO_2 (mmHg)	139.5 (SD 55.5)	147.0 (SD 63.0)	0.99
APACHE II score	27.4 (SD 13.6)	28.4 (SD 11.1)	0.54
pH value	7.40 (SD 0.6)	7.38 (SD 0.5)	0.41
Albumin (g/L)	26.6 (SD 7.9)	27.9 (SD 8.3)	0.88
Time from diagnosis to corticosteroids (days)	5.5 (SD 2.0)	6.0 (SD 2.5)	0.16

Abbreviation: *SD* standard deviation, *NIHSS* National Institutes of Health Stroke Scale, *GCS* Glasgow Coma Scale, *GGOs* ground glass opacities, *APACHE* Acute Physiology and Chronic Health Evaluation, *PaO₂* partial pressure of oxygen in arterial blood, *FiO₂* fraction of inspired oxygen

GGO pattern in chest CT images responded better to corticosteroid therapy than those who did not present that radiologic pattern. Admission NIHSS score, APACHE II score, albumin, and corticosteroid therapy were associated with hospital mortality.

Diagnosing aspiration-related ARDS is a major challenge. Rales on auscultation, tachypnea, and fever are nonspecific signs that cannot be used to identify patients. Conversely, chest CT images are more sensitive for diagnosing ARDS than chest radiographs [16–18]. We found that diffuse GGOs evidenced in CT images had a favorable response to corticosteroid therapy. The GGOs were defined as increased pulmonary attenuation, with preserved bronchial and vascular margins. We consider it advisable to perform

Table 3 Adverse events between patients with and without systemic corticosteroids

	Systemic corticosteroids (n = 47, %)	Without corticosteroids (n = 26, %)	P value
Hyperglycemia with additional glucose-lowering therapy	17 (36.2)	7 (26.9)	0.45
New infection	13 (27.7)	6 (23.1)	0.78
GIB	1 (2.1)	0 (0)	1.00

Abbreviation: *GIB* gastrointestinal bleeding

chest CT timely in order identify aspiration-related ARDS early and to promptly apply proper treatment with the aim of improving the prognosis of our patients. The presence of a GGO pattern can alert the physician that this patient may respond positively to corticosteroid therapy. Thus, a careful assessment of physical symptoms and signs and chest CT images is crucial.

Excessive and protracted inflammation is the pathophysiological basis of ARDS, which would result in multi-organ dysfunction and even death [7, 19, 20]. Corticosteroids are added to the medications because of their important role as anti-inflammatory elements. However, the role of corticosteroids in managing ARDS remains uncertain because of insufficient scientific evidence to provide clinicians with clear and robust guidance [9, 10, 12, 21]. Although existing studies were unable to provide clear evidence of the benefits or harmful effects of corticosteroids, some studies pointed out that patients would benefit patients from steroid administration after the onset of ARDS, particularly to reduce mortality [11]. A systematic review and meta-analysis showed that the use of low-dose corticosteroids was associated with improved mortality and morbidity outcomes without notable side effects [22].

In the present study, corticosteroid therapy was administered in 64.6 % of patients with aspiration-related

Table 4 Determinants of hospital mortality

	Univariate analysis		Multivariate analysis	
	OR (95 % CI)	P value	OR (95 % CI)	P value
Age	0.99 (0.98–1.00)	0.11		
Sex male	1.36 (1.17–1.59)	<0.001		
NIHSS score	4.01 (2.98–5.56)	<0.001	5.04 (1.56–16.28)	0.007
GCS score	0.94 (0.82–1.07)	0.36		
Smoking	1.30 (0.86–1.99)	0.22		
Excess alcohol consumption	1.55 (1.27–1.88)	<0.001		
Pre-existing illnesses				
Hypertension	1.18 (1.01–1.39)	0.03		
Diabetes	1.00 (0.95–1.06)	0.89		
Coronary heart disease	1.09 (0.85–1.67)	0.31		
Kidney disease	1.29 (0.52–3.19)	0.59		
Chest CT				
GGOs	0.49 (0.27–0.86)	0.01		
Consolidation opacities	2.00 (0.92–3.56)	0.09		
Pleural effusions	1.05 (0.65–5.22)	0.25		
Air bronchogram	1.91 (0.54–6.84)	0.32		
PaO_2/FiO_2	0.19 (0.05–0.82)	0.03		
APACHE II score	2.22 (1.90–2.58)	<0.001	1.51 (1.05–2.16)	0.03
pH value	0.99 (0.30–3.31)	0.99		
Albumin	0.94 (0.88–1.00)	0.08	0.88 (0.79–0.97)	0.001
Treatment				
Corticosteroids	0.33 (0.23–0.47)	<0.001	0.50 (0.35–0.70)	<0.001
Non-invasive ventilation	1.69 (0.74–3.88)	0.21		
Invasive ventilation	0.06 (0.01–0.59)	0.02		
Time from diagnosis to corticosteroids treatment	1.28 (0.90–1.82)	0.16		

Abbreviation: *SD* standard deviation, *NIHSS* National Institutes of Health Stroke Scale, *GCS* Glasgow Coma Scale, *GGOs* ground glass opacities, *APACHE* Acute Physiology and Chronic Health Evaluation, *PaO₂* partial pressure of oxygen in arterial blood, *FiO₂* fraction of inspired oxygen

ARDS, among which 66.0 % responded to the treatment. The mean daily dose of methylprednisolone (or its equivalent) was 1.14 (SD 0.47) mg/kg, and the mean duration of treatment was 7.3 (SD 3.8) days. Based on our results, corticosteroid therapy was an independent protective factor for hospital mortality, which suggests that low-dose and short-term corticosteroid use might indeed be beneficial for patients with aspiration-related ARDS. Response to corticosteroid therapy, whether it is ineffective, effective, or toxic, is influenced by the dosage used and duration of the administration [23–25]. The clinical side effects of systemic corticosteroids should not be ignored, such as new infection, hyperglycemia and GIB. One major concern is the high risk of infection, especially aspiration induced lung abscess, secondary to immunosuppression. The adverse events often lead to undesired results. High-dose and long-term corticosteroid therapy may cause serious side effects. In our study, the occurrence of adverse events did not differ between the patients treated with and without the low-dose and short-term corticosteroid schedule. Consequently, in future studies to elucidate the role of corticosteroids in aspiration-related ARDS, it should be taken into account not only which subset of patients can potentially benefit from its administration, but also the optimal dose and duration of corticosteroid therapy. Only in this way, we can achieve the balance between the beneficial and harmful effects of the inflammatory response.

The high mortality observed in this study was also associated with the severity of the illness, which was reflected by NIHSS scores and APACHE II score. Another predictor of hospital mortality was serum albumin, which regulates plasma osmotic pressure. Hypoproteinemia accelerates fluid exudation, promotes alveolar edema, and contributes to ventilation-perfusion imbalance [26]. These suggest that early diagnosis combined with early treatment will benefit the outcome.

Some limitations of this study should be mentioned. First, the analysis was retrospective. The clinical practice and predictive factors of mortality could change substantially. Moreover, we used a single-center design, and the number of patients studied was limited. It is necessary to conduct further multicenter prospective studies to reach more accurate conclusions. Second, the dosage and term of systemic corticosteroids varied for each patient. Timing of corticosteroid administration might also play a critical role in the effects of treatment because the inflammatory response is a dynamic process. Third, adrenocortical function was not evaluated in our study. Elderly stroke patients tend to have a relative adrenal insufficiency [27, 28]. Therefore, the possibility of systemic corticosteroid compensation for adrenal insufficiency should be considered.

Conclusions

Low-dose, short-term corticosteroid therapy may be expected to be effective in reduce hospital mortality in cases of aspiration-related ARDS, without notable side effects. The presence of a GGO pattern in chest CT images obtained in cases of suspected aspiration-related ARDS could translate into an increased possibility of positive response to corticosteroid therapy. However, we are unable to reach an accurate conclusion in terms of defining the optimal dose, timing, and duration of corticosteroid therapy. Definitive treatment recommendations will depend on further larger-scale, randomized, controlled prospective trials.

Abbreviation

AIDS: acquired Immune Deficiency Syndrome; APACHE: Acute Physiology and Chronic Health Evaluation; ARDS: acute respiratory distress syndrome; CI: confidence interval; COPD: chronic obstructive pulmonary disease; CT: computerized tomography; EMR: electronic medical record; FiO_2: fraction of inspired oxygen; GCS: Glasgow Coma Scale; GGOs: ground glass opacities; GIB: gastrointestinal bleeding; IMV: invasive mechanical ventilation; LOS: length-of-stay; MRI: magnetic resonance imaging; NIHSS: National Institutes of Health Stroke Scale; OR: odds ratios; PaO_2: partial pressure of oxygen in arterial blood; RR: respiratory rate; SD: standard deviation; SPO_2: pulse oxygen saturation.

Competing interests

The authors declare that they have no competing interests.

Authors' contributions

JNZ studied and analyzed the data, conducted literature reviews, and drafted the manuscript. HCL designed the study and helped to draft the manuscript. YL carried out the study, collected the data and helped to draft the manuscript. All authors read and approved the final manuscript.

Acknowledgements

We thank the neurology department for providing the data. Funding provided by Science and technology development plan of Shandong Province (Number: 2009GG10002054). The funders had no role in study design, data collection and analysis, decision to publish, or preparation of the manuscript.

Author details

[1]Department of Respiratory Medicine, The First Hospital of Jiaxing, Jiaxing, China. [2]Department of Respiratory Medicine, Shandong Provincial Hospital Affiliated to Shandong University, Jinan, Shandong 250021, China.

References

1. Armstrong JR, Mosher BD. Aspiration pneumonia after stroke: intervention and prevention. Neurohospitalist. 2011;1(2):85–93.
2. Raghavendran K, Nemzek J, Napolitano LM, Knight PR. Aspiration-induced lung injury. Crit Care Med. 2011;39(4):818–26.
3. Marik PE. Aspiration Pneumonitis and Aspiration Pneumonia. N Engl J Med. 2001;344:9–1.
4. MacMahon H, Husain AN, Cardasis JJ. The Spectrum of Lung Disease due to Chronic Occult Aspiration. Ann Am Thorac Soc. 2014;11(6):865–73.
5. Gajic O, Dabbagh O, Park PK, Adesanya A, Chang SY, Hou P, et al. Early identification of patients at risk of acute lung injury: evaluation of lung injury prediction score in a multicenter cohort study. Am J Respir Crit Care Med. 2011;183(4):462–70.
6. de Haro C, Martin-Loeches I, Torrents E, Artigas A. Acute respiratory distress syndrome: prevention and early recognition. Ann Intensive Care. 2013;3(1):11.
7. Matthay MA, Ware LB, Zimmerman GA. The acute respiratory distress syndrome. J Clin Invest. 2012;122(8):2731–40.
8. ARDS Definition Task Force, Ranieri VM, Rubenfeld GD, et al. Acute respiratory distress syndrome: the Berlin Definition. JAMA. 2012;307:2526–33.
9. Sibbald WJ, Anderson RR, Reid B, Holliday RL, Driedger AA. Alveolo-capillary permeability in human septic ARDS. Effect of high-dose corticosteroid therapy. Chest. 1981;79:133–42.
10. Meduri GU, Tolley EA, Chrousos GP, Stentz F. Prolonged methylprednisolone treatment suppresses systemic inflammation in patients with unresolving acute respiratory distress syndrome: evidence for inadequate endogenous glucocorticoid secretion and inflammation-induced immune cell resistance to glucocorticoids. Am J Respir Crit Care Med. 2002;165:983–91.
11. Lee M, Sukumaran M, Berger HW, Reilly TA. Influence of corticosteroid treatment on pulmonary function after recovery from aspiration of gastric contents. Mt Sinai J Med. 1980;47:341–6.
12. Wolfe JE, Bone RC, Ruth WE. Effects of corticosteroids in the treatment of patients with gastric aspiration. Am J Med. 1977;63:719–22.
13. Hoffmann S, Malzahn U, Harms H, Koennecke H-C, Berger K, et al. Development of a Clinical Score (A2DS2) to Predict Pneumonia in Acute Ischemic Stroke. Stroke. 2012;43:2617–23.
14. Westendorp WF, Nederkoorn PJ, Jan-Dirk V, Dijkgraaf MG, van de Beek D. Post-stroke infection: A systematic review and meta-analysis. BMC Neurol. 2011;11:110.
15. Martino R, Foley N, Bhogal S, Diamant N, Speechley M, et al. Dysphagia After Stroke: Incidence, Diagnosis, and Pulmonary Complications. Stroke. 2005;36:2756–63.
16. Rouby JJ, Puybasset L, Nieszkowska A, Lu Q. Acute respiratory distress syndrome: Lessons from computed tomography of the whole lung. Crit Care Med. 2003;31:S285–95.
17. Gattinoni L, Caironi P, Pelosi P, Goodman LR. What has computed tomography taught us about the acute respiratory distress syndrome? Am J Respir Crit Care Med. 2001;164:1701–11.
18. Gattinoni L, Pesenti A, Torresin A. Adult respiratory distress syndrome profiles by computed tomography. J Thorac Imaging. 1986;1:25–30.
19. Levitt JE, Matthay MA. The utility of clinical predictors of acute lung injury: towards prevention and earlier recognition. Expert Rev Respir Med. 2010; 4(6):785–97.
20. Magdalena B, Brandon B, Maureen MC. Acute lung injury and the acute respiratory distress syndrome in the injured patient. Scand J Trauma Resusc Emerg Med. 2012;20:54.
21. Levitt JE, Matthay MA. Clinical review: Early treatment of acute lung injury - paradigm shift toward prevention and treatment prior to respiratory failure. Critical Care. 2012;16:223.
22. Tang BM, Craig JC, Eslick GD, Seppelt I, McLean AS. Use of corticosteroids in acute lung injury and acute respiratory distress syndrome: a systematic review and meta-analysis. Crit Care Med. 2009;37:1594–03.
23. Nafae RM, Ragab MI, Amany FM, Rashed SB. Adjuvant role of corticosteroids in the treatment of community-acquired pneumonia. Egypt J Chest Dis Tuberc. 2013;62(3):439–45.

24. Nawab QU, Golden E, Confalonieri M, Umberger R, Meduri GU. Corticosteroid treatment in severe community-acquired pneumonia: duration of treatment affects control of systemic inflammation and clinical improvement. Intensive Care Med. 2011;37(9):1553–4.

25. Hong-Ryang K, Jae-Ho L, Kyung-Yil L, Jung-Woo R, You-Sook Y, et al. Early corticosteroid treatment for severe pneumonia caused by 2009 H1N1 influenza virus. Critical Care. 2011;15:413.

26. Wang D, Min Y, Hilary M, Liang An H, Gang C, et al. Predictors and outcome of patients with acute respiratory distress syndrome caused by miliary tuberculosis: a retrospective study in Chongqing, China. BMC Infect Dis. 2012;12:121.

27. Kornblum RN, Fisher RS. Pituitary lesions in craniocerebral injuries. Arch Pathol. 1969;88(3):242.

28. Keieger DT. Factors influencing the circadian periodicity of ACTH and corticosteroids. Med Clin N Am. 1978;62:251.

22

Qualitative European survey of patients with idiopathic pulmonary fibrosis: patients' perspectives of the disease and treatment

Anne-Marie Russell[1*], Elena Ripamonti[2] and Carlo Vancheri[3]

Abstract

Background: 'Living with IPF and an exploration of Esbriet® – a new treatment' was an exploratory, qualitative, real-world survey of European patients with idiopathic pulmonary fibrosis (IPF) who were receiving treatment with pirfenidone prior to its commercial availability. The aim of the survey was to probe the impact of IPF on patients' quality of life; the role of healthcare professionals and caregivers; the information needs of both patients and their caregivers; and patients' perceptions of pirfenidone as a new treatment option for IPF.

Methods: Patients from the UK, Germany and Italy, with a diagnosis of IPF (duration >3 months), who were being treated with pirfenidone, were recruited from patient support groups, specialist centres and advocacy groups. Semi-structured, qualitative, in-depth patient interviews of 1-h duration were conducted by an independent researcher. Patients were initially asked about their experiences of living with IPF and then prompted to describe their experiences of taking pirfenidone. Techniques utilised included: the bubble-speech technique; the icon cards projective exercise; and the free association exercise. All interviews were transcribed and analysed by an independent researcher.

Results: Forty-five patients (71 % male) were interviewed (mean age 68.5 years; mean time since diagnosis 3.5 years); 87 % of patients reported that diagnosis took >1 year. Patients reported that IPF had a significant physical and emotional impact on their quality of life. The beneficial role played by caregivers and interstitial lung disease specialist nurses (where available) was specifically highlighted. Although most patients were keen for information on IPF, this was often of poor quality, out of date, or in English only. Patients' perceptions of pirfenidone were largely positive and associated with 'hope' but were also influenced by the level of side effects experienced.

Conclusions: This survey highlights the impact of IPF on patients' lives, and the need to adequately support both patients and their caregivers. These findings demonstrate the value of seeking patients' perspectives of a chronic disease such as IPF and how this information can be used to guide improvements in care, to best support the needs of patients with this devastating condition.

Keywords: Caregiver, Idiopathic pulmonary fibrosis, Impact, Information, Interview, Needs, Patients, Perspectives, Pirfenidone, Survey

* Correspondence: A.Russell@imperial.ac.uk
[1]National Heart & Lung Institute, Imperial College & Royal Brompton Hospital, Respiratory Epidemiology, Occupational Medicine and Public Health, 1b Manresa Road, London SW3 6LR, UK
Full list of author information is available at the end of the article

Background

Idiopathic pulmonary fibrosis (IPF) is a chronic, progressive and irreversible interstitial lung disease (ILD) with a poor prognosis (2–5 years) [1–5]. IPF is predominant in men aged >50 years and, although idiopathic, risk factors may include gastroesophageal reflux, smoking and environmental or occupational exposures [1, 3].

IPF imposes limitations on many daily activities, necessitating a change in lifestyle. In addition to impacts on physical and social function, patients may also experience increased anxiety, depression and a reduced quality of life [6–8]. Increased sleep disruption and a poorer quality of sleep contributes to fatigue, further impacting the emotional and physical well-being of patients [9–11]. The impact of IPF affects not only patients but also caregivers, family and other members of patients' support networks, all of whom have a role to play in helping to manage the burden of the disease [12, 13].

Until recently, the standard of care for patients with IPF was limited to oxygen therapy, pulmonary rehabilitation, palliative care and, in a small minority of patients, lung transplantation [1, 14]. Pirfenidone (Esbriet®), an antifibrotic drug with anti-inflammatory properties, was approved by the European Medicines Agency (EMA) in 2011 for the treatment of adult patients with IPF based on the favourable benefit-risk profile observed in Phase III clinical trials [15, 16]. The US Food and Drug Administration simultaneously approved pirfenidone and a tyrosine kinase inhibitor, nintedanib, for the treatment of patients with IPF in the USA, in October 2014 [17–20]; the EMA subsequently approved nintedanib in January 2015 [21].

Here, we report findings from 'Living with IPF and an exploration of Esbriet® – a new treatment', an exploratory, qualitative, real-world survey of European patients with IPF who were receiving treatment with pirfenidone prior to its commercial availability. The aims of this survey were to: explore patients' experiences of living with IPF and how this impacted on their quality of life; determine the availability and impact of support systems, specifically that of healthcare professionals (HCPs) and caregivers; establish the information needs of both patients with IPF and their caregivers; and explore patients' perceptions of pirfenidone as a new treatment option.

Methods

Design and patients

Patients were invited to enrol through patient support groups (UK), specialist centres (Italy) or an advocacy group (Germany). Eligible patients had a multidisciplinary team-confirmed diagnosis of IPF with disease duration >3 months. All patients were being treated with pirfenidone as part of a Named Patient Program (NPP) under the supervision of an ILD physician.

Patients completed a screening questionnaire to verify their IPF diagnosis and that they were receiving treatment with pirfenidone. Forced vital capacity was not recorded as part of the questionnaire and, while the NPP was in principle limited to patients with mild-to-moderate disease, the decision to ultimately treat each patient was the responsibility of each participating physician, and, therefore, the inclusion of patients with more advanced disease cannot be excluded. All patients provided consent for their participation in the survey and for the future publication of anonymised findings from the survey.

Interviews

Semi-structured, qualitative, in-depth patient interviews of 1-h duration were conducted by an independent researcher at a neutral venue or in the patient's own home, according to preference. Interviews were conducted 1:1, although caregivers could be present at the patient's request. Interviews were audio- and video-recorded (patients were asked not to identify themselves on tape). Patients' experiences of living with IPF, as reported in this manuscript, were discussed initially; patients were then asked about their experiences of taking pirfenidone. The full interview discussion guide is provided (see Additional file 1). The interviews were designed to encourage frank, open discussion and to probe patients' unmet needs and the emotional and rational elements driving their choices and behaviours. Techniques utilised in the interviews included: the bubble-speech technique, to probe patients' expectations of their HCP and their level of satisfaction with the relationship; and the icon cards projective exercise and free association exercise to assess possible new formulations of pirfenidone.

Analysis

All interviews were transcribed verbatim and, where necessary, translated into Italian; transcriptions were anonymised in accordance with local data protection laws and European Pharmaceutical Market Research Association Guidelines. Interview transcriptions were analysed by an independent researcher, and common themes and challenges were extracted and summarised. Disease awareness was determined by motivational and qualitative factors concerning the disease and knowledge of specific terminology. Side effects were reported as per the respondent's spontaneous answers and were not analysed by a physician.

Results

Patients

Forty-five patients (71 % male) from three European countries (UK, Germany and Italy) were interviewed between 24 September and 19 October, 2012. All patients were invited to participate and approximately 80 % of the interviews were conducted with the caregiver present. Mean age was 68.5 years and mean time since diagnosis was 3.5 years at the time of interview. Patients reported that diagnosis frequently involved visits to several different HCPs, and 87 % of patients reported that diagnosis took more than 1 year. Approximately 90 % of patients were receiving oxygen therapy: 55 % used oxygen as needed, for a few hours of the day, while 35 % used continual oxygen therapy.

Impact of IPF on quality of life

Approximately half of the patients reported that IPF had a significant negative impact on their quality of life. The most frequently reported physical symptom of IPF was fatigue (82 % of patients). Other physical symptoms reported by >50 % of patients included loss of appetite (typically in response to feelings of nausea), difficulty in lifting objects (eg, grocery bags), and continuous phlegm and coughing throughout the day.

"Even the simplest things are difficult for me"
(Patient – Italy)

Patients reported that the physical impact of IPF often took an emotional toll, leaving them feeling depressed and often without the emotional strength to fight disease progression. The primary emotional concern reported by patients was fear of the disease progression and its impact on their future (72 % of patients). In addition, 36 % of patients reported feeling frustrated and angry, due to a lack of self-acceptance of their disease and other people's poor knowledge of IPF. Patients also reported feeling isolated (18 %), causing them to withdraw from social relationships.

"I feel really sad; before I was a very cheerful person"
(Patient – Germany)

Patients reported that IPF also impacted on family life. Some patients perceived themselves to be a burden and felt reliant on their family, leading to additional frustration for the patient. Most female patients (90 %) reported a loss of identity as the main family support figure, and some of the male patients (15 %) reported a detrimental impact of IPF on their sex lives, both physically and emotionally. No other gender differences were identified.

"I don't know what type of life I can offer my wife, I don't feel like a man anymore, because of me I am forcing restrictions on myself and other people"
(Patient – Italy)

"My family checks everything I do, I don't feel free"
(Patient - UK)

The initiation of oxygen treatment marked an important stage in disease progression for all patients, due to the perceived limitations it placed on their freedom. Oxygen therapy was associated with less hope for the future and more feelings of shame as their condition became externally visible to others.

"I'm always hooked up to the oxygen, I have a range of movement of 10 m" (Patient – Italy)

The role of HCPs and caregivers

In the UK, 90 % of patients reported that an ILD specialist nurse was their main medical contact for IPF healthcare. Nurses provided information on IPF, patient support organisations and lifestyle advice, as well as helping patients to access medication and manage side effects.

"She [the nurse] is everything for me, she is a shoulder to cry on, she answers any question I ask her, I hope she never leaves!" (Patient – UK)

In Germany, patients reported that physicians were their main contact, particularly concerning treatment efficacy and side effects, whereas nurses played a more marginal role in their care. In Italy, patients perceived IPF as a rare condition requiring specialist knowledge; they reported that nurses were not involved in their care and that they generally interacted exclusively with their physician.

"I am one of many patients; it is not easy to build a relationship" (Patient –Germany)

"The doctor is my reference; he is the person I call, definitely not the nurse who does not know much" (Patient – Italy)

Most patients reported feeling that they lacked the psychological support necessary to face their IPF-related difficulties, with only one-fifth of patients having received professional psychological support.

"The doctors helped me, but I have never received any psychological support, I really need it" (Patient – Germany)

More than half of the patients felt they needed a caregiver in their household. Patients reported several important roles that were fulfilled by caregivers, including reminding patients to take medications, accompanying patients to medical appointments and researching information on IPF. Many caregivers present during the interviews demonstrated a greater knowledge of IPF than the patient.

Information needs of patients and their caregivers

The level of disease awareness varied widely amongst patients, but approximately one-third of patients felt inadequately aware of or informed about IPF. Patients in the UK and Germany largely understood the severity of their IPF and their prognosis, as well as the available treatments, whereas patients in Italy generally reported being less well-informed about IPF and mostly relied only on information provided by their physician.

"No idea about the name of this disease, I call it lung infection" (Patient –Italy)

Most patients (74 %) reported searching for information about IPF. However, many patients described issues with what they found, including poor-quality and out-of-date information, which was only available in English.

"It's imperative to have information about this disease" (Patient – Germany)

Patients in the UK and Germany preferred to receive information about IPF online – most frequently via the Pulmonary Fibrosis Foundation, British Lung Foundation (BLF) and LungenFibrose websites – whereas Italian patients preferred printed materials. The main areas of patient interest included information on IPF, the use of pirfenidone, and updates on new research and therapy (Table 1). Emerging needs spontaneously reported by patients concerned a lack of expert advice relating to lifestyle (51 %), diet (38 %), oxygen treatment (38 %) and physical exercise (18 %). Many patients reported that they would like to receive practical information about lifestyle changes that would help them manage their disease. Patients also expressed an interest in knowing how many other people in their area were affected by IPF and wanted the general public to be better informed about the disease.

Caregivers reported feeling inadequately prepared for the caregiving role. Caregivers stressed a need to receive adequate psychological support to accept the disease and better relate to the patient; a need for strategies to manage the everyday life of a patient with IPF; and a need for more background information on IPF.

"It is difficult for us to help them, we would like to have more information about what we should do at home" (Caregiver – UK)

Patients' perceptions of pirfenidone

Patients' perceptions of pirfenidone were largely positive, scoring 7.4 on a scale of 0 (not satisfied) to 10 (very satisfied). Satisfaction was influenced by the level of side effects experienced by patients, with an average satisfaction score of 6.1 ($n = 25$) for patients with side effects and 8.3 ($n = 20$) for patients with no side effects. Side effects, including nausea and photosensitivity, were reported to have a negative psychological impact on patients who perceived little awareness of their treatment working. Patients with side effects also reported a general deterioration in their quality of life, which they perceived to be related to pirfenidone. Furthermore, if a patient was experiencing side effects, they often attributed all of these effects to pirfenidone, even if any correlation between the two was unconfirmed.

'I have so many problems, such as nausea, itchy legs and backache' (Patient – Germany)

Patients without side effects reported feeling that their condition had stabilised with the use of pirfenidone, which in turn gave them a sense of hope and the feeling they were being taken care of by HCPs. Patients reported feeling reassured when HCPs confirmed their disease had stabilised (according to clinical parameters), which gave them greater confidence for the future.

"I feel I'm taking something that can really halt this disease and make me live longer" (Patient – Germany)
"Ever since I started taking pirfenidone, I feel more protected" (Patient – Italy)

Discussion and conclusions

IPF is a devastating disorder and the findings of this qualitative survey of UK, German and Italian patients with IPF add to the existing body of knowledge regarding the substantial impact IPF has on the lives of patients and their caregivers [6–11]. In agreement with recent literature [12, 22], these findings also identify the need to more adequately support patients with IPF in terms of disease awareness, lifestyle management, psychological support

Table 1 Patients with IPF indicated clear needs for information in three areas

IPF	Pirfenidone	Updates on new research and therapies
Greater knowledge about IPF, the causes of the disease and the number of people affected	More data regarding the efficacy and tolerability of pirfenidone, including how to practically manage tolerability issues	Information on the new drugs that are being studied for IPF, including results from clinical trials

IPF idiopathic pulmonary fibrosis

and management of medication side effects, as well as emphasising the important role played by the HCP in having primary contact with the patient and their family.

Approximately one-third of patients in the survey were identified as being unaware of and/or uninformed about IPF, and most patients wanted a better understanding of the disease. However, sources of information on IPF were frequently of poor quality, out of date or not available in the patients' native language. In the UK and Germany, patients predominantly used online sources when looking for further information about their condition, while Italian patients reported a preference for printed materials; however, it was unclear whether this was actually due to preference or to a lack of web-based IPF information in Italian. In general, however, when diagnosed with a chronic disease such as IPF, many patients now turn to online sources of health information as this allows them a degree of autonomy, and the ability to examine and digest information at their leisure [23]. The findings of this study support the need for good-quality, freely available, online information on IPF in multiple languages, to support patients in learning more about the practical management of their disease. It is also interesting to note that many patients expressed a desire for better understanding of IPF among the general public. The recent US EXPLORE survey found that patients with IPF often felt isolated, embarrassed and stigmatised [24], and patients with other chronic respiratory diseases, such as chronic obstructive pulmonary disease, often also report feeling stigmatised [25].

The findings of this survey also emphasise the important role played by the HCP who is the primary contact for a patient, whether they are a physician or a specialist nurse. In the UK, specialist nurses were reported to play an important role in supporting patients with many aspects of disease management and patients clearly felt this was beneficial. However, the UK is quite unique in having advanced ILD specialist nurses who are able to play a significant role in helping patients understand the disease and coordinate their care [22]. In a recent report by the BLF, 50 % of English healthcare trusts reported allocating an ILD specialist nurse within 6 months of a patient's diagnosis [22]. Furthermore, UK clinical guidelines state that all patients with IPF should have an ILD specialist nurse allocated to them and that any centre that wants specialist status must employ a specialist ILD nurse [26]. UK clinical guidelines also recommend that the ILD specialist nurse should provide accurate and clear information to patients and their families, regarding diagnosis and management of IPF, and support the patient at all stages of the care pathway to facilitate transitions in care and advise on symptom management [26, 27]. In Germany and Italy, nurses were less involved in patient care. Specialist nurses for IPF care

may warrant consideration by German and Italian healthcare authorities due to their ability to provide a holistic programme of care.

Caregivers were present in 80 % of the interviews conducted for this survey and provided a useful source of information. However, it should be acknowledged that the presence of caregivers during the interview may have inhibited responses from some patients. Nevertheless, the findings of this survey support the difficulties faced by caregivers in looking after patients with IPF and are in agreement with the literature. The caregivers of patients with IPF have reported hardships throughout the course of a loved one's disease, including emotional devastation at the initial diagnosis and difficulties living with a loved one because of their limitations [28, 29]. Furthermore, providing additional support to caregivers of patients with IPF has been demonstrated to provide some positive benefits. For example, caregivers who attended a 6-week nurse-led group intervention programme on IPF management, alongside their loved ones with IPF, reported significantly lower stress levels post-intervention compared with those who did not attend the intervention programme [29].

Pirfenidone was the first medication approved for the treatment of European patients with IPF, and the positive feedback reported in this survey suggests it provides hope and reassurance to patients. However, the findings of this survey also highlight the need for guidance on how to identify and mitigate the side effects experienced by some patients during treatment with pirfenidone, such as the nausea and loss of appetite reported as symptoms of IPF in this study, which may have been related to pirfenidone therapy [16, 17] rather than to IPF itself. It should be noted that this survey was conducted in 2012, prior to the launch of pirfenidone in some European countries (including the UK). At this time, HCPs would have been less familiar with pirfenidone and its side-effect profile than they are at present. Recent reports from real-world studies suggest that the tolerability issues with pirfenidone can be well managed, with no new safety signals identified versus the clinical trial programme [16, 17, 30, 31]. However, there remains a need to provide patients with lifestyle guidance when they are taking pirfenidone to minimise the risk of treatment side effects. Some strategies that have proved successful include using sun protection to avoid photosensitive skin reactions and taking pirfenidone during or after a meal to alleviate effects on gastric motility [32].

While this survey reports the impact IPF has on patients' lives and supports the need to address the unmet needs of patients' and their caregivers, several limitations must be addressed. The survey was not designed to exclusively evaluate patients' experiences of

IPF. No formal measure of quality of life was implemented and patients were not randomly selected for participation in the survey. Furthermore, the sample size was small, although this is typical of other surveys that have been conducted in patients with IPF [2, 6, 11].

Developments in IPF management and disease awareness

As a result of surveys such as this one, many aspects of care for patients with IPF in Europe have changed since 2012. In 2013, the patient support initiative 'IPF Care' was established in eight European countries, to provide help and education for patients treated with pirfenidone through frequent discussions with ILD specialist nurses. The benefits of the programme are already receiving recognition, such as in the UK where 66 % of patients who reported an adverse event during the 'IPF Care' programme remained on maintenance therapy [13], and in Austria, where 96 % of patients who started pirfenidone with the support of 'IPF Care' remained on treatment for ≥3 months compared with only 64 % of patients who were not enrolled in the programme [13]. The success of 'IPF Care' demonstrates the value that patient support programmes can offer as a tool for complementing and enhancing the support provided by healthcare systems, and as a forum within which to discuss patients' worries. Other initiatives include IPF World Week, established in 2012, to raise awareness of the disease through its 'Blowing Bubbles' campaign in several European countries [33], and the European IPF Patient Charter, established to support equal access to IPF treatment and care standards in Europe [34].

In the UK specifically, there have been many advances in IPF, including the launch of two patient advocacy groups (Pulmonary Fibrosis Trust in 2011 [35] and Action for Pulmonary Fibrosis in 2013 [36]), which provide information and support to patients, and the launch of a clinical pathway for IPF in early 2015 [37]. Furthermore, the BLF has supported the development of many projects, including an IPF Patient Charter (supported by multidisciplinary IPF experts, patients and caregivers) [38], a survey evaluating patients' experiences in England [22] and numerous sources of patient information. The BLF is also contemplating the development testing the feasability of a personal organiser for patients with IPF in the UK.

In Italy, general awareness of IPF is slowly improving; for example, there are several patient associations, including RespiRARE in Sicily, dedicated to rare lung diseases [39] and Ama Fuori dal Buio, which is very active in supporting patients and providing them with disease information [40]. The Observatory for Rare Disease conducted a successful social-media campaign inviting people to post pictures or videos of them trying not to breathe, to raise awareness of IPF [41], and in 2013, a patient- and caregiver-specific website was launched

with disease information in Italian [42]. Italian clinical guidelines for IPF were also recently published [43]. In Germany, the patient association Lungenfibrose e.V is also very active in supporting patients and providing disease information [44], and clinical guidelines for IPF were launched in 2013 [45].

Future directions in IPF management and disease awareness

Nevertheless, more work is still needed to improve the diagnosis and management of IPF. In this study, most patients reported a delayed diagnosis and this is not uncommon for IPF and other rare diseases [46], as demonstrated by the results of the BLF's recent survey where many patients with IPF in England reported struggling to obtain a diagnosis [22]. Patients in the BLF survey also reported not having access to information about IPF that they could understand, having to navigate their own care pathway, and a lack of access to an ILD specialist nurse. We should, therefore, continue to seek each patient's perspective on their disease and treatment, so that the information and care they receive can be tailored to their specific needs, thereby providing the support they and their families require to live with IPF.

Abbreviations
BLF: British Lung Foundation; EMA: European Medicines Agency; HCP: healthcare professional; ILD: interstitial lung disease; IPF: idiopathic pulmonary fibrosis; NPP: Named Patient Program.

Competing interests
Anne-Marie Russell has received educational grants and consultancy fees from InterMune and Roche; and consultancy fees from Novartis. She is also a member of the British Lung Foundation IPF Advisory Board and has received a travel scholarship from Action for Pulmonary Fibrosis UK. Elena Ripamonti has no conflicts of interest to declare. Carlo Vancheri was previously part of the InterMune scientific board. He is now part of the Roche scientific board.

Authors' contributions
All authors were involved in the design of this study. AMR and CV were involved in the selection and management of patients . ER coordinated a team of researchers from Elma Research S.R.L in preparing the interview discussion guide, facilitating the interviews and summarising interview outcomes. All authors contributed to the manuscript from the outset and read and approved the final draft.

Acknowledgements
The authors acknowledge the contribution of Christopher Giot of InterMune International AG, Muttenz, Switzerland, now a wholly owned Roche subsidiary. Medical writing support was provided by Lauren Donaldson on behalf of Complete Medical Communications Ltd, funded by F. Hoffmann-La Roche Ltd.

Funding
This survey was funded by InterMune International, AG, which became a wholly owned subsidiary of F. Hoffmann-La Roche Ltd in 2014.

Author details

[1]National Heart & Lung Institute, Imperial College & Royal Brompton Hospital, Respiratory Epidemiology, Occupational Medicine and Public Health, 1b Manresa Road, London SW3 6LR, UK. [2]Elma Research S.R.L, Viale Tunisia 41, 20124 Milan, Italy. [3]Regional Referral Centre for Rare Lung Diseases, Department of Clinical and Experimental Medicine, University of Catania, via S. Sofia 78, 95123 Catania, Italy.

References

1. Raghu G, Collard HR, Egan JJ, Martinez FJ, Behr J, Brown KK, et al. An official ATS/ERS/JRS/ALAT statement: idiopathic pulmonary fibrosis: evidence-based guidelines for diagnosis and management. Am J Respir Crit Care Med. 2011;183:788–824.
2. Schoenheit G, Becattelli I, Cohen AH. Living with idiopathic pulmonary fibrosis: an in-depth qualitative survey of European patients. Chron Respir Dis. 2011;8:225–31.
3. King Jr TE, Pardo A, Selman M. Idiopathic pulmonary fibrosis. Lancet. 2011;378:1949–61.
4. Kim DS, Collard HR, King Jr TE. Classification and natural history of the idiopathic interstitial pneumonias. Proc Am Thorac Soc. 2006;3:285–92.
5. Meltzer EB, Noble PW. Idiopathic pulmonary fibrosis. Orphanet J Rare Dis. 2008;3:8.
6. De Vries J, Kessels BL, Drent M. Quality of life of idiopathic pulmonary fibrosis patients. Eur Respir J. 2001;17:954–61.
7. Elfferich MD, De Vries J, Drent M. Type D or 'distressed' personality in sarcoidosis and idiopathic pulmonary fibrosis. Sarcoidosis Vasc Diffuse Lung Dis. 2011;28:65–71.
8. Giot C, Maronati M, Becattelli I, Schoenheit G. Idiopathic Pulmonary Fibrosis: an EU patient perspective survey. Curr Respir Med Rev. 2013;9:112–9.
9. Krishnan V, McCormack MC, Mathai SC, Agarwal S, Richardson B, Horton MR, et al. Sleep quality and health-related quality of life in idiopathic pulmonary fibrosis. Chest. 2008;134:693–8.
10. Mermigkis C, Stagaki E, Amfilochiou A, Polychronopoulos V, Korkonikitas P, Mermigkis D, et al. Sleep quality and associated daytime consequences in patients with idiopathic pulmonary fibrosis. Med Princ Pract. 2009;18:10–5.
11. Swigris JJ, Stewart AL, Gould MK, Wilson SR. Patients' perspectives on how idiopathic pulmonary fibrosis affects the quality of their lives. Health Qual Life Outcomes. 2005;3:61.
12. Duck A, Spencer LG, Bailey S, Leonard C, Ormes J, Caress AL. Perceptions, experiences and needs of patients with idiopathic pulmonary fibrosis. J Adv Nurs. 2015;71:1055–65.
13. Duck A, Pigram L, Errhalt P, Ahmed D, Chaudhuri N. IPF Care: A support program for patients with idiopathic pulmonary fibrosis treated with pirfenidone in Europe. Adv Ther. 2015;32:87–107.
14. Adamali HI, Anwar MS, Russell AM, Egan JJ. Non-pharmacological treatment of idiopathic pulmonary fibrosis. Curr Respir Care Rep. 2012;1:208–15.
15. European Medicines Agency. European public assessment report for Esbriet® pirfenidone 2015. http://www.ema.europa.eu/ema/index.jsp?curl=pages/medicines/human/medicines/002154/human_med_001417.jsp&mid=WC0b01ac058001d124. Accessed 10 Sep 2015.
16. Noble PW, Albera C, Bradford WZ, Costabel U, Glassberg MK, Kardatzke D, et al. Pirfenidone in patients with idiopathic pulmonary fibrosis (CAPACITY): two randomised trials. Lancet. 2011;377:1760–9.
17. King TE, Bradford WZ, Castro-Bernardini S, Fagan EA, Glaspole I, Glassberg MK, et al. A phase 3 trial of pirfenidone in patients with idiopathic pulmonary fibrosis. N Engl J Med. 2014;370:2083–92.
18. Richeldi L, du Bois RM, Raghu G, Azuma A, Brown KK, Costabel U, et al. Efficacy and safety of nintedanib in idiopathic pulmonary fibrosis. N Engl J Med. 2014;370:2071–82.
19. Genentech. Esbriet prescribing information. 2014. http://www.gene.com/download/pdf/esbriet_prescribing.pdf. Accessed 10 Sep 2015.
20. Boehringer-Ingelheim. Ofev prescribing information. 2014. http://bidocs.boehringer-ingelheim.com/BIWebAccess/ViewServlet.ser?docBase=renetnt&folderPath=/Prescribing+Information/PIs/Ofev/ofev.pdf. Accessed 19 Jun 2015.
21. European Medicines Agency. EU/3/13/1123: Public summary of opinion on orphan designation: Nintedanib for the treatment of idiopathic pulmonary fibrosis. 2015. http://www.ema.europa.eu/ema/index.jsp?curl=pages/medicines/human/orphans/2013/05/human_orphan_001201.jsp&mid=WC0b01ac058001d12b. Accessed 10 Sep 2015.
22. British Lung Foundation. IPF report: Lost in the system. 2015. http://www.blf.org.uk/Page/IPF-report-Lost-in-the-System. Accessed 10 Sep 2015.
23. Mahler DA, Petrone RA, Krocker DB, Cerasoli F. A perspective on web-based information for patients with chronic lung disease. Ann Am Thorac Soc. 2015;12:961–5.
24. Boehringer Ingelheim. Explore IPF Survey. 2015. https://www.lungsandyou.com/ipf/what_is_ipf/explore_ipf. Accessed 10 Sep 2015.
25. Berger BE, Kapella MC, Larson JL. The experience of stigma in chronic obstructive pulmonary disease. West J Nurs Res. 2011;33:916–32.
26. National Institute of Health and Care Excellence. Idiopathic pulmonary fibrosis: The diagnosis and management of suspected idiopathic pulmonary fibrosis. 2015. http://nice.org.uk/guidance/cg163. Accessed 10 Sep 2015.
27. Russell AM. Idiopathic pulmonary fibrosis: care standards. Nursing Times. 2015;111:23–5.
28. Belkin A, Albright K, Swigris JJ. A qualitative study of informal caregivers' perspectives on the effects of idiopathic pulmonary fibrosis. BMJ Open Respir Res. 2014;1, e000007.
29. Lindell KO, Olshansky E, Song MK, Zullo TG, Gibson KF, Kaminski N, et al. Impact of a disease-management program on symptom burden and health-related quality of life in patients with idiopathic pulmonary fibrosis and their care partners. Heart Lung. 2010;39:304–13.
30. Wuyts W, Bondue B, Slabbynck H, Schlesser M, Gusbin N, Compere C, et al. PROOF-Registry: a prospective observational registry to describe the disease course and outcomes of idiopathic pulmonary fibrosis patients in a real-world clinical setting. Poster presented at the American Thoracic Society, Denver, Colorado, USA, 15–20 May, 2015.
31. Koschel D, Cottin V, Skold M, Tomassetti S, Azuma A, Giot C, et al. Real-life experience with pirfenidone: A post-authorisation safety registry (PASSPORT) - Interim analysis. Poster presented at the European Respiratory Society, Munich, Germany, 6–10 September, 2014.
32. Costabel U, Bendstrup E, Cottin V, Dewint P, Egan JJ, Ferguson J, et al. Pirfenidone in idiopathic pulmonary fibrosis: expert panel discussion on the management of drug-related adverse events. Adv Ther. 2014;31:375–91.
33. World IPF. IPF World Week. 2015. http://www.ipfworld.org/ipf-world-week.html. Accessed 10 Sep 2015.
34. F.Hoffmann-La Roche Ltd. European Idiopathic Pulmonary Fibrosis (IPF) Patient Charter. 2015. http://www.ipfcharter.org/the-charter/. Accessed 10 Sep 2015.
35. Pulmonary Fibrosis Trust. Pulmonary Fibrosis Trust. 2015. www.pulmonaryfibrosistrust.org. Accessed 10 Sep 2015.
36. Action for Pulmonary Fibrosis. Action for Pulmonary Fibrosis. 2015. www.actionpulmonaryfibrosis.org. Accessed 10 Sep 2015.
37. National Clinical Guideline Centre (UK). NICE pathway for idiopathic pulmonary fibrosis. 2015. http://pathways.nice.org.uk/pathways/idiopathic-pulmonary-fibrosis. Accessed 10 Sep 2015.
38. British Lung Foundation. IPF Patient Charter. 2015. https://www.blf.org.uk/Page/IPF-patient-charter. Accessed 10 Sep 2015.
39. RespiRare. RespiRARE. 2015. www.respirare.eu. Accessed 10 Sep 2015.
40. Fuori dal Buio. 2015. http://fuoridalbuio.it/. Accessed 10 Sep 2015.
41. Observatory for Rare Disease. Senzafiato campaign. 2015. http://www.senzafiato.org/. Accessed 10 Sep 2015.
42. Malattie Rare Polmone Sicilia. Malattie Rare Polmone Sicilia. 2015. www.malattierarepolmonesicilia.it. Accessed 10 Sep 2015.
43. Tomassetti S, Albera C, Aronne D, Confalonieri M, Harari S, Luisetti M, et al. Documento AIPO-SIMeR sulla Fibrosi Polmonare Idiopatica, Rassegna di Patologia dell'Apparato Respiratorio. 2015.
44. Lungenfibrose e.V. 2015. http://www.lungenfibrose.de/. Accessed 10 Sep 2015.
45. Behr J, Günther A, Ammenwerth W, Bittmann I, Bonnet R, Buhl R, et al. German guideline for diagnosis and management of idiopathic pulmonary fibrosis. Pneumologie. 2013;67:81–111.
46. Spagnolo P, du Bois RM, Cottin V. Rare lung disease and orphan drug development. Lancet Respir Med. 2013;1:479–87.

Permissions

The contributors of this book come from diverse backgrounds, making this book a truly international effort. This book will bring forth new frontiers with its revolutionizing research information and detailed analysis of the nascent developments around the world.

We would like to thank all the contributing authors for lending their expertise to make the book truly unique. They have played a crucial role in the development of this book. Without their invaluable contributions this book wouldn't have been possible. They have made vital efforts to compile up to date information on the varied aspects of this subject to make this book a valuable addition to the collection of many professionals and students.

This book was conceptualized with the vision of imparting up-to-date information and advanced data in this field. To ensure the same, a matchless editorial board was set up. Every individual on the board went through rigorous rounds of assessment to prove their worth. After which they invested a large part of their time researching and compiling the most relevant data for our readers.

The editorial board has been involved in producing this book since its inception. They have spent rigorous hours researching and exploring the diverse topics which have resulted in the successful publishing of this book. They have passed on their knowledge of decades through this book. To expedite this challenging task, the publisher supported the team at every step. A small team of assistant editors was also appointed to further simplify the editing procedure and attain best results for the readers.

Apart from the editorial board, the designing team has also invested a significant amount of their time in understanding the subject and creating the most relevant covers. They scrutinized every image to scout for the most suitable representation of the subject and create an appropriate cover for the book.

The publishing team has been an ardent support to the editorial, designing and production team. Their endless efforts to recruit the best for this project, has resulted in the accomplishment of this book. They are a veteran in the field of academics and their pool of knowledge is as vast as their experience in printing. Their expertise and guidance has proved useful at every step. Their uncompromising quality standards have made this book an exceptional effort. Their encouragement from time to time has been an inspiration for everyone.

The publisher and the editorial board hope that this book will prove to be a valuable piece of knowledge for researchers, students, practitioners and scholars across the globe.

List of Contributors

Ferran Morell
Vall d´Hebron Institut de Recerca (VHIR), Respiratory Department, Hospital Universitari Vall d´Hebron and CIBER in Respiratory Diseases, Passeig de la Vall d'Hebron, 119-129, 08035 Barcelona, Spain

Dirk Esser, Jonathan Lim and Susanne Stowasser
Boehringer Ingelheim, Binger Str. 173, 55216 Ingelheim am Rhein, Germany

Diana Nieves, Max Brosa and Alba Villacampa
Oblikue Consulting S.L., Avenida Diagonal 514, 3°-3a, 08006 Barcelona, Spain

Brynja Jónsdóttir and Olle Melander
The Department of Clinical Sciences Malmo, Faculty of Medicine, Lund University, Lund, Sweden

Åsa Jaworowski and Brynja Jónsdóttir
Department of Lung- and Allergy Medicine, Skåne University Hospital, Malmö, Sweden

Carmen San Miguel, Olle Melander and Brynja Jónsdóttir
Department of Internal Medicine and Emergency Medicine, Skåne University Hospital, Malmö, Sweden

Toby M. Maher and Anne-Marie Russell
NIHR Respiratory Biomedical Research Unit, Royal Brompton Hospital and Fibrosis Research Group, National Heart and Lung Institute, Imperial College London, London, UK

Maria Molina-Molina
University Hospital of Bellvitge, Institut d'Investigacions Biomèdiques de Bellvitge (IDIBELL), Barcelona, and Centro de Investigación Biomédica en Red Enfermedades Respiratorias (CIBERES), Barcelona, Spain

Francesco Bonella
Ruhrlandklinik, University Hospital Essen, Essen, Germany

Stéphane Jouneau
Hôpital Pontchaillou, IRSET UMR 1085, Université de Rennes 1, Rennes, France

Elena Ripamonti
Elma Research S.R.L, Milan, Italy

Judit Axmann
F. Hoffmann-La Roche Ltd., Basel, Switzerland

Carlo Vancheri
Regional Referral Centre for Rare Lung Diseases, University of Catania, Catania, Italy

Toby M. Maher
Fibrosis Research Group, Inflammation, Repair and Development Section, NHLI, Sir Alexander Fleming Building, Imperial College London, London SW7 2AZ, UK

Marcin Kurzyna, Justyna Norwa and Adam Torbicki
Department of Pulmonary Circulation, Thromboembolic Diseases and Cardiology, Centre of Postgraduate Medical Education, European Health Centre Otwock, Borowa 14/18, 05-400 Otwock, Poland

Tatiana Mularek-Kubzdela and Katarzyna Małaczyńska-Rajpold
1st Department of Cardiology, University of Medical Sciences, Poznan, Poland

Andrzej Koteja
Department of Anesthesiology and Intensive Care, European Health Centre Otwock, Otwock, Poland

Agnieszka Pawlak
Department of Invasive Cardiology, Central Clinical Hospital of the Ministry of the Interior and Administration, Warsaw, Poland

Łukasz Chrzanowski
Department of Cardiology, Medical University of Lodz, Lodz, Poland

Michał Furdal
Department of Cardiology, Provincial Specialist Hospital in Wroclaw, Research and Development Centre, Wrocław, Poland

Zbigniew Gąsior
Department of Cardiology, SHS, Medical University of Silesia, Katowice, Poland

Wojciech Jacheć
2nd Department of Cardiology, School of Medicine with Dentistry Division, Medical University of Silesia, Zabrze, Poland

Bożena Sobkowicz
Department of Cardiology, Medical University of Bialystok, Białystok, Poland

Tatsuya Nitawaki, Yoshihiko Sakata, Kodai Kawamura and Kazuya Ichikado
Division of Respiratory Medicine, Saiseikai Kumamoto Hospital, 5-3-1 Chikami, Kumamoto 861-4193, Japan

Meng-Yu Wu, Yu-Sheng Chang and Pyng-Jing Lin
Department of Cardiovascular Surgery, Chang Gung Memorial Hospital and Chang Gung University, Taoyuan, Taiwan

Meng-Yu Wu
School of Traditional Chinese Medicine, Chang Gung University, Taoyuan, Taiwan

Chung-Chi Huang
Department of Thoracic Medicine, Chang Gung Memorial Hospital and Chang Gung University, Taoyuan, Taiwan

Tzu-I Wu
Department of Obstetrics and Gynecology, School of Medicine, College of Medicine, Taipei Medical University, Taipei, Taiwan
Department of Obstetrics and Gynecology, Wan Fang Hospital, Taipei Medical University, Taipei, Taiwan

Yosuke Tanaka and Mitsunori Hino
Department of Respiratory Medicine, Nippon Medical School, Chiba
Hokusoh Hospital, 1715 Kamagari, Inzai, Chiba 270-1694, Japan

Akihiko Gemma
Department of Pulmonary Medicine and Oncology, Graduate School of Medicine, Nippon Medical School, 1-1-5 Sendagi, Bunkyo-ku, Tokyo 113-8603, Japan

Ji Eun Park, Chi Young Kim, Moo Suk Park, Joo Han Song, Young Sam Kim and Song Yee Kim
Division of Pulmonology, Department of Internal Medicine, Severance Hospital, Institute of Chest Diseases, Yonsei University College of Medicine, 50-1, Yonsei-ro, Seodaemun-gu, Seoul, Republic of Korea

Hyo Chae Paik and Jin Gu Lee
Department of Thoracic and Cardiovascular Surgery, Severance Hospital, Yonsei University College of Medicine, Seoul, Republic of Korea

Ji Eun Park
Department of Pulmonary and Critical Care Medicine, Ajou University School of Medicine, Suwon, Republic of Korea

Takeshi Terashima, Taro Shinozaki, Eri Iwami, Takahiro Nakajima and Tatsu Matsuzaki
Department of Respiratory Medicine, Tokyo Dental College Ichikawa General Hospital, 5-11-13, Sugano, Ichikawa, Chiba 272-0824, Japan

Thomas Radtke and Susi Kriemler
Epidemiology, Biostatistics and Prevention Institute (EBPI), University of Zurich, Zurich, Switzerland

Holger Dressel, Marion Maggi-Beba and Thomas Radtke
Division of Occupational and Environmental Medicine, University of Zurich and University Hospital Zurich, Zurich, Switzerland

Peter Fischer, Lukas Böni and Peter Bohnacker
Department of Health Science and Technology, ETH Zurich, Zurich, Switzerland

Christian Benden
Division of Pulmonology, University Hospital of Zurich, Zurich, Switzerland

Pablo Altman
Novartis Pharmaceuticals Corporation, East Hanover, NJ, USA

Luis Wehbe
Instituto Ave Pulmo, Fundación Enfisema, Mar del Plata, Argentina

Juergen Dederichs, Miguel Cardenas Moronta and Pankaj Goyal
Novartis Pharma AG, Basel, Switzerland

Tadhg Guerin
Novartis Ireland Limited, Dublin, Ireland

Brian Ament
Novartis Pharmaceuticals Corporation, San Carlos, California, USA

Andrea Valeria Pino
Novartis Argentina S.A, Buenos Aires, Argentina

Fen Yang, Yuncui Wang, Hui Hu and Zhenfang Xiong
School of Nursing, Hubei University of Chinese Medicine, Wuhan, China

Chongming Yang
Research Support Center, Brigham Young University, Provo, UT, USA

Dante A. Suffredini, Jason M. Elinoff and Michael A. Solomon
Critical Care Medicine Department, National Institutes of Health Clinical Center, Bethesda, MD, USA

Jung-Min Lee
Women's Malignancies Branch, Center for Cancer Research, National Cancer Institute, National Institutes of Health, Bethesda, USA

Cody J. Peer
Clinical Pharmacology Program, Center for Cancer Research, National Cancer Institute, National Institutes of Health, Bethesda, USA

Drew Pratt and David E. Kleiner
Laboratory of Pathology, Center for Cancer Research, National Cancer Institute, National Institutes of Health, Bethesda, USA

Michael A. Solomon
Cardiovascular Branch, National Heart, Lung, and Blood Institute, National Institutes of Health, Bethesda, USA

Eric W. Tsang
The Laboratory of Neuroscience for Education, Faculty of Education, The University of Hong Kong, Hong Kong, China

Henry Kwok and Chetwyn C. H. Chan
Department of Rehabilitation Sciences, The Hong Kong Polytechnic University, Hung Hom, Kowloon, Hong Kong, China

Aidan K. Y. Chan
Department of Life Science, Imperial College of London, London, UK

Kah Lin Choo
Department of Medicine, North District Hospital, Hong Kong, China

Kin Sang Chan
Department of Medicine, Haven of Hope Hospital, Hong Kong, China

Kam Shing Lau
Department of Medicine, Ruttonjee Hospital, Hong Kong, China

George Bardsley, Janine Pilcher, Steven McKinstry, Philippa Shirtcliffe, James Fingleton and Richard Beasley
Capital and Coast District Health Board, Wellington, New Zealand

James Berry, Richard Beasley, James Fingleton, Philippa Shirtcliffe, Steven McKinstry, Janine Pilcher and George Bardsley
Medical Research Institute of New Zealand, Wellington, New Zealand

Richard Beasley, Steven McKinstry and Janine Pilcher
Victoria University Wellington, Wellington, New Zealand

James Berry and Mark Weatherall
Wellington School of Medicine and Health Sciences, University of Otago Wellington, Wellington, New Zealand

George A. Margaritopoulos, Athina Trachalaki, Eirini Vasarmidi, Eleni Bibaki, George Papastratigakis, Nikos Tzanakis and Katerina M. Antoniou
Respiratory Medicine Department, University Hospital of Heraklion, Crete, Greece

Athol U. Wells and George A. Margaritopoulos
Interstitial Lung Disease Unit, Royal Brompton Hospital, London, UK

Stathis Detorakis
Radiology Department, University Hospital of Heraklion, Crete, Greece

Yonghua Bi, Zepeng Yu, Jianzhuang Ren, Gang Wu and Xinwei Han
Department of Interventional Radiology, the First Affiliated Hospital of Zhengzhou University, Zhengzhou, China

Jindong Li
Department of Thoracic Surgery, the First Affiliated Hospital of Zhengzhou University, Zhengzhou, China

Holger Woehrle
Sleep and Ventilation Center Blaubeuren, Respiratory Center Ulm, Ulm, Germany

Michael Arzt
Department of Internal Medicine II, University Hospital Regensburg, Regensburg, Germany

Andrea Graml
ResMed Science Center, ResMed Germany, Martinsried, Germany

Ingo Fietze
Charité – University Medical Center Berlin, Center for Cardiovascular and Vascular Medicine, Interdisciplinary Sleep Medicine Center, Berlin, Germany

Peter Young
Clinic for Sleep Medicine and Neuromuscular Diseases, University Hospital Münster, Münster, Germany

Helmut Teschler
Department of Pneumology, Ruhrlandklinik, West German Lung Center, University Hospital Essen, University Duisburg-Essen, Essen, Germany

Joachim H. Ficker
Department of Respiratory Medicine, Allergology and Sleep Medicine, General Hospital Nuremberg, Nuremberg, Germany
Paracelsus Medical University, Nuremberg, Germany

George Giannakoulas, Panagiotis Savvoulidis, Sophia-Anastasia Mouratoglou, Haralambos Karvounis and Stavros Hadjimiltiades
Department of Cardiology, AHEPA University Hospital, Aristotle University of Thessaloniki, Stilp. Kiriakidi 1, Thessaloniki 54637, Greece

Vasilios Grosomanidis
Department of Anesthesiology and Intensive Care Medicine, AHEPA University Hospital, Aristotle University of Thessaloniki, Stilp. Kiriakidi 1, Thessaloniki 54637, Greece

Isabelle Delanote, Wim A. Wuyts, Jonas Yserbyt, Geert M. Verleden and Robin Vos
Department of Respiratory Diseases, Interstitial Lung Disease and Lung Transplant Unit, University Hospitals Leuven, Leuven, Belgium

Geert M. Verleden, Robin Vos and Wim A. Wuyts
KULeuven, Department of Clinical and Experimental Medicine, Division of Respiratory Diseases, Laboratory of Respiratory Diseases, Lung Transplantation Unit, KU Leuven, Herestraat 49, B-3000 Leuven, Belgium

Eric K. Verbeken
KULeuven, Department of Histopathology, Leuven, Belgium

Jiang-nan Zhao
Department of Respiratory Medicine, The First Hospital of Jiaxing, Jiaxing, China

Yao Liu and Huai-chen Li
Department of Respiratory Medicine, Shandong Provincial Hospital Affiliated to Shandong University, Jinan, Shandong 250021, China

Anne-Marie Russell
National Heart and Lung Institute, Imperial College and Royal Brompton Hospital, Respiratory Epidemiology, Occupational Medicine and Public Health, 1b Manresa Road, London SW3 6LR, UK

Elena Ripamonti
Elma Research S.R.L, Viale Tunisia 41, 20124 Milan, Italy

Carlo Vancheri
Regional Referral Centre for Rare Lung Diseases, Department of Clinical and Experimental Medicine, University of Catania, via S. Sofia 78, 95123 Catania, Italy

Index

www.ingramcontent.com/pod-product-compliance
Lightning Source LLC
Chambersburg PA
CBHW080244230326
41458CB00097B/3166